Drugs, Development, and
Cerebral Function

Drugs, Development, and Cerebral Function

Compiled and Edited by

W. LYNN SMITH, Ph.D.

Director
Cortical Function Laboratories
Porter Memorial Hospital
Denver, Colorado
and
White Memorial Medical
Center
Los Angeles, California

With a Foreword by

Marcel Kinsbourne, M.D., Ph.D.

Associate Professor of Pediatrics and Neurology
Lecturer in Psychology
Duke University Medical Center
Durham, North Carolina

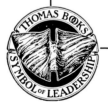

CHARLES C THOMAS · PUBLISHER
Springfield · Illinois · U.S.A.

Published and Distributed Throughout the World by
CHARLES C THOMAS • PUBLISHER
Bannerstone House
301-327 East Lawrence Avenue, Springfield, Illinois, U.S.A.
Natchez Plantation House
735 North Atlantic Boulevard, Fort Lauderdale, Florida, U.S.A.

© *1972, by* CHARLES C THOMAS • PUBLISHER
ISBN 0-398-02417-0
Library of Congress Catalog Card Number 72-165900

With THOMAS BOOKS *careful attention is given to all details of
manufacturing and design. It is the Publisher's desire to present books
that are satisfactory as to their physical qualities and artistic possibilities and appropriate for their particular use.* THOMAS BOOKS *will
be true to those laws of quality that assure a good name and good will.*

Printed in the United States of America
N-1

Contributors

Martin W. Adler, Ph.D.

Associate Professor of Pharmacology
Department of Pharmacology
Temple University College of Medicine
Philadelphia, Pennsylvania

Louis A. Barker, Ph.D.

USPHS Postdoctoral Fellow
Department of Psychology
Queens College of the City University of New York
Flushing, New York

Robert Bittman, Ph.D.

Associate Professor of Chemistry and Biochemistry
Department of Psychology
Queens College of the City University of New York
Flushing, New York

Joseph E. Bogen, M.D.

Senior Neurosurgeon
Ross-Loos Medical Group
Los Angeles, California

Charles W. Burklund, M.D.

Chief, Neurosurgery Section
Veterans Administration Hospital
Associate Professor of Surgery
University of Nebraska College of Medicine
Omaha, Nebraska

C. Keith Conners, Ph.D.

Director, Child Development Laboratory
The Massachusetts General Hospital
Boston, Massachusetts
Associate Professor of Psychology
Harvard University Medical School
Cambridge, Massachusetts

D. Hywel Davies, M.D.

Associate Professor of Medicine
University of Colorado Medical School
Chief, Cardiology Services
Veterans Administration Hospital
Denver, Colorado

David M. Engelhardt, M.D.

Professor of Psychiatry
Director, Psychopharmacology Research Unit
Downstate Medical School
Brooklyn, New York

Walter B. Essman, Ph.D.

Professor of Psychology and Biochemistry
Department of Psychology
Queens College of the City University of New York
Flushing, New York

Rachel Gittelman-Klein, Ph.D.

Research Associate
Hillside Hospital
Glen Oaks, New York

Turan M. Itil, M.D.

Professor of Psychiatry
Associate Chairman—Research
Missouri Institute of Psychiatry
University of Missouri School of Medicine
St. Louis, Missouri

Marvin E. Jaffe, M.D.

Neurologist, Stroke Research Center
Philadelphia General Hospital
Instructor in Neurology
Jefferson Medical College
Philadelphia, Pennsylvania

Kent Jordan, M.D.

Assistant Professor of Psychiatry
University of Colorado Medical Center
Denver, Colorado

Seymour S. Kety, M.D.

Professor of Psychiatry
Harvard University Medical School
Director, Psychiatric Research Laboratories
Massachusetts General Hospital
Boston, Massachusetts

Donald F. Klein, M.D.

Medical Director—Evaluation
Hillside Hospital
Glen Oaks, New York

Marcel Kinsbourne, M.D., Ph.D.

Associate Professor of Pediatrics and Neurology
Lecturer in Psychology
Duke University Medical Center
Durham, North Carolina

Jack B. Lowrey, M.D.

Internist
Porter Memorial Hospital
Denver, Colorado

Lawrence C. McHenry, Jr., M.D.

Director, Stroke Research Center
Philadelphia General Hospital
Instructor in Neurology
Jefferson Medical College
Philadelphia, Pennsylvania

Frank J. Menolascino, M.D.

Associate Professor
Departments of Psychiatry and Pediatrics
University of Nebraska Medical Center
Omaha, Nebraska

David R. Metcalf, M.D.

Director of EEG Research
Associate Professor of Psychiatry
University of Colorado Medical Center
Denver, Colorado

Bernd Salatu, M.D.

Research Associate
Missouri Institute of Psychiatry
University of Missouri School of Medicine
St. Louis, Missouri

Raymond U. Seale, Ph.D.

Assistant Professor of Anatomy
Department of Anatomy
University of Colorado Medical Center
Denver, Colorado

Aaron Smith, Ph.D.

Director, Neuropsychological Laboratory
Department of Physical Medicine and Rehabilitation
University of Michigan Medical School
Ann Arbor, Michigan

W. Lynn Smith, Ph.D.

Director, Cortical Function Laboratories
Porter Memorial Hospital
Denver, Colorado
White Memorial Medical Center
Lon Angeles, California

George A. Ulett, M.D., Ph.D.

Professor and Chairman
Missouri Institute of Psychiatry
University of Missouri School of Medicine
St. Louis, Missouri
Director, Missouri Division of Mental Diseases

To
MY BROTHER AND SISTER
and to
OUR PARENTS
WHO
GREW UP WITHOUT THEIRS

Foreword

IN ANY BIOLOGICAL FIELD of inquiry, more is known of the fully developed adult organism of the relevant species than of its young, or of its adult in their declining days. This is necessarily so, as biological mechanisms are more amenable to study in that temporarily stable state, than against the shifting backdrop of developing and dissolving structure and function. Yet it is the latter more involved study which is ultimately the more significant. In any species, and most emphatically in the human, the adult represents the peak of function, interesting to measure, but hardly to be improved upon. The developmental origins of that capability, so sensitive to vagaries of heredity and environment, and its dissolution, so varied in the emphasis of its impact, are the greater challenge for those of us who are social and scientific activists (as we all are nowadays). This is where our best ideas will bear best fruit.

Developmental studies have legitimate claim to first priority. This will in time be acknowledged. Today the need is first to advance those studies, but second, also to propagandize their intellectual challenge and their breathtaking potential. This purpose is best fulfilled by the scientific communications of outstanding merit. But where developmental scientists are gathered together, the resulting debate may offer a perspective beyond that offered by any single approach. This is least likely to happen when the group is one of old friends (or enemies) who wander from meeting to meeting, picking up at each the thread of an endless recursive conversation. It has the best prospect of succeeding when the group is various, drawn from many disciplines, but of a single mind as to the goal to be achieved. Dr. Lynn Smith brought such a group together. This volume reports what they said to each other. The reader, looking in on their reflections, should find, beyond the obvious diversity of approach, unusual and tantalizing intimations of present and impending understanding. I, at any rate, as participant, neither said what I usually say, nor heard what I usually hear. It was a rare pleasure to take one's scientific notions for a trot. The reader also may find some cobwebs well and truly blown away.

MARCEL KINSBOURNE

Introduction

DRAMATIC PROGRESS is being made in the development of new drugs as well as in new application of existing drugs which is bringing about untold benefits in behavioral changes for both young and old. Drugs are being sought to influence perceptual and cognitive functions; to help those with emotional disorders, those with memory, learning, and thinking disorders; to integrate and control emotional responses; to monitor and influence specific behavior.

Along with these scientific advances the revolution in psychopharmacotherapy is accompanied by increasingly more complex investigative procedures with every conceivable level of biological organization and disorganization being studied in an effort to learn not only more about drugs which influence brain/behavior but what specific drug action can do toward clarifying brain mechanisms.

In the latter part of June of 1970 a group of distinguished professionals assembled for four days in Denver, Colorado, the home of the Annual Cerebral Function Symposium, for its second meeting. "Drugs, Development, and Cerebral Function" is the second public record in this series of annual meetings. The third meeting will narrow its focus to hemisphere deconnection and cerebral function. Like the first meeeting, "Drugs and Cerebral Function," the edited procedings by the same writer and publisher, this second meeting was a continuation in format except with a developmental emphasis, i.e. the six areas focused on included psychoactive drugs, drugs that facilitate learning in the young and memory and orientation in the elderly, the areas of biochemicals; neuroanatomical/behavioral considerations. In the latter area is the promising electroencephalographic study approach to drug action and the Xenon injection method for radioisotope monitoring of regional blood flow which provides a much needed outside criterion to anchor neuropsychological findings in studying the elderly.

Further studies were presented in biochemical processes of various biogenic amines underlying various mental functions as memory and learning. Subcortical-cortical functional relationships in cerebral excitability were reported, such as the limbic system and cerebellar functions, resulting in violent-aggressive and autistic-depressive behavior. This year's focus on methodological problems in developmental study evinced many clinical-experimental dilemmas and some answers to them, as well as what to expect clinically from EEG ontogenetic studies in normal children. The section on hemispherectomy emphasizes the critical importance of the "coalescence of neurology and psychology" as urged by Lashley as well as the other disciplines represented here, over whose borders the problem of human brain/behavior relationships overlap. A panel of selected participants discussed their drug researches and the immediate problems and prospects within these studies.

The twenty-one distinguished professionals who gave papers comprised a most heterogenous, multidisciplinary group which included neuropsychologists, psychiatrists, child psychiatrists, neurologists, pediatric neurologists, neurosurgeons, anatomists, biochemists, and pharmacologists. The second meeting's success again was due to the remarkable extent to which a useful exchange was achieved among its members which was a reflection of their ability to cross interdisciplinary barriers and stimulate discussion.

The excellence of the presentations by the panel participants is evident in the papers of this volume. In keeping with the purpose of the Annual Cerebral Function Symposium, the papers satisfy the widespread need for continuity in expanding developments as well as bringing forth research either previously unpublished or, if published, made current.

W. LYNN SMITH, *Chairman*

Acknowledgments

I WANT TO EXPRESS my gratitude to the panelists for their fine papers and to my staff who handled the details of this meeting so efficiently. My sincere thanks also go to the fifteen pharmaceutical companies who helped defray some of the costs of this meeting: Abbott Laboratories, Ciba Pharmaceuticals, Hoffmann-La Roche, Inc., Ives Laboratories, Inc., The Lilly Research Laboratories, Marion Laboratories, McNeil Laboratories, Inc., Mead Johnson, Merck, Sharp and Dohme Postgraduate Program, The William S. Merrell Co., Riker Laboratories, Sandoz Pharmaceuticals, E. R. Squibb and Sons, Inc., Wallace Pharmaceuticals, and Wyeth Laboratories.

W. L. S.

Contents

PART I
NEUROANATOMICAL/BEHAVIORAL CORRELATES, HEMISPHERECTOMY

PART II
CEREBRAL BLOOD FLOW

PART III
DEVELOPMENTAL AND METHODOLOGICAL APPROACHES TO DRUG STUDY

PART VI
SYMPOSIUM PANEL: "NEUROPSYCHOPHARMACOLOGY TODAY"

Drugs, Development, and Cerebral Function

PART I

NEUROANATOMICAL/BEHAVIORAL CORRELATES, HEMISPHERECTOMY

Chapter 1

Introduction to Hemispherectomy

JOSEPH E. BOGEN

D R. LYNN SMITH HAS CHARGED ME with the responsibility of initiating this part of the Symposium; he has advised that I begin, in his words, "with a few half-wit jokes." So I would like to tell you about a lady friend of mine (G. E.), briefly described in a previous publication.[1] She had her right hemisphere removed because of a tumor which first put in its appearance when she was twenty-eight years old. When I first met her she was still in the hospital receiving physiotherapy and doing quite well. She could walk up and down stairs using a cane and wearing a light brace on the left ankle to keep her toe from scuffing. After I entered her room and introduced myself, she asked, "Have you come to take Dr. S's place?" This took me aback a little as Dr. S. was the junior resident who had just been transferred elsewhere and I was still somewhat proud of my position as Assistant Professor. My chagrin may have shown on my face for she continued, "Do you think you can fill his shoes? Or maybe you would like to fill his pants?"

Now, the psychiatrists among us may feel that this lady's query evidenced a certain "looseness of associations" so that her mental status was not entirely normal in spite of her alertness, excellent orientation, and lively affect. However, a certain looseness of association is probably prerequisite to all humor, half-wit or otherwise. It is a surprising thing, in view of the many papers already published on hemispherectomized people, that no one has specifically investigated whether the sense of humor is different in persons with one hemisphere than in those with two.

Whatever we may think of G. E.'s sense of humor, she certainly provided good evidence for what A. L. Wigan said in 1844,[2] "It only takes one hemisphere to have a mind." Wigan so concluded after attending an autopsy where one cerebral hemisphere was clearly absent although the deceased had seemed essentially normal only a few days before. Similar preservation of the person in spite of the loss of one hemisphere from natural causes has been observed by others.[3,4] Moreover, Wigan's conclusion has been repeatedly supported by the experimental removal of one hemisphere in the laboratory animal. The first experimental hemispherectomies in mammals were done by Goltz.[5] He wrote in 1888:

Beginnen will ich mit der mitteilung eines Versuches wie ich hoffe, von allen wirklichen Freunder wahrer Forschung gewurdigt werden wird.

Reading this to you in German is perhaps another half-witted joke; fortunately von Bonin[6] has provided us with an English translation:

> I will begin by relating an experiment which I hope will be acclaimed by all true friends of science.

Goltz continued,

> I succeeded in observing for 15 months an animal in which I had taken away the whole left hemisphere. (p. 118)

He then described at some length the behavior of this preparation, concluding:

> We have seen that a dog without a left hemisphere can still move voluntarily all parts of his body and that from all parts of his body, action can be induced which can only be the consequence of conscious sensation. This is incompatible with that construction of centers which assumes that each side of the body can serve only those conscious movements and sensations which concern the opposite half of the body. (p. 130)

Toward the end of his essay, Goltz went so far as to say:

> Finally, as far as Man is concerned, the fact that a dog after an extirpation of a whole hemisphere shows essentially the same personality with only slightly weakened intelligence might make it possible to take out even very large tumors if they are confined to one-half of the brain. (p. 158)

Subsequent experimental hemispherectomy[7-17] has confirmed Goltz in the main. But what of the human for whom the concept of Mind was invented? Following McKenzie[18] and Krynauw[19] the removal of an entire hemisphere from the human as a treatment for certain kinds of epilepsy became relatively common.* And it has been noted over and over again, as Glees[20] wrote:

> Even the removal of a complete hemisphere (about 400 grams of brain substance) may be said to have little effect on intellectual capacity or social behavior, producing at most a lessened capacity for adaptability and a more rapid mental exhaustion.

With respect to "cerebral dominance" it is particularly interesting that of the 150 cases reviewed by H. H. White[21] and the 35 cases reviewed by Basser[22] approximately one half involved the left hemisphere, and one half, the right hemisphere. And following the removal of one hemisphere (or brain, Wigan would say), there remained a "person," no matter which hemisphere was removed.

It can be argued that hemispherectomy for epilepsy is done in a setting of abnormal maturation and that the crucial test comes with hemispherectomy in a normally developed adult. We recall that Goltz suggested hemispherectomy for tumors; Dandy[23] carried out such operations as have others especially his student Dr. Burklund.

---

*See the papers by Doctors Burklund and Smith for further references.

Perhaps the papers which follow in this section will tell us as to what extent Wigan was correct. He may have been at least half right when he asserted that only one hemisphere is needed to sustain "the emotions, sentiments and faculties which we call in the aggregate, mind."

REFERENCES

1. Bogen, J. E.: The other side of the brain. I: Dysgraphia and dyscopia following cerebral commissurotomy. *Bull Los Angeles Neuorl Soc, 34*:73-105, 1969.
2. Wigan, A. L.: *The Duality of the Mind.* London, Longman, 1844.
3. Bodey, Atrophy of one-half of the encephalon. *Amer J Med Sci, 7*:224, 1830.
4. Weiss, S., Levy, I., Smith, S., and O'Leary, J. L.: Loss of right hemisphere due to natural causes. *Electroenceph Clin Neurophysiol, 8*:682-684, 1956.
5. Goltz, F.: Über die Verrichtungen des Grosshirns. *Pflüger's Arch Physiol, 42*:419-467, 1888.
6. Von Bonin, G.: *Some Papers on the Cerebral Cortex.* Springfield, Thomas, 1960.
7. Karplus, J. P., and Kreidl, A.: Ueber total—extierpation einer und beider Grosshirn Hemispharen an Affen. *Arch f anat u Physiol, 14*:155-212, 1914.
8. Bazett, H. C., and Penfield, W. G.: A study of the Sherringtonian decerebrate animal in the chronic as well as the acute condition. *Brain, 45*:185-265, 1922.
9. Tsang, Y.-C.: Maze learning in rats hemidecorticated in infancy. *J Comp Psychol, 24*:221-254, 1937.
10. Walker, A. E., and Fulton, J. F.: Hemidecortication in chimpanzee, baboon, macaque, potto, cat and coati: A study in encephalization. *J Nerv Ment Dis, 87*:677-700, 1938.
11. Mettler, F. A.: Extensive unilateral cerebral removals in the primate: Physiologic effects and resultant degeneration. *J Comp Neurol, 79*:185-245, 1943.
12. Kennard, M. A.: Reactions of monkeys of various ages to partial and complete decortication. *J Neuropath Exp Neurol, 3*:289-310, 1944.
13. White, J. R., Schreiner, L. H., Hughes, R. A., Mac Carty, C. S., and Grindlay, J. H.: Physiologic consequences of total hemispherectomy in the monkey. *Neurology, 9*:149-159, 1959.
14. Pasik, P., Pasik, T., and Bender, M. B.: Oculomotor function following cerebral hemidecortication in the monkey. *Arch Neurol, 3*:298-305, 1960.
15. Bogen, J. E., and Campbell, B.: Total hemispherectomy in the cat. *Surg Forum, 11*:381-383, 1960.
16. Kruper, D. C., Koskoff, Y. D., and Patton, R. A.: Delayed alternation in hemicerebrectomized monkeys. *Science, 133*:701-702, 1961.
17. Wenzel, B. M., Tschirgi, R. D., and Taylor, J. L.: Effects of early postnatal hemidecortication on spatial discrimination in cats. *Exp Neurol, 6*:332-339, 1962.
18. McKenzie, K. G.: The present status of a patient who had the right cerebral hemisphere removed. *Zbl Neurochir, 14*:42-50, 1954.
19. Krynauw, R. A.: Infantile hemiplegia treated by removing one cerebral hemisphere. *J Neurol Neurosurg Psychiat, 13*:243-267, 1950.
20. Glees, P.: *Experimental Neurology.* London, Oxford University Press, 1961, p. 486.
21. White, H. H.: Cerebral hemispherectomy in the treatment of infantile hemiplegia. *Confin Neurol, 21*:1-50, 1961.
22. Basser, L. S.: Hemiplegia of early onset and the faculty of speech with special reference to the effects of hemispherectomy. *Brain, 85*:427-460, 1962.
23. Dandy, W. E.: Removal of right cerebral hemisphere for certain tumors with hemiplegia. *JAMA, 90*:823-825, 1928.

Chapter 2

Cerebral Hemisphere Function in the Human: Fact Versus Tradition

CHARLES W. BURKLUND

For here we are not afraid to follow truth wherever it may lead, nor to tolerate error so long as reason is left free to combat it.

THOMAS JEFFERSON

INTRODUCTION

REPORTS of removal of an entire cerebral hemisphere in the human have occurred periodically since Dandy's report in 1928. The majority of reports have been concerned with the removal of a cerebral hemisphere for lesions occurring during infancy or adolescence. Various degrees of recovery of motor and sensory functions and improvement of behavior and intellectual functions have been reported in the patients subjected to hemispherectomy for lesions that occurred in childhood. Language was not usually affected and developed normally, irrespective of whether right or left hemisphere was involved in the patients with the lesions occurring in the early periods of life.

A much smaller number of patients have been reported in whom the hemisphere was removed for lesions occurring after full maturation and establishment of function. Articles concerning the removal of a cerebral hemisphere after maturity have concerned themselves generally with the clinical considerations. The clinical application of this procedure for lesions occurring in adult life have remained unchanged since Dandy's first report, primarily being reserved for those lesions unresectable by any other means and in the patients who desire life in spite of the handicap under which they will be forced to live.

Observations relative to cerebral physiology and speculations regarding the neuroanatomic implications have usually been brief and appear to have been of secondary concern. Subjects to be reported in this chapter have been viewed as clinical problems; however, observations were also made preoperatively and postoperatively with an objective of elucidating information relative to function of the cerebral hemisphere.

The present study spans a period of over twenty years. The early observations were made with the assistance of the late Dr. Frederick Hesser of the Albany Medical Center, Albany, New York. More recently clinical studies have been complemented by neuropsychological studies in association with

Dr. Aaron Smith of the University of Michigan Neuropsychological Laboratory. A small number of studies have been made on other primates (Macaque species) and relevant material will be included. The present report attempts to present the material as a physiologic study separating, in so far as possible, the factual observations from the interpretations and speculations of the author.

MATERIALS AND METHODS

The material consists of twelve mature human males (Table 2-I) who, as far as could be determined, had developed normally until the onset of their disease in adult life and four mature Macaque monkeys.

TABLE 2-I

Number	Year Of Operation	Age	Hemisphere*	Length of Survival or last Examination
1	1952	29	right	15 years (continues to survive)
2	1952	43	right	1 day
3	1952	28	right	5 months, 1 day
4	1953	54	left	1 month, 19 days
5	1954	21	left	7 months, 16 days
6	1956	31	right	2 months, 11 days
7	1957	44	right	2 days
8	1960	38	left	2 days
9	1965	47	left	2 years, 4 days
10	1966	48	left	7 months
11	1967	42	right	3 days
12	1968	47	left	6 months, 2 days

*Left hemisphere dominant in all subjects.

The cerebral hemisphere was removed in humans and monkeys in as close to the same manner as technically feasible. Following exposure of the entire cerebral hemisphere (in the humans, verification of the necessity and feasibility of the operation), the carotid, middle cerebral, and anterior cerebral arteries were identified, clipped, and divided. All of the bridging veins from the surface of the cortex to the superior longitudinal sinus were either coagulated or clipped and divided. The corpus callosum was then sectioned in its entire length exposing the interior of the lateral ventricle. The foramen of Monro was identified and an incision from its anterior superior border to the stria terminalis was made. The choroid plexus was coagulated and removed from the floor of the lateral ventricle, and an incision was made in the line of the stria terminalis posteriorly; this continued anteriorly and medially to include the anterior and dorsomedial nuclei of the thalamus, and it entered the posterior border of the foramen of Monro. The incision was extended into the depths of the brain posteriorly with the electrosurgical unit attempting to stay in the internal capsule posteriorly. The posterior cerebral artery was encountered, clipped, and divided distal to the branch to the geniculate ganglion. The incision anteriorly was continued adjacent to the stria terminalis until the anterior and posterior cuts joined and the entire cerebral hemisphere, including all of the basal ganglia and the anterior dorsal portions of the thalamus, was removed (Fig. 2-1, 2-2, and 2-3). The posterior dorsal portions of the thalamus were excluded from the resection (Fig. 2-4 and 2-5).

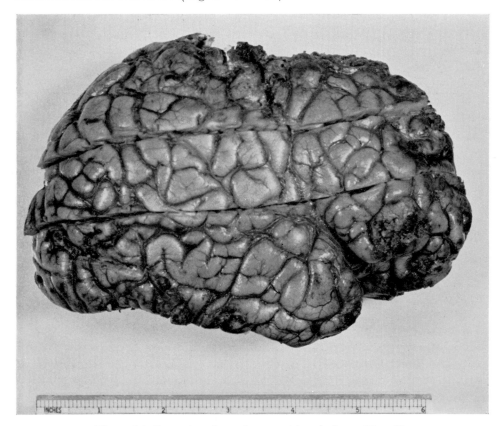

Figure 2-1. Lateral surface of resected hemisphere (Case 1).

OBSERVATIONS

Motor

Flexion of the wrist, fingers, elbow, hip, and knee; abduction of the shoulder and hip; and extension of the knee were performed by the affected extremities during the immediate postoperative period in all but numbers five, seven, and eight. The movements were carried out on command fol-

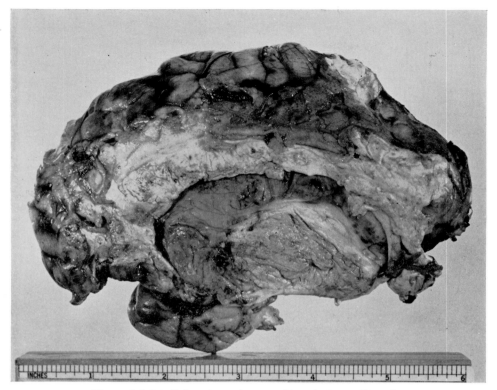

Figure 2-2. Medial surface of resected hemisphere (Case 3).

lowing nondominant hemisphere removal in all but number six. Painful stimulation was required to demonstrate the motor function after dominant hemisphere removal during the early postoperative period and also in number six. Initially, elbow flexion, shoulder abduction, hip flexion, and knee extension were of sufficient strength to overcome gravity, but not to resist counter-pressure. The remaining movements described were accomplished only in a neutral position. The extremities were maintained in a position of mild flexion of the upper extremity and extension of the lower extremity. The wrist was maintained in a flexed position, and the foot, in ventriflexion with complete loss of ability to extend the wrist or foot. Subjects five, seven, and eight extended and internally rotated the upper extremity and extended the lower extremity on painful stimulation.

The movements described during the immediate postoperative period disappeared between two and twenty-four hours later in subjects two, four, ten, eleven, and twelve. Subjects two, four, and eleven flexed the elbow, abducted the shoulder sufficiently to raise the paretic arm from the bed, and flexed the knee and thigh raising the leg from the bed for twenty-four hours.

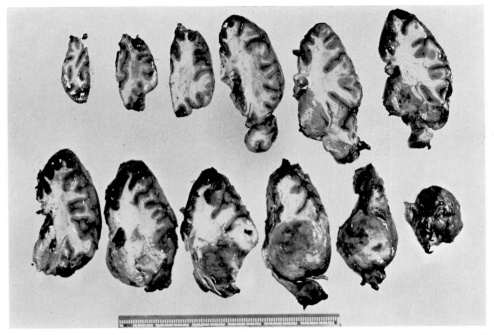

Figure 2-3. Cross section of resected hemisphere demonstrating basal ganglia and anterior superior thalamus (Case 3).

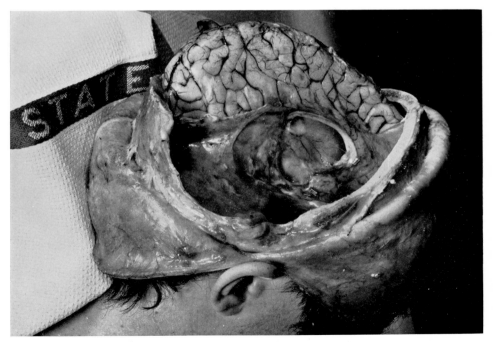

Figure 2-4. Postmortem photograph demonstrating intact posterior and superior thalamus remaining (Case 3).

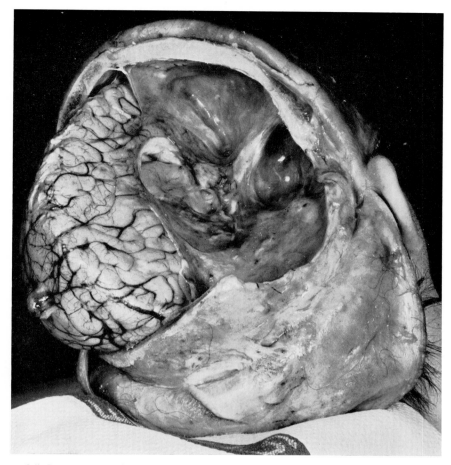

Figure 2-5. Postmortem photograph demonstrating intact posterior and superior thalamus remaining (Case 3).

The described movements disappeared at the intervals mentioned and did not return. The integrated movements were replaced by extension and internal rotation of the upper extremity and extension of the lower extremity obtained only by painful stimulation.

Number six continued the movements described until immediately prior to death, but failed to demonstrate improvement. Improvement of function in subject one continued over a period of two years, then stabilized, and remains present at the time of this report. Subjects three and nine continued to perform the described movements with steady improvement until evidence of recurrence of the primary disease. Subjects one, three, and nine were all ultimately able to ambulate, one with a short leg brace, one with a long leg brace, and one totally unassisted. The gait was one of circumabduction of the lower extremity with the arm and hand held in flexion and with both the arm and leg moving in unison. Ventriflexion of the foot was present. Subjects one and three recovered strength and coordination in the affected extremities to the extent of performing functions useful to them in their daily life. Only two movements were totally and permanently absent in all subjects observed. Extension of the wrist and fingers and dorsiflexion of the foot and toes were never observed. Movements of individual digits of either the upper or lower extremity were also not observed.

Subject three recovered sufficient control and strength to perform gross functions, but he did not use them routinely. Subject number one recovered control and strength of the affected extremities sufficiently for him to use them routinely. Examination fifteen years postoperatively revealed he was able to abduct the shoulder and raise his arm to bring his hand to the back of his head (Fig. 2-6) and to grasp objects with strength enough to hold and lift them (Fig. 2-7, 2-8, and 2-9). At the time of the last examination he

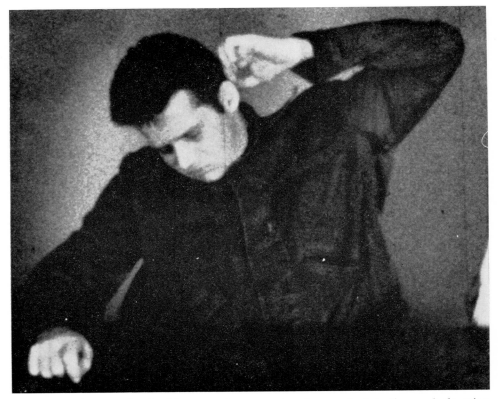

Figure 2-6. Photograph of subject one demonstrating degree of abduction and elevation of upper extremity.

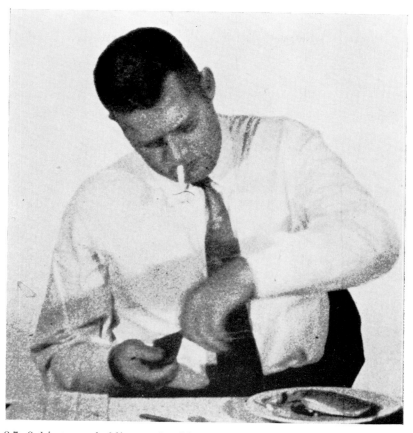

Figure 2-7. Subject one holding pack with paretic hand while extracting cigarette with right hand.

played gin rummy with the examiner, holding cards in the paretic hand and playing the cards with the unaffected hand.

Subject twelve, who was operated upon under local anesthesia, moved the affected extremities spontaneously and voluntarily on the operating table following removal of the cerebral hemisphere and during the period of closure of the wound. He demonstrated the above described integrated movements to painful stimulation for two hours postoperatively. He did ultimately learn to ambulate with a long leg brace and a three point cane, but exhibited only very weak abduction and flexion of the hip and no voluntary movements of the upper extremity.

Two subjects exhibited improvement of motor function immediately following hemisphere removal. Number one had been unable to elevate either the affected arm or leg from the bed for over one month preopera-

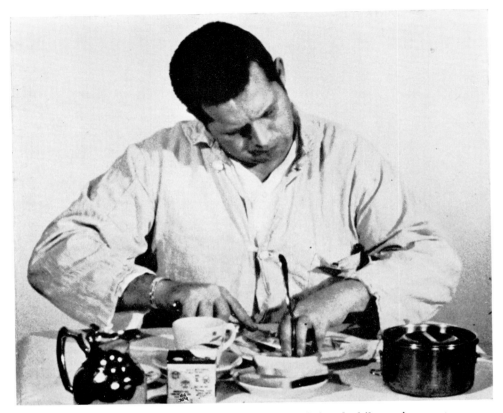

Figure 2-8. Subject one holding fork with paretic hand while cutting meat.

tively. Immediately upon recovery from anesthesia he was able to lift his arm to the level of his head and to elevate the leg from the bed (Fig. 2-10). Number four had exhibited extensor and internal rotation movements of the affected extremities in response to painful stimulation, but spontaneously lifted his arm from the bed within a few hours postoperatively.

Muscle tone was increased in the affected extremities but to a lesser degree than usually observed in a severe hemiplegic. The extremities were easily moved through the full range of motion, and tone was the same throughout the entire range. Muscle tone was slightly greater in the flexors of the upper extremities and the extensors of the lower extremities except for the foot where ventriflexor tone was greater than dorsiflexor tone.

All subjects exhibited weakness and flatness of the affected side of the face with normal movements of the muscles of the forehead. All subjects who maintained function beyond twenty-four hours postoperatively held the head tilted toward the affected side with the chin turned slightly in

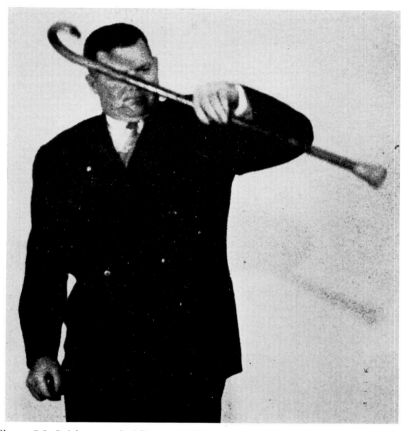

Figure 2-9. Subject one holding and lifting cane with paretic upper extremity.

that direction. If the head was placed in a midline position, this posture was maintained until the attention of the subject was diverted, and then the head slowly deviated back to the original position. The tongue, when protruded, deviated very slightly to the affected side without evidence of loss of strength or coordination.

Sensory

Responses to deep pain stimulation, over the entire side, were present immediately postoperatively in all subjects and continued to be present throughout the length of observation. Response to pin prick was sufficiently retained to obtain a response in all subjects save over the hand and foot.

Subjects one, three, and nine were subjected to detailed sensory examination, and the findings were as follows: Pin prick was recognized over the trunk and both extremities except for the foot and hand during the im-

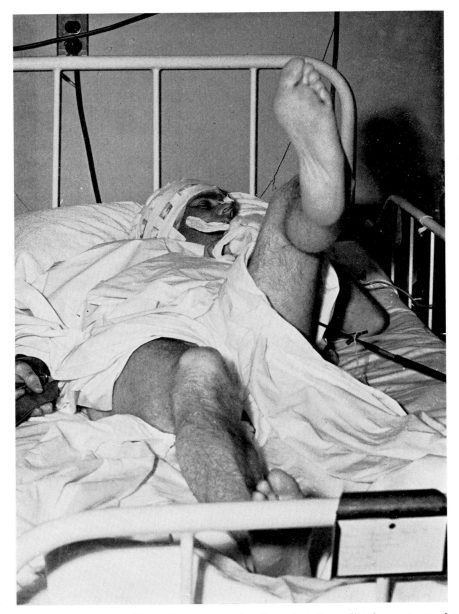

Figure 2-10. Subject one lifting lower extremity from bed immediately postoperatively. He had been unable to lift the leg from the bed for three months prior to operation.

mediate postoperative period, and this continued. During the early post-operative period painful stimulation was often interpreted as a burning itching sensation, and perception of the stimulus persisted for several seconds following its discontinuation.

After approximately three months perception of pin prick stabilized and remained unchanged for the remaining period of observation. Pin prick perception, after three months, was perceived over the entire trunk and extremities, but was reduced as compared to the unaffected side and was reduced over the hands and feet on the affected side as compared with the remaining part of the body on that side. Localization of the site of pin prick stimulation was grossly accurate, but tended to be displaced toward the midline.

Reliable responses to touch perception were not obtained prior to about three months. At three months subjects one and three had absence of touch perception over the hand and foot up to the carpal and tarsal joints and perceived them accurately with grossly normal localization over the remainder of the affected side. Again, the location of the stimulus tended to be displaced proximally. Subject nine was unable to perceive touch beyond the upper third of the arm, but perceived touch all the way to the toes in the lower extremity.

Position sense in the immediate postoperative period was denied by all three subjects. It was observed in subject one, six hours following operation, that while he verbally denied recognition of changes of position of the extremities in space, when they were painfully stimulated, following the placing of the extremity in a new position, he reached for the extremity and scratched it in its new position while continuing to deny verbally that it had been moved. Position sense returned in all three subjects after three months postoperatively, and changes in position of the extremities were recognized except for movement of the digits. Greater range of motion of the extremity was required on the affected side than the unaffected side.

Two-point discrimination was absent in all three subjects in the immediate postoperative period, but returned after several months and required only one to two millimeters greater separation between the two points on the affected side than on the unaffected side for them to be identified properly. Two-point discrimination was not possible over the hands or feet. Recognition of double simultaneous stimulation of either the two upper or two lower extremities or the upper extremity and the cheek were absent in the immediate postoperative period in subjects one and three, but again this phenomenon disappeared after a few months. Vibratory sense was perceived equally on the affected and unaffected side proximal to the ankle and wrist.

All modalities of sensation were intact over the face on the affected side in all three subjects. Perception of sensory stimuli over the face was minimally reduced compared with the unaffected side.

Reflexes

Myotatic reflexes were increased on the affected side in both extremities to the same degree as is usually seen in severely hemiplegic patients. The plantar response was dorsiflexor, but differed from that usually seen in the hemiplegic patient by a wider variation from time to time of examination. On occasion plantar response was neutral in all subjects. The dorsiflexor plantar responses was increased by turning the head toward the affected side. A forced grasp reflex was noted only in subject one and only for a very short period of time. The grasp reflex was increased by turning the head toward the affected side. Optokinetic nystagmus was tested only in subject nine. Optokinetic nystagmus was produced by rotating the drum either from right to left or left to right, but was greatest when rotating the drum from right to left or in other words when coming from the hemianopic field to the normal field.

Autonomic

Marked increase in perspiration was noted over the face and upper extremity and at times down to the nipple line on the involved side (contralateral to the cerebral lesion) in all subjects. The pupil of the eye on the paretic side was enlarged one and one-half to twice the diameter of the other pupil in all subjects. The pupil responded normally to light and in accommodation. Case three developed disturbances in sodium and water metabolism and an elevated blood pressure. He had been normotensive prior to hemispherectomy, but postoperatively developed elevated blood pressure, both systolic and diastolic, which persisted for the remainder of his life. The blood pressure, which prior to operation had been in the range of 120 to 130 systolic and 80 to 90 diastolic was consistently elevated in the range of 160 to 170 systolic and 110 diastolic postoperatively. The serum sodium was elevated postoperatively (range 152 mEq to 158 mEq), and the urinary sodium output was increased during the immediate postoperative period. The serum potassium level remained in the normal range. Cortical steroids were administered, and the serum sodium and sodium excretion returned to the normal range. Nineteen days following the return to a normal level the serum sodium again became elevated (high of 177 mEq). Cortical steroid therapy was discontinued eighteen days following recurrence of the serum sodium elevation. Following discontinuation of steroids, the serum sodium level gradually receded to within the normal range over a period of two weeks. Following stabilization in the normal range, the patient was given an abnormal salt load, and he again exhibited an abnormally elevated serum sodium for several days and then gradually receded to normal limits. Mild diabetes insipidus was present for one week postoperatively and then disappeared. The electrolyte disturbances, elevation of blood pressure, and diabetes insipidus were not observed in any of the other subjects.

Subjects one, nine, and twelve were able to live for varying periods of time in the home environment; and one, nine, and twelve reported normal sexual libido and potentia. The normalcy of sexual function was confirmed by the spouse in all three instances. We were unable to obtain any information relative to the sexual functions of subject ten.

Language

Language dysfunction on routine clinical tests was not detected in subjects one, two, three, or seven following removal of the nondominant hemisphere. Case one did not demonstrate any language dysfunction with the usual clinical testing, but when examined fifteen years following hemispherectomy, his speech revealed frequent slurring, gross mispronunciations, and inability to recall common words. Oral, picture vocabulary, and other tests indicated various defects in expressive and receptive language functions. He replied to some questions, "I can't think of the word." Verbal comprehension, as measured by Peabody's Picture Vocabulary test in subject one fifteen years postoperatively, revealed subnormal scores of ninety-five and nintey-three.

Case four, for one year prior to hemisphere resection, had shown ability to respond properly to simple commands, and to smile and laugh appropriately at jokes, but demonstrated no ability to express himself. Following removal of the dominant cerebral hemisphere the language functions were unchanged until only a few days prior to his death. Case eight revealed no response to verbal commands during the two days he survived postoperatively. Case ten and twelve demonstrated ability to comprehend and carry out simple commands for twenty-four and four hours, respectively, following which they demonstrated no ability to understand either verbal or written commands during the entire period of observation. Subjects ten and twelve fed themselves, shaved themselves, were able to get about the ward in wheelchairs and case twelve, as noted above, ultimately could stand and ambulate with a leg brace and three-pointed cane. Case ten was tested only with simple commands and did not respond to any of them. Case twelve was tested not only with simple commands, but also with more complex requests and failed likewise to respond to any verbal or written stimulus.

Case nine responded to simple commands from the first day postoperatively, and continued to improve in his receptive ability for eighteen months. One year after operation his score on the Peabody Picture Vocabu-

lary test was ninety-eight. Six months prior to his death progressive deterioration of language ability developed, and the last two months of his life he
showed no response to verbal commands. Some improvement in expressive
ability was observed in case nine during the same period that there was
improvement in his receptive abilities, but never to the same degree. His
expressive language was confined to a few appropriate words and on rare
occasions a single simple sentence which was coherent and appropriate.
However, he was able to sing "America" and "Home on the Range" rarely
missing a word and with nearly perfect enunciation. During the first six
months postoperatively case nine appeared to understand commands to perform purposeful movements with the unaffected left arm, but was intermittently unable to accomplish the requested movement. Occasionally he was
unable to flip a coin with the thumb of his left hand either when command-
ed to do so or in an act of mimicry, or to blow out a match either by mimicry
or upon command. He performed similar movements, however, during the
course of normal daily activities. Inability to carry out purposeful movements with the unaffected left extremities and the mouth gradually disappeared after six months except for his inability to protrude the tongue on
command, although he frequently protruded the tongue spontaneously.

EVALUATION

Motor

The three subjects (five, seven, and eight) who failed at any time during
the postoperative period to demonstrate any purposeful movements of the
paretic side had either clinical or postmortem evidence of bilateral involvement. Postmortem examination was not obtained on subject five, but absence of purposeful movement was noted bilaterally with bilateral spasticity,
increased reflexes, and extensor plantar response. Subjects seven and eight,
both of whom survived only two days, exhibited at postmortem examination
extensive thrombosis and infarction of the thalamus and upper brain stem
bilaterally. Subjects two, four, ten, eleven, and twelve had purposeful
movements and then lost them between two and twenty-four hours later.
Subject two survived only one day, and reexploration of the operative
wound demonstrated occlusion of the vein of Galen. Autopsy was not obtained. Subject four developed staphylococcal infection of the operative
site forty-eight hours postoperatively, and his general physical condition was
so precarious during the one month and nineteen days he survived that
neurological evaluation was not valid. Subject ten had gross involvement of
the posterior thalamus and upper brain stem at the time of the hemispherectomy necessitating carrying the surgical resection much farther caudad than
desirable. Number twelve did not at any time evidence bilateral involve-

ment nor did the tumor involve more caudal structures. Unfortunately request for a postmortem examination was denied. The remainder of the subjects, all of whom continued to show purposeful action of the paretic extremities, only one (number six) failed to demonstrate improvement of motor function. Number six never demonstrated any response to his environment other than painful stimulation, and at postmortem examination infarction of the dorsal rostral brain stem bilaterally was noted. Subjects three and nine demonstrated improvement over periods of four months and one year, respectively, postoperatively and then developed signs of regression with ultimate decerebrate behavior. Autopsy revealed extensive involvement in the opposite hemisphere and in case nine extension into the upper brain stem. Case one continues to survive, and functional activity of the paretic extremities continues.

Sensory

It will be noted from the observations and the clinical and autopsy information presented under "Motor" that only patients one, three, and nine were at any time capable of being examined sufficiently to determine any more than the responses to painful stimulation. The sensory recovery in patients two and nine ceased, and a period of regression, to the point of responding only to painful stimuli, occurred concurrently with the deterioration in other neurological function.

Autonomic

The unusual disturbances of water and electrolyte metabolism and the elevation of blood pressure described in subject three appeared to be related to the destruction of the hypothalamus in the right rostral portion. The brain of subject three was sent to a neuroanatomist for detailed study; unfortunately the specimen was lost before detailed neuroanatomic studies could be carried out.

Language

Subjects five, eight, ten, and twelve had removal of the dominant hemisphere and demonstrated no language function, either expressive or receptive. Subject five, as already noted above, had evidence of bilaterality and never responded to stimulation other than pain. Subject eight survived only two days and responded only to painful stimulation. Subject ten, as noted above, had gross involvement of the thalamus necessitating much farther caudal resection than was desirable. Subject twelve was able to comprehend and carry out simple commands for a brief period postoperatively and then never again demonstrated any receptive or expressive language ability.

Subject four developed an intracranial infection and was too ill for several days prior to his death to expect responses to verbal stimuli. He had evidenced comprehension of language, unchanged from the preoperative level, prior to the onset of the fatal complication.

Subject nine demonstrated excellent comprehension and some ability of language expression until the last two months of his life. At autopsy the neoplasm had recurred along the line of resection, replaced the entire subcortical tissue of the right hemisphere, and had extensively invaded the thalamus, mesencephalon, and cerebellum (Fig. 2-11, 2-12, 2-13, and 2-14).

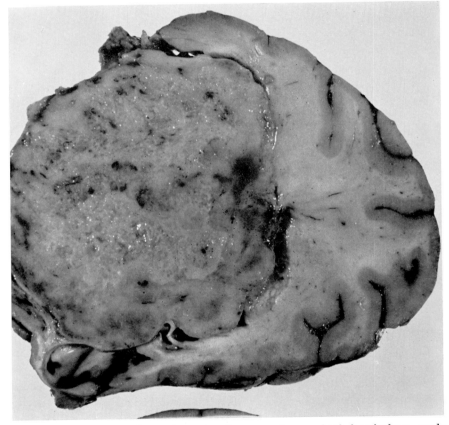

Figure 2-11. Recurrence of neoplasm in the opposite cerebral hemisphere replacing subcortical white matter (Case 9).

INTERPRETATION AND SPECULATION

Motor

The quantity and quality of movement in the paretic extremities and the loss of movements after relatively short periods of time postoperatively

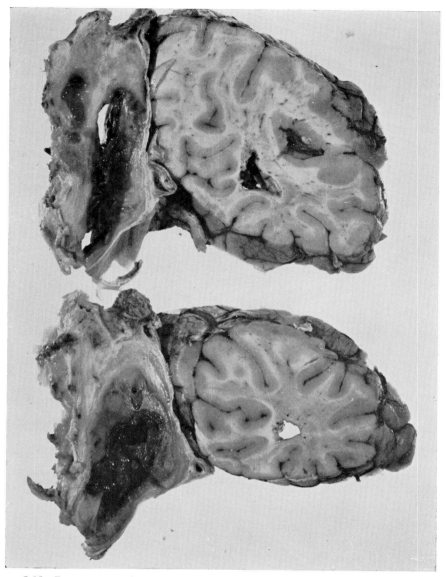

Figure 2-12. Recurrence of neoplasm in the posterior-dorsal thalamus and opposite hemisphere (Case 9).

in the majority of the subjects are of considerable interest. The quality and quantity of movement appears to be much greater following removal of an entire cerebral hemisphere, including the basal ganglia, than in excisions involving only a portion of the cerebral hemisphere, especially lesions of the sensorimotor strip. Traditionally any movements present in the in-

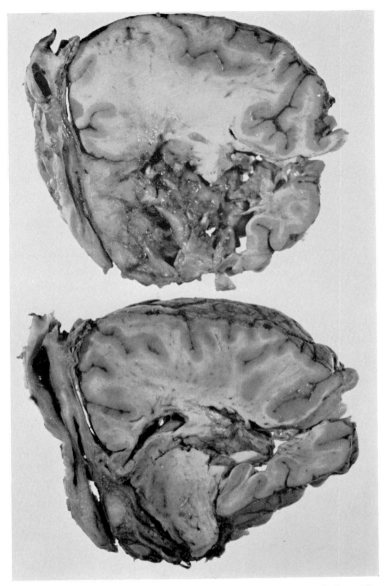

Figure 2-13. Recurrence of neoplasm involving rostral mesencephalon (Case 9).

volved extremities have been attributed to function of the basal ganglia or
the opposite hemisphere. Our observations cast serious doubt upon, if they
do not indeed completely refute, this explanation. Certainly the origin of
the movements is not in the caudate nucleus, globus pallidus, or putamen
since these structures were removed at the time of operation (Fig. 2-3, 2-4,

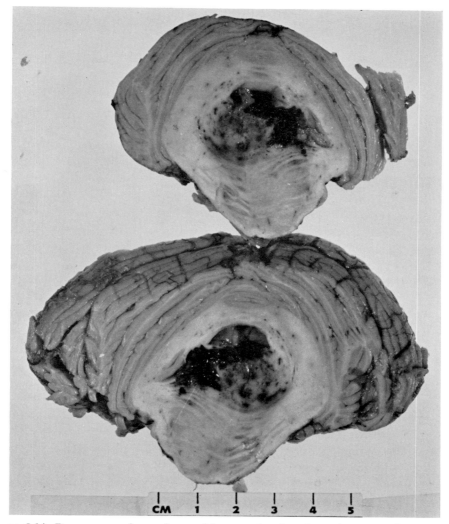

Figure 2-14. Recurrence of neoplasm with extensive invasion of pons and cerebellum (Case 9).

and 2-5). The presence of integrated movements in the immediate post-operative period followed by the loss within a short period of time, in our opinion, implicates caudal structures contiguous to the line of resection and not contralateral homologous areas. Absence of any ipsilateral dysfunction occurring at the time of loss of function is also more consistent with involvement of caudal homolateral areas.

Patterns of normal motor function in mammalia change concurrently with complexity of cerebral cortical development. Animals with the least cortical development (e.g. ungulates and carnivores) have patterns of motor function with rather marked differences of strength. Antigravity muscles are grossly stronger than their antagonists. Herdsmen and animal curators, for generations, have taken advantage of the relative differences of motor strength in handling their charges. The weakest of all muscle groups are the extensors of the carpal and tarsal joints. The absent or very poorly developed digits do not allow for well-integrated movements and only mass movements are present.

Primates, especially anthropoid apes and humans, have more nearly equal strength of agonist and antagonist muscle groups. The digits increase in size and complexity of function in the primate to the ultimate opposing thumb of the human.

Cerebral size increases simultaneously with the change to more uniform muscle strength. Furthermore the relative proportion of cortical representation increases in areas responsible for the movements of the most distal portions of the extremities and especially the digits.

Concurrently with increasing cortical representation, the structure of the nucleus ruber alters. The nucleus ruber in the animals with less cortical development is composed of large cells (pars magnocellularis) with a relatively small and poorly differentiated pars parvacellularis. Contrarily, in primates, the nucleus ruber has a relatively smaller pars magnocellularis and larger and highly differentiated pars parvacellularis. Furthermore the rubrospinal tract is a well-developed and discreet tract in the mammals with less encephalization and a very insignificant structure in the primates. Terminations in the spinal cord of rubrospinal fibers correspond, for the most part, with terminations of the corticospinal fibers.

The anatomical change of the nucleus ruber from a structure composed largely of large motor type cells to one composed, for the most part, of small intergrative type of cells would make one expect even greater degrees of variation of strength of agonist and antagonist in the primate when forced to carry out motor activity with this nucleus. It is apparent that the observations we have reported fit the expected pattern.

Assuming the correctness of our speculation, that the retained and/or regained functions are arising from the nucleus ruber and associated structures, the deficit would be expected to be less in primates with poorest cortical organization. Our observations in the four Macaques mentioned in the material, demonstrated much less deficit. The monkeys were able to ambulate within seventy-two hours and were climbing on the cage within one week postoperatively, only occasionally slipping with the affected hand and foot. Removal of a cerebral hemisphere by the same operative technique was accomplished in several dogs. The motor function of the dogs, within only a few days postoperatively, revealed only a very mild spasticity and differences of motor function between the two sides were discerned only by very careful observation. Travis and Woolsey have reported similar observations of motor function retained and regained following bilateral neocortical removal in the monkey. However, the qualitative and quantitative differences of retained and regained function between the species and between the immature and mature animal may not be entirely correlated with phylogenic and/or ontogenic encephalization. Our observation, that motor function is present immediately postoperatively and then disappears, suggests that part of the difference of function is related to the technical problem of removing the larger adult human brain as compared with the relatively smaller less complex monkey brain or the atrophic undeveloped cerebral hemisphere of the infantile hemiplegic.

The improvement occurring immediately following operation in two of the observed subjects establishes existence of structures located in the cortex and/or basal ganglia which suppress the function of structures responsible for the retained and regained movements.

Sensory

Sensory examination of the only three subjects with sufficient period of survival and quality of response to allow careful evaluation, demonstrates that, with the exception of olfaction and vision, sensory perception is not cortically dependent. Olfactory function was not tested since the olfactory nerve is removed with the hemisphere.

We are skeptical of the cortical dependency of vision. Damage to the geniculate ganglion or optic tracts in the process of removal of the hemisphere is technically difficult to avoid in the adult human. Attempts to stimulate with a small discreet light only the heminopic portion of the retina gave a much reduced pupillary response indicating the possibility at least that damage to one or the other of these structures had occurred. However, we attempted localized retinal stimulation in only one patient. Removal of the visual cortex bilaterally in the monkey by Klüver, Weiskrantz, and Pribram demonstrated at least limited ability in light discrimination. Bender and Krieger have reported the ability of humans to perceive a highly luminescent target in the hemianopic field.

The pattern of retained or regained function of sensory perception, as in the motor system, follows the phylogenetic development. The mammals with less encephalization are snout-oriented and face-oriented in their tactile exploration. Tactile perceptions in the paws of the carnivore are poorly developed and of little significance in the exploration of their environment. Contrarily, tactile perception with the face and snout is highly developed (e.g. whiskers of the upper lip). Tactile sensation in the ungulate, with hooved feet, approaches zero. Sensory capabilities, similar to motor function, following loss of the cerebral hemisphere, have their greatest deficiency in the modalities and body areas poorly developed in mammals with a less degree of encephalization. Structural differences between the mesencephalic-diencephalic sensory areas in carnivores and primates have not been recognized.

Autonomic

Increased pupillary size and increased hidrosis of the arm and face on the affected side do not establish cortical control of these functions since at least limited involvement of the contiguous hypothalamus would be expected. The severe water and electrolyte and blood pressure disturbances in one patient would appear to be very definitely related to hypothalamic damage.

Language

Tradition locates expressive speech in the frontal lobe and receptive speech in the temporal parietal regions of the "dominant" hemisphere. Removal of the frontal lobe, and in one instance a lesion confined to the inferior frontal convolution, has in our experience always resulted in only a temporary loss of expressive speech. Following recovery, the only discernible dysfunction of speech, is at most, a mild insignificant dysarthria. Localized removals of the temporal lobe or temporoparietal regions, when the lesions have not extended medial to the ventricular system, in the dominant hemisphere result in a severe, permanent defect of expressive speech (Fig. 2-15). Receptive language dysfunction has been temporary, but improvement has not resulted in complete receptive speech function.

Receptive language function in subject nine improved to a level approaching his preoperative ability and was continuing up to the time at which other evidence of the recurrence of the neoplasm occurred. Isolated, this observation could be attributed to an individual variation or indeed to bilaterality of language function in a particular individual. However, review of the reports by other observers following resection of a dominant hemisphere closely approximate the observations made in subject nine. Therefore, it is a total loss of language function without evidence of bilateral involvement either at the time of operation or clinically in subjects ten and twelve that are unusual. The pulvinar was found to be involved with tumor and was removed at the time of resection in case ten. The pulvinar was left intact, as is usually intended, in subject twelve, but it must be noted that receptive language function was observed on the operating table following resection of the cerebral hemisphere and continued for a period of several hours postoperatively.

We have observed a patient with infiltrating glioma of the dominant

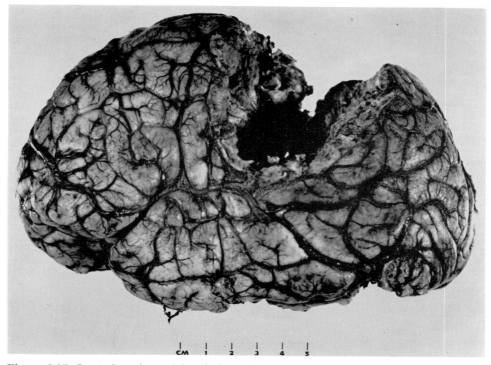

Figure 2-15. Lateral surface of hemisphere demonstrating location of biopsy involving posterior temporal and parietal areas. Subject, under local anesthesia, became unable to speak, but continued to obey simple commands coincident with the biopsy (Case 12).

temporal parietal lobe which extended deep to the ventricular system and was incompletely excised. The patient's language function postoperatively demonstrated almost perfect diction, but the words were not placed in the appropriate locations in the sentence. Syntax, except for very brief periods, was completely lacking. The psychological tests were interpreted as indicating bilateral cerebral hemisphere involvement with the reservation that the defect might be a postoperative phenomenon and might decrease. Repeated observations of this patient, over a period of nearly a year, did not result in improvement but rather in gradual regression of receptive function. The patient's diction continued to be very good until he entered a phase of gradually reduced responses to his environment. Postmortem examination of the brain revealed no bilateral involvement but extensive replacement of the dorsal thalamus with neoplastic tissue, only a very thin rim remaining intact (Fig. 2-16). The brain stem and cerebellum were likewise invaded by neoplasm on the homolateral side (Fig. 2-17).

We therefore speculate that expressive language is a function of the

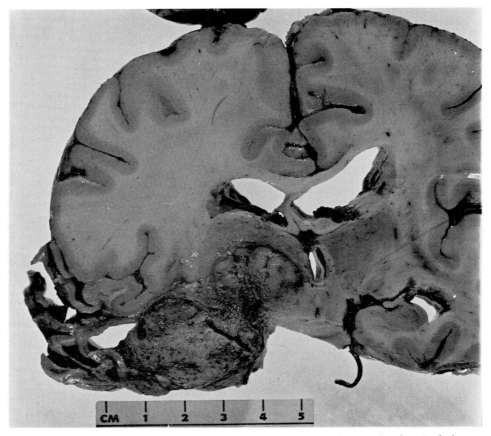

Figure 2-16. Postmortem specimen demonstrating invasion of posterior-dorsal thalamus.

cerebral cortex, bilaterally represented but with a predominance in one hemisphere, usually the left. We conclude that expressive language function is much more dependent upon the posterior temporal and parietal regions, especially the supra-angular and marginal gyri, but some elements of expressive language functions are dependent upon other cortical structures. We speculate that receptive language function does not reside in the cerebral cortex, but is a function of more caudad structures, one of which is the pulvinar. It would appear that perhaps a predominance of one side of the brain over the other may also occur at the diencephalic-mesencephalic level. The predominance of one side is in no way proven since one cannot conclude that a tumor involving only the thalamus on one side has not, in some way, altered the function of a structure so closely approximated as the opposite pulvinar. Van Buren and Borke have implicated the pulvinar in language function.

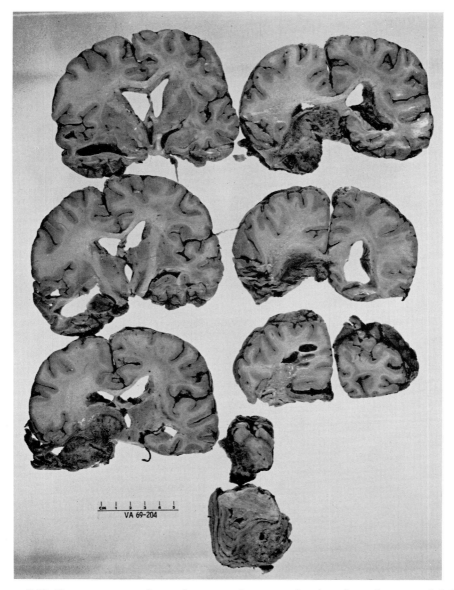

Figure 2-17. Postmortem specimen demonstrating extensive invasion of temporal lobe, thalamus, mesencephalon, and cerebellum confined to the left side.

Nonlanguage Psychological Function

We have noted elsewhere a defect of recent recall in at least one of our patients. It is interesting that the four monkeys, following excision of the cerebral hemisphere, all exhibited this phenomenon. The monkeys, when introduced into the testing chamber following recovery from hemispherectomy, all behaved as though the test situation was a completely new experience. Their behavior toward the test situation was similar to their first experience when arriving in the laboratory.

The monkey's ability to relearn to respond to the visual stimuli in the postoperative period was at the same rate and to the same degree of accuracy and retention as observed in the preoperative state. The ability to regain verbal and nonverbal skills in the postoperative period by our patients has appeared to be related in a similar way to their preoperative abilities although much of the evaluation of the patient's preoperative ability must be by inference from his level of education and type of employment pattern.

Subject twelve, who demonstrated no language ability after the first few hours postoperatively, developed the ability to perceive nonverbal cues to the extent that he often deceived observers into thinking he was comprehending what they were saying. A student nurse became irate at our statement that he was unable to comprehend language, and it was only with considerable effort that we were able to demonstrate to her that, when she requested him to get up and walk, it was the nonverbal cue involving the three-pointed cane, and not her words, which was responsible for his response. Subject twelve was, while home on leave with his wife, able to tell lunch time by the position of the clock hands. He had always apparently been a stickler for prompt meals and would point to the clock at noon time when his wife did not have lunch prepared. He was also capable of operating the elevator to get to the proper locations although repeated attempts on our part to demonstrate any ability to understand numbers themselves met with failure. We assume that the locations of the elevator buttons and clock hands, rather than the numbers, were the cues which allowed him to recognize their significance. Testing of subject twelve with the object assembly test resulted on several occasions in his ability to assemble or nearly completely assemble the hand and the mannequin. It was interesting to observe the subject in his approach to the problem. After demonstrating to him what was required he appeared as though he did not in any way recognize the object which he was assembling, but achieved his objective by painstakingly matching piece after piece. In other words, his assembling of the hand and of the mannequin was similar to the behavior of an individual putting together a jig saw puzzle with the picture side turned down.

Tradition has told us for so long that language and intellectual functions, indeed all "higher" functions reside in the cerebral cortex. The constant repetition and teaching of the traditional view have made us like a snake who, about to shed his skin, can no longer see through the opaque scales of his eyes. It appears to us rather obvious that much of what we have observed, and for the most parts corroborated by other observers, does not conform to the traditional view.

We do not have an answer to the question, "What is the function of the cerebral hemisphere?" It is interesting to speculate that the cerebral cortex which develops phylogenetically in concurrence with the cerebellum may have a very similar function. Perhaps the cerebral hemisphere is only a giant motor system as the cerebellum is considered to be. Perhaps the sensory input into the cerebral hemisphere serves only the purpose of initiating the motor response and has nothing to do with the perception of the sensory stimulus. The difference between a man and his dog or the philosopher and the plowman may not be one of greater perception and comprehension but only of more complex motor response.

Our speculation is difficult to prove since we are dependent upon the patient's responses either verbally or by some other motor activity for our interpretation as to whether he perceives a stimulus or understands a language. Sperry's observation of emotional response to a verbally denied visual image is very similar to our observation of appropriate proprioceptive response to painful stimulation of an extremity, which has been moved, with verbal denial of the knowledge that the extremity had been moved. Such observations make painfully evident the difficulties of observing, much less interpreting, functions of perception and/or awareness.

To know that I know not is to know.
Confucius

EPILOGUE

Far too long have man's thought been regimented and his view of himself distorted by the yoke of tradition. Tradition has its highest development and exerts the greatest mischief in man's religions, but unfortunately pervades every aspect of his existence. We should like to plead for a renaissance in which we return intellectually to our earliest childhood inclinations, observing man, including ourselves, as objectively as possible and with as little prejudice as we are capable.

To the neurophysiologist and the psychologist we make a plea to consider man as a member of the living species with similarities to and differences from the other members; but in no way "unique." To the behaviorist we register a plea to observe human action objectively. Behavior, in common with all other biological activity, follows the lambda curve. One extreme represents action incompatible with social life. The other extreme represents subjugation of self to the welfare of the social structure. Can we delete, from the language of behavioral study, the terms (e.g. philanthropist, psychopath, martyr) implying value judgement of behavior? Can we somehow more objectively observe man's neurophysiological and psychological function, including his behavior, as it is and not in the framework of some preconceived notion of what it ought to be?

> The secret waits for the insight
> Of eyes unclouded by longing,
> Those that are filled with desire
> See only the outward container.

Bhagavad-Gita

REFERENCES

1. Austin, G. M., and Grant, F. C.: Physiologic observations following total hemispherectomy in man. *Surgery, 38:*239-258, 1955.
2. Bender, M. B., and Krieger, H. P.: Visual function in perimetrically blind fields. *Arch Neurol Psych, 65:*72-79, 1951.
3. Crockett, H. G., and Estridge, N. M.: Cerebral hemispherectomy. A clinical, surgical and pathologic study of four cases. *Bull Los Angeles Neurol Soc, 16:*71-87, 1951.
4. Dandy, W. E.: Removal of right cerebral hemisphere for certain tumors with hemiplegia; preliminary report. *JAMA, 90:*823-825, 1928.
5. Gardner, W. J., Karnosh, L. J., McClure, C. C., and Gardner, A. K.: Residual function following hemispherectomy for tumour and for infantile hemiplegia. *Brain, 78:*487-502, 1955.
6. Hillier, W. F.: Total left cerebral hemispherectomy for malignant glioma. *Neurology, 4:*718-721, 1954.
7. Klüver, H.: Visual functions after removal of the occipital lobe. *J Psychol, 11:*23-45, 1941.
8. Pribram, K. H., Spinelli, D. N., and Reitz, S. L.: The effects of radical disconnexion of occipital and temporal cortex on visual behavior of monkeys. *Brain, 92:*301-312, 1969.
9. Smith, A.: Speech and other functions after left (dominant) hemispherectomy. *J Neurol Neurosurg Psychiat, 29:*467-471, 1966.
10. Smith, A., and Burklund, C. W.: Dominant hemispherectomy. *Science, 153:*1280-1282, 1966.
11. Smith, A., and Burklund, C. W.: Nondominant hemispherectomy. In *Proceedings 75th Annual Convention, APA.* 1967, pp. 103-104.
12. Sperry, R. W.: Hemisphere deconnection and unity in conscious awareness. *Amer Psychol, 23:*723-733, 1968.
13. Van Buren, J. M.: Alterations in speech and the pulvinar—a serial section study of cerebro-thalmic relationships in cases of acquired speech disorders. *Brain, 92:*255-284, 1969.
14. Weiskrantz, L.: Contour discrimination in a young monkey with striate cortex ablation. *Neuropsychologia, 1:*145-165, 1963.
15. Nyberg-Hansen, R., and Brodal, A.: Sites and mode of termination of rubrospinal fibers in the cat. An experimental study with silver impregnation methods. *J Anat (Lond), 98:*235-253, 1964.
16. Hongo, T., Jankowska, E., and Lundberg, A.: Effects evoked from the rubrospinal tract in cats. *Experienta (Basel), 21:*525-526, 1965.

Chapter 3

Dominant and Nondominant Hemispherectomy

AARON SMITH

M Y APPRECIATION for the important implications of hemispherectomy
developed through a close association with Dr. Burklund and collab-
orative studies of his cases with hemispherectomy for tumor beginning in
1964. Since then, thanks to the kind cooperation of many neurosurgeons and
a grant from the National Institute of Mental Health, I have been engaged
in locating and examining children and adults with hemispherectomy for
infantile hemiplegia (IH) as well as for tumor.

Use of a standardized neuropsychological test battery, designed to differentiate language, sensory, motor, and mental defects, provided uniform
measures of twenty-four patients with hemispherectomy for IH* and five
for tumor who have been examined thus far.

Previous studies (Gros and Vlahovitch, 1953; Gardner *et al.,* 1955) indicated various similarities and differences between initial and later effects of
removal of a right or left hemisphere diseased or damaged in early life and
the removal of a hemisphere that had developed normally in an adult until
the occurrence of a lesion. Detailed comparisons of effects of hemispherectomy for tumor and for IH will be presented elsewhere. This report will
focus on salient findings in the data accumulated thus far bearing on certain historical controversies. Although the voluminous literature cannot be
reviewed here, selected references may provide a context for evaluating and
comparing the results of the present study with those of earlier studies of
similar patients with hemispherectomy and others with lateralized brain
lesions.

THE DEVELOPMENT OF CEREBRAL LOCALIZATION AND "DOMINANCE"

Until a century ago, the established beliefs of human brain functions
were based on extrapolations of the results of animal experiments by
Haller, Flourens, and others (McHenry, 1969). Thus, it had been believed
that all parts of the brain were functionally equivalent. Flourens, the outstanding authority for most of the nineteenth century, had "established"
that the cerebral hemispheres were incapable of producing any movement.

---

*Includes one patient (the only aphasic) examined after talk on June 24, 1970; among the
twenty-three others, one was blind and another was Spanish-speaking.

Experimental hemispherectomies of twin-brained animals by Flourens (1824), Vulpian (1866), and Goltz (1888) supported the view that the two great cerebral hemispheres in man were functional as well as anatomical duplicates.

Generalizations of many of the findings in experimental animal studies to man were later shown to be in error. However, certain observations by Vulpian and later by Goltz (1888) anticipated not only the development of hemispherectomy in man but the significant differences between effects of hemispherectomy for IH (usually in children) and for tumor (usually in adults).

Vulpian reported, "When one attempts an experiment of this sort (hemispherectomy) on mammals, it is necessary whenever possible to make use of very young animals, for on the one hand, these support operation well, and on the other, the functional relations between the different parts of the encephalon are not yet as narrowly circumscribed *as they later become;* to such effect, that ablation from the brain has less influence on the action of other parts than in the adult animal." (Vulpian, 1866; translated by Kennard and Fulton, 1942, p. 595, italics added.)

Goltz observed the similarity in initial and residual effects of right and left hemisphere removals in dogs. Since "personality" was unchanged and loss of intelligence and other functions in the dog was "amazingly small," Goltz suggested that hemispherectomy might be feasible for removal of large lateralized tumors in man. (The first case of successful diagnosis, localization, and excision of a concealed intracranial tumor, however, had been reported only three years earlier [Bennett and Godlee, 1885]. Since surgical treatment of brain tumors was widely considered dangerous and ineffectual, Goltz's proposal was ignored.)

Accumulating studies of aphasics in the nineteenth century led to Broca's (1865) eventual claim that speech was localized in the third left frontal convolution. Although Jackson and others rejected the equation of localization of defects with the localization of functions, Jackson emphasized one of the most striking findings in studies of aphasics. "Damage to but one hemisphere will make a man speechless." Thus, the neat, rational dogma that man's twin brains were functional as well as anatomical duplicates was shattered forever.

Comparative studies had consistently failed to reveal any differences in the functions of the two cerebral hemispheres in infrahuman species. However, in addition to the special role of the life hemisphere in language, the asymmetry of human hemispheric functions was reflected in handedness. In contrast to random preference for either upper extremity in lower species, preference for the right hand in 90 percent of all normal adults also attested to the special status of the left hemisphere.

The suddenly elevated status of the left hemisphere thus invited detailed clinicoanatomical correlation studies of its component structure in efforts to "localize" other language and nonlanguage functions. Reports of defects in auditory comprehension, reading, writing, calculation, general intelligence, and other nonlanguage functions following variously situated lesions in the left hemisphere, and the absence of such defects in cases with corresponding right hemisphere lesions were cited as evidence of the existence of specific "centres" for the functions within the left hemisphere. Although based on correlations of impairment in visual ideation following right posterior lesions, Jackson's (1876) description of the right hemisphere as leading in "higher" non-language reasoning capacities was largely ignored.

At the beginning of the twentieth century, Liepmann (1905) reported that the left hemisphere controlled the right in execution of purposeful left-hand movements. This added investiture of a directional role in nonlanguage functions further enhanced the already elevated status of the hemisphere. Subsequent references to it as "dominant," "major," and "leading" reflected widespread views that man's left hemisphere was superior to the right in all functions. The "nondominant," "minor," and "subordinate" right hemisphere, or to use the apt title of the review by Bogen (1969a), "The Other Side of The Brain," was relegated to a vague, undefined, but unquestionably inferior role.

Thus, the concept of cerebral "dominance" developed as an offshoot of early claims of cerebral localization based on comparisons of patients with comparable lateralized brain lesions. Although even Broca had declared that the right hemisphere participated in comprehension, many writers subsequently localized all language functions exclusively in the left hemisphere (Smith, 1971). Commenting on Dandy's (1928) report of normal mental capacities following right hemispherectomy for tumor, Lhermitte (1928) pointed out that previous studies had long established that the left was "l'hémisphère intellectuèlle." Until recently, "it was possible to say that animals below man have two 'right' hemispheres, one on each side" (Teuber, 1967, p. 212). Thus, man's proud perch atop the highest rung on the phyletic scale-ladder he constructed was solely due to his speaking, intelligent "dominant" hemisphere.

THE DEVELOPMENT OF HEMISPHERECTOMY FOR BRAIN TUMOR

The development of hemispherectomy by Dandy for otherwise incurable and inevitably fatal gliomas was based on his observations in surgical treatment of cerebral tumors. He reported that since each of the lobes in the right hemisphere could be removed without apparent mental impairment, it was logical to expect that the entire right cerebral hemisphere might be removed "with little if any change in the mentality of a right-handed patient" (Dandy, 1928, p. 823).

In his initial report on five cases, Dandy (1928) noted that apart from relieving preoperative mental symptoms, removals of the entire right cerebral hemisphere for tumor had no discernible effects on language, general intelligence, or personality.

Since two subsequent similar cases also failed to reveal any mental abnormalities, Dandy might have cited his findings as confirmation of his expectation. However, if removals of the normally developed abult right hemisphere resulted in only the same left-sided sensory and motor deficits observed after limited right-sided lesions, what functions did the much larger areas of the right hemisphere not involved in sensory and motor functions serve? Was the right hemisphere a vestige organ that, apart from "lower" level sensory and motor functions, did not contribute to or participate in any "higher" intellectual or psychological functions?

Dandy probably pondered these questions between his 1928 and 1933 reports. For although he presented clinical studies demonstrating normal mental capacities in his 1933 report, Dandy was now also unwilling to say that right hemispherectomy had no effect on mentality, but rather that his cursory mental examinations and referrals "to the best available talent" had failed to disclose any abnormalities (Dandy, 1933).

Lhermitte (1928) had also called attention to the heuristic significance of Dandy's pioneer studies and emphasized the importance of hemispherectomy for evaluating prevailing notions of cerebral localization of motor, sensory, and mental functions. In addition to providing the first detailed studies of neurological functions following removals of the entire right cerebral hemisphere that had developed normally in right-handed adults until the growth of a malignant tumor, Dandy's cases demonstrated that continuing survival with but one cerebral hemisphere was possible in the human adult, albeit with obviously more profound motor defects than those resulting from hemispherectomy in lower species.

In light of historical controversies on the exclusive localization of language and intellectual functions in the adult left hemisphere, Dandy's preoccupation with possible undisclosed psychological abnormalities following right hemispherectomy for tumor is understandable. It is especially interesting to note, therefore, that standardized procedures for removal of *either the right or left* hemisphere for infantile hemiplegia were subsequently developed as much to alleviate *psychological disorders* as well as intractable seizures in children with early extensive lateralized brain damage.

HEMISPHERECTOMY FOR INFANTILE HEMIPLEGIA

Following isolated cases by McKenzie (1938) and Williams and Scott (1939), Krynauw (1950) demonstrated the feasibility of hemispherectomy for IH in a report on twelve cases (10 left and 2 right hemispherectomy) with but a single operative death. Krynauw cited Osler's emphasis of the mental enfeeblement often following IH. He noted that many parents sought help for the mental state rather than hemiplegia or epilepsy. In these twelve patients with age at operation from eight months to twenty-one years, Krynauw reported that following removal of the entire left hemisphere in an infant, language functions developed normally without any apparent speech difficulties. Following left hemispherectomy in a nine-year-old girl, ability to use the right arm was only slightly impaired compared to the situation before operation, and she could speak, understand speech, read, and write without difficulty. In two cases, speech actually improved markedly after hemispherectomy.

Right or left hemispherectomy caused no more than a transient increase in hemiparesis. "Although return of function and power to the preoperative level was predicted and expected in these cases, improved tone and function beyond this level has ben a happy by-product of this operation, and is perhaps a little difficult to explain" (Krynauw, 1950, p. 267).

Krynauw noted that EEG abnormalities (a nonspecific dysrythmia) in IH were not confined to the pathological hemisphere. Following its removal, however, EEG tracings over the remaining hemisphere rapidly settled to normal limits, presumably for the first time since onset of IH. This indicated that radiation of effects from the pathological hemisphere had disrupted the natural physiological activities of the anatomically normal side, "particularly those more especially concerned with the highest intellectual integration" (Krynauw, 1950, p. 245). In cases with limited surgical excisions, the remaining portions of the diseased hemisphere could continue to disrupt the anatomically normal side. Thus, Krynauw concluded, it was necessary to remove the entire pathological hemisphere.

Epilepsy, which had been present in ten of the eleven cases surviving hemispherectomy, ceased, and without requiring sedative medication. Personality and behavior disorders were markedly improved. Krynauw also observed that improvement in the mental sphere *"presupposes, and is dependent upon, the integrity of the remaining hemisphere and its ability to function normally once it has been released from abnormal influences from the pathological side"* (Krynauw, 1950, pp. 266-267, italics added).

Since no apparent defects in language were observed in any of the ten cases with left and one case with right hemispherectomy, Krynauw reasoned "hemispheric dominance had adjusted itself before removal of the affected hemisphere, and that it was the minor hemisphere which was removed in all cases" (Krynauw, 1950, p. 267). Another observation is especially pertinent in considering preoperative disabilities and recovery of functions following hemispherectomy for tumor and for IH. "In the past many of our clinical deductions regarding localization and function in the central nervous system have been based on the concept of nonfunction and negative activity of areas of pathology, and due regard has not always been given to the fact that these areas may often be the site of increased, albeit distorted activity; in other words, zones of dysfunction rather than nonfunction." (Krynauw, 1950, p. 245.)

COMPARISONS OF HEMISPHERECTOMY FOR TUMOR AND FOR INFANTILE HEMIPLEGIA

In a report on an adult with right hemispherectomy for tumor, Mensh *et al.* (1952) reviewed the findings in forty-one previously reported cases of hemispherectomy for tumor and for IH. They cited the diverse and often contradictory descriptions of psychological effects of hemispherectomy and emphasized the need for systematic studies with standardized psychological techniques. Noting that previous reports emphasizing the absence of psychological impairment had been based on clinical studies, they summarized the results of repeated postoperative examinations with psychological tests. "The examination data reflect wide variations in functioning, with concreteness and perseveration of ideas, confused and psychotic-like thinking. . . . Also seen are premorbid levels of superior vocabulary and verbal facility and extremely compulsive behavior" (Mensh *et al.*, 1952, p. 796) .

In the first comparison of hemispherectomy for IH and for lesions occurring in the adult brain, Gros and Vlahovitch (1953) reported that the only difference was the capacity for transfer of cerebral dominance in IH cases to the remaining hemisphere. In a summary of the results in Gardner's ten tumor cases, Gardner *et al.* (1955) compared residual motor, sensory, language, and psychological functions with those reported by others in hemispherectomy for tumor and for IH. "When the functioning of the patients operated upon for brain tumour is compared with that reported in patients operated upon for infantile hemiplegia, it is apparent that, if one hemisphere is impaired, whether by developmental anomaly, birth trauma, or some disease process occurring shortly after birth, other parts of the brain do, *to some extent,* acquire the functions which otherwise would be performed by the parts that have failed to develop. In the adult nervous system, where physiological centres and pathways and engrams already have been laid down, other areas cannot "take over" the function of parts destroyed. In other words, the immature cortex of one hemisphere can acquire functions which nature planned for the cortex of the other side, but (with the possible exception of speech) once a function has become established in the cortex, it cannot be transferred. Since corticalization of function is an ontogenetic as well as phylogenetic phenomenon, the infant can part with his cortex with less resulting functional deficit than can an adult" (Gardner *et al.*, 1955, p. 501, italics added) .

The fact that less than fifty cases of hemispherectomy for brain tumor have been reported since 1928 reflects widespread doubts on the feasibility of hemispherectomy as a possible treatment for otherwise incurable malignant cerebral neoplasms (e.g. Pool, 1968), and extreme reluctance to attempt removals of a left "dominant" hemisphere in adults (Smith and Burklund, 1966) . The reports reflect high operative mortality rates and, in most cases, death from recurrence of the tumor shortly after surgery. Although two adults (R_2 and R_3 in Table 3-I) survived after right hemispherectomy for tumor for fifteen and thirty years, respectively, the quality of postoperative survival was generally poor. Only one patient (case #9, Gardner *et al.*, 1955) was able to return to self-supporting work, albeit in a less responsible job.

Reviews of over five hundred cases of hemispherectomy for IH (White, 1961; Basser, 1962; Ignelzi and Bucy, 1968; Wilson, 1970), however, show a relatively low operative mortality rate (about 7%) with approximately equal proportions of left and right hemispherectomy. Although Wilson (1970) reported a high long-term mortality rate largely because of later occurring intracranial hemorrhages, Falconer and Wilson (1969) pointed out that, with prompt, correct diagnosis, these long term postoperative complications are remediable. Wilson also observed, "Although the better the original substrate the better the achievement after hemispherectomy, nevertheless roughly 42 percent of the patients assessed before operation as being of borderline or severely subnormal intellect proved to some degree educable or employable after hemispherectomy." (Wilson, 1970, p. 154.)

In general, the results of hemispherectomy for IH consistently show elimination or reduction of severe intractable seizures and/or severe behavior disorders in the overwhelming majority of cases followed removals of either hemisphere. Thus recent findings (White, 1961; Ignelzi and Bucy, 1968; Wilson, 1970) support earlier conclusions (e.g. Krynauw, 1950; Cairns and Davidson, 1951) that in properly selected cases of IH, hemispherectomy may be considered the treatment of choice.

Although many generalizations of the results of twin-brained animal experiments led to erroneous conclusions, certain findings reported by Vulpian (1866) were confirmed in comparisons of hemispherectomy for IH and for tumor. Despite the obvious differences in the underlying morbid anatomy, the markedly lower operative mortality rate in IH cases may reflect the younger age at operation as well as possibly less surgical difficulty in removing an atrophic hemisphere than one containing a neoplasm. The diverse and usually diffuse lesions resulting in IH (White, 1961, p. 3) occur before, at, or shortly after birth. In a review of 420 cases, Ignelzi and Bucy (1968) reported brain damage occurred before birth in 75 percent; in the remaining 25 percent, onset occurred in infancy or very early childhood. Hemispherectomy for IH is therefore usually performed in early life (e.g. in 148 cases reviewed by White, mean age at operation was 12.9 years, range 7 months to 38 years).

Except for a fourteen-year-old boy (Hillier, 1954) and two girls aged nine and ten (Gardner *et al.*, 1955), all reported cases of right or left hemispherectomy for tumor were adults in whom the brain had matured normally until the development of a cerebral neoplasm. The reported age in thirty-one such cases listed in the literature ranged from twenty-three to sixty-seven, with a mean of forty years. (All three children survived 20 or more months postoperatively before death of recurrence of the tumor in 2 reported cases, the third not being reported.) The markedly lower operative mortality rate in approximately five hundred IH cases thus confirms Vulpian's observation for experimental hemispherectomy studies that younger subjects "support operation well."

Vulpian also pointed out that hemispheric ablations in older animals result in more marked disabilities because in younger animals the functions are not yet as narrowly circumscribed as they later become. He thus anticipated the concept of "chronogenic localization" enunciated by von Monakow (1911), and the striking differences between effects of lesions occurring at different stages in the development of the right or left hemisphere in man.

ASYMMETRY OF ADULT HEMISPHERIC FUNCTIONS

In an introduction to the *Handbook of Clinical Neurology,* Critchley called attention to the continuing diversity of current concepts of cerebral localization. "Neurological thinking today is still divided between localizers, half-hearted localizers, and nonlocalizers" (Critchley, 1969, p. 4). This might suggest that there have been few if any significant advances in efforts to define specific brain structure—function relationships within and between the two hemispheres since the development of the principles of cerebral localization a century ago. Although Patterson and Zangwill (1944, 1945) confirmed Jackson's findings that the right hemisphere plays a leading role in visual spatial and ideational functions, until recently their findings were also largely ignored. However, in a review of "Handedness and Cerebral Dominance," Subirana affirmed the need "to re-evaluate the role of the so-called 'minor' hemisphere in light of the new ideas of hemispheric specialization" (Subirana, 1969, p. 269).

As Lhermitte (1928) had pointed out, studies of hemispherectomy in man provided opportunities for evaluating traditional concepts of cerebral localization and of similarities and differences in the functions of the right and left hemispheres. Early cases of right hemispherectomy for tumor revealed no apparent mental defects. However, the first reported case of left hemispherectomy for tumor (Zollinger, 1935) revealed that speech was present immediately after operation. Although the patient died seventeen days postoperatively, improvement of expressive and receptive language functions continued throughout the short period of survival. Thus, Lereboullet pointed out, "From a physiologic point of view, this case proves that the dogma of localization in the left hemisphere of word centers is not absolute and that the right hemisphere contributes to this function" (Lereboullet, 1936, p. 360) .

The marked differences between effects of right and left hemispherectomy for tumor with respect to the readily apparent severe aphasia immediately after left hemispherectomy, have been observed in all subsequent reported cases (Smith, 1966) .

Failures in early studies of similar cases of right hemispherectomy or of adults with right-sided lesions to reveal any characteristic defects or to indicate any special role of the adult nondominant hemisphere in intellectual functions reflected the difficulties in dislodging the old popular concept of the left brain as "l'hémisphère intellectuèlle," as well as emphasis on verbal reasoning and language functions in clinical studies.

Standardized intelligence tests like the Stanford-Binet had been developed on the widely accepted rationale that "Language, essentially, is the shorthand of the higher thought processes, and the level at which this shorthand functions is one of the most important determinants of the level of the processes themselves" (Terman and Merrill, 1936, p. 5) . Thus, it is not surprising that Rowe (1937) reported that a preoperative Stanford-Binet IQ of 115 was unchanged six months after right hemispherectomy, and that similar IQ tests based on the rationale that intellectual processes are carried on and expressed in verbal symbols would frequently reveal no evidence of intellectual deficits following extensive lesions, or indeed total removals of the right hemisphere.

Early clinical studies by Jackson and others (Bogen, 1969b) had indicated that the right hemisphere played a leading role in nonverbal or visual ideational and constructional functions. Although subsequent psychometric studies (Weisenburg and McBride, 1935; Weisenburg, McBride, and Roe, 1936; Hebb, 1939) increasingly reported impairment in objective nonverbal reasoning tests, until recently (e.g. Strong and Elwyn, 1943) , authoritative neurological textbooks continued to maintain that apart from sensory and/or motor disturbances, lesions of the right "nondominant" hemisphere produced no recognizable disturbances.

Use of a standardized neuropsychological battery of more recently developed psychological tests in studies of adults with hemispherectomy for tumor, however, revealed that, although language and verbal reasoning capacities were not appreciably impaired, removal of an adult right hemisphere that had developed normally until the growth of a tumor resulted in a consistent pattern of marked impairment in nonverbal reasoning and visual ideational capacities. In a comparison of effects of right and left hemispherectomy for tumor in adults, Smith (1969) reported:

1. Adult hemispheric functions differ quantitatively rather than qualitatively, with a markedly greater role of the left hemisphere in speech, reading and writing (but not verbal comprehension) than that of the right in nonlanguage or visual ideational functions.
2. Each adult hemisphere alone is capable of performing in more limited and varying degrees those functions in which the opposite hemisphere specialized.
3. The absence of the opposite hemisphere has little effect on the specific functions in which the remaining hemisphere specialized.

Table 3-I below includes data for three previously reported cases of right hemispherectomy (R_1, R_2, R_3) and partial data for a fourth similar patient (R_4) kindly furnished by Dr. Julius Wishner (case #3, Austin and Grant, 1955). Continuing studies of the patient with a left hemispherectomy (L_1) previously reported by Dr. Burklund and myself (Smith and Burklund, 1966) provided additional data on long-term effects of "dominant" hemispherectomy, and on the effects of recurrence of the tumor on language and nonlanguage functions before death two years after operation.

Despite marked differences in age, education, and postoperative intervals (from 10 days to 30 years), the Wechsler Verbal Subtest scores of all four patients with right hemispherectomy are within the normal range, with Verbal IQ's of 85 for R_2 (with the least education) fifteen years after right hemispherectomy, to 103 for R_4 only ten days postoperatively, and 99 for R_3 thirty years after nondominant hemispherectomy. This suggests that verbal reasoning, early acquired information, calculation, immediate auditory retention, and vocabulary are usually not diminished either ten days or thirty years after removal of a right hemisphere that has matured normally.

Comparisons of nonlanguage tests of visual ideational, spatial, constructional, and memory functions, however, reveal marked initial and enduring impairment in all four patients. Since normal visual acuity was indicated in ability to perceive small missing details in the Picture Completion Subtest, the subnormal scores in all other nonlanguage tests suggest the underlying disorder is not a "lower level" visual perceptual loss (e.g. a selective impairment of spatial attributes in the visual fields) but an impairment of "higher level" integrative functions unique to the mediation and pro-

TABLE 3-I

RIGHT AND LEFT HEMISPHERECTOMY FOR BRAIN TUMORS

	Right				Left		
	R$_1$ (GE)	R$_2$ (DB)	R$_3$ (JP)	R$_4$ (JH)	L$_1$ (EC)		
Postop Interval	1 yr	15 yrs	30 yrs	10 days	13 mos	19 mos	20 mos
Age/Education (Years)	29/15	44/9	66/11	48/12	....	....	....
	Raw/Weighted Score (WAIS)			(WBI)	(WAIS)		
Information	17/11	13/9	17/11	14/10	....	....	....
Comprehension	21/13	13/7	13/7	12/11	....	....	....
Arithmetic	7/7	8/7	9/8	6/7	12/11	1/1	3/3
Similarities	13/10	12/9	9/8	8/7	....	....	....
Digit Span	10/9	8/6	10/9	10/7	(6/2)	0/0	0/0
Vocabulary	....	24/7	40/10	27½/13	....		
Digit Symbol	29/6	3/0	0/0	0/0	3/0	0/0	0/0
Picture Completion	9/7	7/6	4/4	5/3	14/10	14/10	4/4
Block Design	18/6	8/3	8/3	3/3	36/11	28/9	8/3
Picture Arrangement	16/7	10/5	10/5	0/0	20/9	24/10	0/0
Object Assembly	21/6	11/4	6/2	0/0	29/9	29/9	0/0
Verbal IQ	99	85	99	103	....	....	....
Performance IQ	77	63	73	68	110	108	56
Full Scale IQ	89	74	87	84	....	....	....
Peabody Picture Vocab	125	95	109	....	98	91	....
Visual Memory	2	2	0	....	6	2	1
Copying Designs	10	4	5	....	10	....	0
Colored Matrices	18	8	14	....	32	27	18
Visual Organization	29	10½	7	....	29	22	....
SDMT Written	25	0	0	....	4	7	0
SDMT Oral	35	0	0	....	....	....	0
Porteus Maze	....	5½	6	....	15	14	....
DSS (Face-Hand)	normal	bilateral	bilateral	....	right sensory	right sensory	bilateral

cessing of visual information. The marked discrepancies between Wechsler Verbal IQ's (ranging from 85 to 103) and Performance IQ's (ranging from 63 to 77) in the four cases of adult hemispherectomy were consistent with prorated IQ's reported by Bruell and Albee (1962) in a similar case (Verbal IQ, 121, Performance IQ, 76). Moreover, nonverbal analagous reasoning capacities or the ability to abstract in visual systems of thought as measured by the Raven Coloured Progressive Matrices, and visual memory as measured by the Visual Retention Test, in R$_1$, R$_2$, and R$_3$ one to thirty years after right hemispherectomy were inferior to those of average eight-year-old children.

The markedly subnormal scores by all four right hemispherectomy cases (with left hemiplegia and homonymous hemianopsia) in nonlanguage tests standardized on adults with normal vision and bilateral manual dexterity might be interpreted as evidence of "lower level" sensory and motor defects, rather than impairment in the "higher level" visual ideational processes. However, despite right hemiplegia, right homonymous hemianopsia, and severe speech, reading, and writing defects, the same nonlanguage tests of visual ideational, constructional, and memory functions thirteen months after left hemispherectomy revealed no changes in the normal or above normal capacities demonstrated in preoperative tests by L_1.

The marked differences in effects of left hemispherectomy for tumor were apparent in the severe aphasia immediately after surgery. Although all language functions were profoundly impaired, speech was not abolished, and ability to follow simple verbal commands revealed some comprehension of speech. In our brief reports on this patient, an observation in preoperative and postoperative studies of speech and hearing by Professor John Wiley is noteworthy. In L_1's attempts to answer questions immediately after surgery, he could produce isolated words, but after struggling to organize a meaningful reply, he uttered expletives and short emotional "nonpropositional" phrases. He also spontaneously articulated words and short phrases, but could not communicate an idea in speech. Speech slowly improved, and though still severely impaired a year after surgery, his ability to communicate in short spoken sentences had increased significantly. However, Professor Wiley (1968) noted that although L_1's speech had been dysarthric before hemispherectomy, despite the severe persisting aphasia, postoperative studies of language functions revealed no dysarthria.

The marked differences between effects of left and right hemispherectomy for tumor in all reported cases of children and adults thus reflect the increasing specialization of language functions in the adult left hemisphere. But this does not appear to be a totally exclusive or irrevocable assumption of all four language functions by the left hemisphere. Although severely impaired, L_1 demonstrated varying degrees of recovery in speech, reading, and writing. However, the ability to comprehend speech, which was least impaired initially, showed striking and continuing improvement until recurrence of the tumor. The marked recovery of auditory comprehension to nearly normal levels was reflected in clinical studies and in increasing scores in Peabody Picture Vocabulary Tests (98 at 13 months versus 85 at 7 months postoperatively, surpassing a score of 95 by R_2 15 years after right hemispherectomy). Other functions, variously dependent on comprehension of speech and auditory memory, showed marked improvement during the same period. His score in the Digit Span Subtest rose from 2 at 7 months to 6 at 13 months; in Arithmetic, from 4 to 12.

Thus, as Dr. Burklund and I have reported, and as the ingenious studies of patients with commissurotomy by Sperry, Bogen, and Gazzaniga (Sperry *et al.*, 1969) have also indicated, the right hemisphere alone is apparently able to sustain auditory comprehension and arithmetic reasoning.

In contrast to the marked initial and residual impairment in visuoideational functions and apparently intact language functions after right hemispherectomy for tumor, although speech, reading, and writing are profoundly impaired by similar left hemispherectomy, visuoideational functions are relatively intact. In fact, L_1's prorated WAIS performance IQ (110) thirteen months postoperatively places him in the 75th percentile of the general population in nonverbal reasoning capacities.

Increasing clinical signs suggesting recurrence of the tumor were noted by Dr. Burklund some time after thirteen months postoperative tests. Since the removal of the right hemisphere is all four similar cases resulted in the previously described defects in nonlanguage tests, the marked and increasing declines in comparisons of nonlanguage test scores at thirteen, nineteen, and twenty months suggest the increasing dysfunction of the right hemisphere. The marked decrements in nonlanguage tests (for example from a PIQ of 110 to 56; Visual Retention from 6 to 1; Design Copying from 10 to 0) reflect marked impairment in visual constructional, spatial, ideational, and memory functions comparable to that of the right hemispherectomy patients. The progressive deterioration was also shown in the almost total loss of speech and markedly reduced comprehension, and was reflected in marked decrements in language as well as nonlanguage test scores.

Thus, removals of a left or right hemisphere that has matured normally in man reveal systematic differences. Following left hemispherectomy, although nonlanguage mental functions remain intact, all language functions are initially profoundly impaired and subsequently show varying degrees of recovery, with only comprehension approximating normal levels one year postoperatively. (Although speech, reading, and writing had shown less recovery until tumor recurrence, the extent to which they may have improved with continuing survival remains unknown). It should also be pointed out that since the degree of hemispheric specialization in language function varies, all language functions may not be necessarily impaired after left "dominant" hemispherectomy.

Immediately following right hemispherectomy, although language functions were not noticeably impaired, nonverbal—visual ideational or reasoning, spatial, constructional, and memory capacities were severely impaired. Continuing severe nonlanguage defects in R_2 fifteen years postoperatively and in R_3 thirty years postoperatively do not indicate any capacity for other remaining structures (either in the left hemisphere or those remaining on the right side after hemispherectomy) to significantly amplify previously smaller contributions to these functions.

It is especially noteworthy that despite the severe residual language versus nonlanguage defects observed in one adult with left versus three with right hemispherectomy for tumor, *there was no evidence of psychosis, bizarre*

*behavior, or impairment of volition or will. None of the patients revealed
any suggestion of prosopagnosia, anosognosia, color agnosia, word deafness,
complete constructional apraxia, sympathetic dyspraxia, sensory or motor
amusia, or other total defects variously described in cases with restricted
lesions in either hemisphere.*

In some earlier reported cases of right hemispherectomy for tumor, findings based on psychological tests and on clinical observations were apparently confounded by effects of unsuspected recurring tumors which resulted
in death not long after examination. For example in the first detailed psychological study of effects of right hemispherectomy for tumor (Mensh *et
al.*, 1952), eight examinations from 18 to 134 days postoperatively showed
generally declining scores in the later tests. However, the early recurrence
and increasing invasion of the neoplasm were indicated in the appearance of
seizures in the 6th postoperative month, and death 6.5 months after surgery.
Marked mental changes (suicidal ideas) were reported with recurrence of
the tumor 18 months after right hemispherectomy in a nine-year-old girl
(case #9, Gardner *et al.*, 1955), followed by death 20 months postoperatively.

Another similar patient (Bruell and Albee, 1962) underwent hemispherectomy on November 24, 1954, was examined in March, 1955, and
died in April, 1955, also apparently because of recurrence of the tumor.
This is the only reported case I have discovered in the literature with bizarre
behavior and a transient episode of anasognosia following right hemispherectomy for tumor. (Although psychological testing was necessarily
limited, Bruell and Albee were the first to report the marked contrast between intact language and above normal verbal reasoning (prorated Wechs-
ler-Belleview Verbal, IQ 121) and gross impairment in nonverbal reasoning
(prorated Performance, IQ 76) capacities following adult right hemipherec-
tomy for tumor.)

Thus, although psychotic or bizarre behavior has been occasionally noted after right hemispherectomy for tumor, the emergence of behavioral abnormalities was associated with the recurrence of the tumor. The consistent
pattern of marked initial and enduring impairment in visual ideational,
constructional, and memory functions associated with normal capacities in
verbal reasoning and language functions following removals of a right hemisphere that had matured normally in three right-handed and one left-handed adult supports Jackson's (1876) conclusion that just as the left hemisphere plays "a leading" role in language functions, the right hemisphere
plays a similar role in visuoideational processes.

"STOCK-BRAINEDNESS" AND "PLASTICITY" OF HEMISPHERIC FUNCTIONS

Early reports of aphasia following right-sided lesions in left-handed adults had initially been interpreted as evidence that right or left hemisphere "dominance" for language systematically varied with handedness. Bramwell (1899) and Kennedy (1916), however, called attention to the "crossed aphasias," i.e. aphasias resulting from right-sided lesions in right-handed adults and from left-sided lesions in left handed adults. Since the "crossed aphasias" clearly contradicted the assumption that language was systematically localized in the cerebral hemisphere opposite to the preferred hand, Kennedy proposed that right or left hemisphere dominance for language was hereditary and that "stock-brainedness" was independent of handedness.

The relationship between handedness and hemispheric specialization in language, however, has remained a source of historical controversy (e.g. Zangwill, 1967; Subirana, 1969; Smith, 1971). Roberts (1969) has concluded that "Dominance of the left cerebral hemisphere for speech is inherited." He also reported that, although the left hemisphere was dominant for speech in 95 percent of all dextrals and in two thirds of all sinistrals, the exact relationship between "stock-brainedness" and handedness (which also may be inherited) is unknown.

Early definitions of relationships between cerebral dominance and handedness were based on studies of patients with focal lateralized lesions. They reflected the view that in addition to intelligence, all language functions were localized exclusively in one "dominant" hemisphere. Citing reports of the absence of aphasia following left or right hemispherectomy for IH, Zangwill observed that "at birth the two hemispheres are virtually equipotential in regard to the acquisition of language and that dominance may be readily shifted in consequence of early brain injury" (Zangwill, 1960, p. 2). However, in the normally developed brain, Zangwill described dominance as "a graded characteristic, varying in scope and completeness from individual to individual. Its precise relation to handedness and its vicissitudes still remains to be ascertained" (Zangwill, 1960, p. 27). Thus, as Gardner *et al*, (1955) and Zangwill (1960) have suggested, individual variations in hemispheric specialization in language and nonlanguage functions may be inherited and thus be a significant determinant of the results of hemispherectomy for tumor or for IH.

Early reports of improvements or development of language and mental functions following left or right hemispherectomy for IH were consistently cited as evidence that the hemisphere removed had been the "nondominant" one (Krynauw, 1950; Obrador, 1951; Gros and Vlahovitch, 1953;

French et al., 1955; Feld, 1953). However, these findings had been largely based on clinical observations and were limited to relatively short postoperative intervals. In a review of 150 reported cases, White (1961) noted general agreement that language was either acquired or improved following left or right hemisphere removals. He also observed that in contrast to disorders of spatial thought, body image, constructional apraxia, and other defects reported in adults with parietal lesions, mental capacities were not adversely affected. "Functional sites, in the same manner as mobility and sensibility, for speech, praxis and gnostic modalities have been 'reallocated' to other (healthy) areas of the brain in the course of development of IH. The transference of function can be spontaneously accomplished only before cerebral dominance is established. The age of establishment of cerebral dominance and the degree to which this dominance occurs are, without doubt, extremely variable among individuals." (White, 1961, p. 37.)

Although the extensive subsequent literature cannot be reviewed here, later studies using standardized psychological tests reported findings variously confirming and qualifying those of earlier clinical studies.

The reported differences between effects of hemispherectomy for IH and for tumor raise several critical questions. Gardner *et al.* (1955) suggested that following early lateralized brain insult, with the possible exception of speech, functions which would otherwise be performed by parts of the brain that failed to develop are to some extent "acquired" by the remaining presumably intact hemisphere. Like White (1961) and Lenneberg (1967), they also indicated that once a function has been "corticalized" or "established" in the right or left hemisphere, it cannot be transferred. To what extent may a specific function which later becomes "established" in either hemisphere be "transferred" to the opposite hemisphere following early lateralized brain damage?

The significance of age at time of brain insult and of the rate of "chronogenic localization" was also suggested by Teuber,". . . we need to approach the problem in developmental terms; it is still not known how early the differentiation between hemispheres arises, whether before birth or soon after, whether predominantly as an effect of genetic factors, or as a result of use. We are all appreciative of the alleged plasticity of the infant brain, but we do not seem to have any strong evidence to suggest that the lateralization of different functions can really be reversed with complete impunity. One obvious task is to perform much more extensive studies than heretofore on childhood hemiplegia, since there is the strong possibility (we have some preliminary data) that right-hemisphere and left-hemisphere lesions, even in early infancy, produce reciprocally different syndromes, with right hemiplegia being associated with retarded language development and diminished ultimate language competence, while left hemiplegics show spatial and constructional difficulties." (Teuber, 1967, p. 213).

In light of the specialization in language and verbal reasoning capacities by the left hemisphere, and in visual ideational, spatial, and constructional functions by the right hemisphere in the adult, it is logical to ask "Can a single hemisphere, either left or right, develop the normal levels of both language and nonlanguage capacities of the average adult with two intact cerebral hemispheres? If not, are there systematic differences in the subsequent development of these capacities as a function of the side removed?"

Based on comparisons of preoperative and postoperative IQ tests of twenty-eight cases of hemispherectomy and nine of partial lateralized excisions for IH, McFie (1961) reported a greater increase in postoperative scores by the hemispherectomy group. However, he noted that the increased IQ's occurred exclusively in hemispherectomized cases who had sustained injuries in the first year of life, regardless of the side removed or age at time of operation. McFie also reported that although patients with normal EEG's in the remaining hemisphere showed the greatest increase, the majority of unoperated patients with IH demonstrated". . . a verbal deficit, amounting in some cases to dysphasia, irrespective of hemisphere damaged. . . ," and ". . . these results indicate a limit to the capacity of the remaining hemisphere, imposed by the mediation of the normal functions of both hemispheres by one hemisphere alone" (McFie, 1961, p. 249). According to McFie, "by the end of the first year, it appears likely that the conventional partition of functions into right and left hemispheres has begun, and that subsequent injury to a hemisphere does not entirely dislodge its functions to the other side, with the result that removal of a hemisphere removes a certain amount of functioning tissues". The limitation of a single right or left remaining hemisphere "may bear particularly heavily upon language as opposed to nonlanguage functions."

Subsequent studies of similar populations, however, reported different findings. Griffith and Davidson (1966) presented comparisons of preoperative, initial postoperative, and four-year to fifteen-year postoperative IQ's in three cases with right and eight with left hemispherectomy for IH. The remarkable outcome in Griffith's case #1 warrants individual consideration. Following onset of seizures at the age of ten, hemiplegia at twelve, a right hemispherectomy was performed by Mr. Huw Griffith of Oxford, England at the age of nineteen. He subsequently obtained a university diploma. Tests fifteen years after the operation revealed a WAIS Full Scale IQ of 109 (Verbal IQ of 121 and Performance IQ of 91 versus a Verbal IQ of 101 and Performance IQ of 63 before surgery at the age of 19). Moreover, this thirty-four-year-old man was continuing successfully in a responsible administrative position with a local authority. (This might be of special interest to one editorial writer in a southern newspaper who, on learning of the normal nonverbal mental capacities reported in Dr. Burklund's patient #9 (L_1) with left hemispherectomy for tumor, published the suggestion that L_1 might be better suited for an administrative post in the Federal Government than many of the incumbents at the time.)

Since this young man and a second patient with right hemispherectomy had higher verbal than nonverbal reasoning capacities, and two similar patients with left hemispherectomy had higher nonverbal than verbal skills, Griffith and Davidson cited these findings as evidence that the transfer of intellectual faculty from one hemisphere to another after infantile hemiplegia or hemispherectomy for early lateralized lesions "may be incomplete, as it is for somatic functions." Although Griffith and Davidson recognized that this pattern was observed in only four of the eleven reported cases, they proposed that it was more easily detectable in the more intelligent patient. And, although these findings indicated subsequent development of language functions in all eight patients with left and three with right hemispherectomy, they also raised the question about earlier conclusions that the side removed was always "nondominant," regardless of whether it was the left or right hemisphere.

In contrast to earlier studies based primarily on clinical observations, standardized psychological tests in the above studies suggest systematic differences in effects of early lateralized lesions or hemispherectomy on the development of language and verbal reasoning versus nonverbal reasoning, visual ideational, spatial, and constructional capacities. However, other studies also using standardized tests reported different findings.

In comparisons of effects of IH on speech in 102 cases (54 left versus 48 right hemiplegics) and of effects of hemispherectomy in thirty-five of these patients, Basser (1962) reported no significant differences in preoperative verbal intelligence between right and left hemiplegics and no such differences after left and right hemispherectomy. Thus, Basser concluded ". . . speech was maintained and developed in the intact hemisphere and in this respect the left and right hemisphere were equal" (Basser, 1962, p. 451). Although handedness is necessarily determined by the pathological involvement of either hemisphere, Basser noted the equipotentiality of the two hemispheres obtains irrespective of stockhandedness (and presumably, of stock-brainedness).

In the previously cited follow-up study of thirty cases with right and twenty with left hemispherectomy for IH (Wilson, 1970), earlier psychometric studies in the first thirty-four cases had been the bases for the findings by McFie (1961) described above. However, Wilson's later follow-up studies indicated different findings. Preoperatively, speech had been acquired or had developed in all but the two youngest patients. Patients "who were hemiplegic before the acquisition of speech had no gross clinical disturbance of speech after hemispherectomy, irrespective of which hemisphere was removed. When the hemiplegia had followed the acquisition of speech, removal of the dominant left hemisphere led to failure of speech functions, but with later recovery in all but one instance" (Wilson, 1970, p. 166).

With respect to general intelligence, Wilson observed, "The influence of hemispherectomy upon IQ levels has proved difficult or impossible to assess with accuracy." In the few patients with repeated postoperative tests ". . . changes were rarely more than a few points either way on the IQ scale" (Wilson, 1970, p. 168). However, as noted above, he also attributed the level of residual functions to the quality of the substrate before hemispherectomy.

McFie's conclusions of impairment in verbal functions in left and right infantile hemiplegics before and after right or left hemispherectomy were tested in a study of sixteen patients with hemispherectomy for IH and matched unoperated controls by Carlson *et al.* (1969). However, in addition to standardized IQ (Wechsler and Stanford Binet) tests, their testing battery included specific language tests for assessment of dysphasic disorders as well as tests of nonlanguage functions. In a summary of the overall findings, they reported no differences between effects of right and left hemispherectomies, and ". . . we have been unable to demonstrate any disturbance of language functions as measured by the tests we have used. Thus, not only have we been unable to confirm McFie's findings, but our patients have shown significantly higher verbal than performance IQ's when compared to the control group." (Carlson *et al.,* 1969, p. 201.) Although this pattern was also evident in comparisons of three patients with hemispherectomy before the age of six months and thirteen with hemispherectomy after two years of age, the mean IQ of the three early operated cases[78] was significantly higher than that of the thirteen operated upon after the age of two years.[61] Thus, their findings of greater residual language and nonlanguage functions in the early operated group are consistent with the report by McFie of larger increases in IQ in cases undergoing hemispherectomy for brain insults sustained in the first year of life.

Just as in psychological studies of "brain damaged" populations, the diverse findings in studies of hemispherectomy suggest inherent difficulties in precise definitions of the two fundamental variables, structure and function (Smith, 1962). Comparisons of effects of hemispherectomy for tumor are qualified by differences in the following: neurosurgical procedures and the extent of hemispheric removals; associated pathophysiological reactions, such as increased intracranial pressure, disturbances in the vascular supply, and radiation of effects to the opposite hemisphere which are often relieved by surgery; postoperative complications; age; postoperative intervals and secondary necrosis; individual variations in premorbid capacities and in the extent to which specialized functions have developed in each hemisphere; the absence of premorbid measures, as well as methods of testing; and, as noted above, the presence of unsuspected recurring gliomas which increasingly attenuate the functions of the remaining hemisphere.

Although preoperative studies contribute to definitions of effects of hemispherectomy for IH, the diverse reported findings suggest uncontrolled effects of the above and other factors. Assessments of effects based on comparisons of preoperative and postoperative studies may be confounded by the effects of prolonged large doses of anticonvulsant drugs which, while failing to eliminate seizures, may significantly reduce cerebral functions. Instead of the recurrence of tumors, the findings in earlier studies of operated and unoperated cases of IH are often similarly qualified by unsuspected damage to the presumably intact hemisphere, either concomitant with—or subsequent to —the initial early brain insult.

In most IH cases with severe seizures, hemispherectomy is performed only after prolonged efforts to control severe seizures have failed. Cairns, however, wrote, "it seems well established that fits can produce additional cerebral hemorrhages or infarctions" (Cairns, 1951, p. 41). Carlson *et al.* (1968) urged early operation "to free the undamaged hemisphere from the disruptive influences of the damaged one and, more important, avoid the cerebral damage which occurs as a result of recurrent seizures" (Carlson *et al.*, 1968, p. 201).

Ignelzi and Bucy (1968) reported that EEG evidence alone of abnormal activity on the side opposite the obviously damaged hemisphere does not contraindicate surgery unless other findings indicate bilateral lesions. This view is compatible with Krynauw's (1950) observation that, following hemispherectomy, abnormal EEG tracings over the remaining hemisphere rapidly returned to normal. McFie's (1961) report of the presence of abnormal EEG's over the remaining hemisphere in eighteen of thirty-one cases, however, suggested that preoperative damage had not been confined to a single hemisphere in approximately 60 percent of these early cases. It is therefore not surprising that the fifteen with lowest postoperative IQ's (ranging from 19 to 59) included fourteen of the eighteen with abnormal postoperative EEG's.

As indicated above, the methods of examination are also of critical importance. Early psychological studies of adults with right hemispherectomy for tumor failed to reveal any characteristic mental deficits because of the prevailing emphasis on projective tests such as the Rorschach as well as on tests of verbal reasoning capacities. The limited value of projective tests in such studies was also clearly indicated in the report by Bruell and Albee (1962). However the marked differences in their patient's scores in the two nonlanguage tests also demonstrated that aggregate IQ scores in omnibus intelligence tests like the Wechsler scales may obscure specific defects resulting in markedly impaired performances in certain subtests.

Thus, in addition to possibly significant differences in individual natural endowment and other above cited factors, the wide variations in intellectual capacities in all reported studies of right or left hemispherectomy for IH may reflect differences in the tests used to assess mental functions as well as differences in the frequency and extent of unsuspected preoperative damage to the residual hemisphere.

It is therefore not surprising that in contrast to the pattern of systematic differential impairment of language versus nonlanguage capacities following "dominant" and "nondominant" hemispherectomy, neuropsychological tests of fourteen patients with left and ten with right hemispherectomy for IH showed wide individual variations in these capacities regardless of the hemisphere removed. A detailed report of the overall results will be presented elsewhere. However, to illustrate the marked differences between right and left hemispherectomy for tumor in adults and for lesions in early infancy resulting in IH, Table 3-II presents the scores of two of fourteen *adults* with hemispherectomy for IH tested thus far.

As noted above, earlier studies had cited the subsequent development of normal language and improvement of mental functions as evidence that the hemisphere removed in IH, whether left or right, was the nondominant one. However, McFie (1961) reported language and verbal reasoning deficits before and after right or left hemispherectomy for IH indicated greater attenuation in the development of language than nonlanguage functions. And Gardner *et al.* (1955) Griffith and Davidson (1966) and Teuber (1967), suggested that in such cases, transfer of (left hemisphere) verbal and (right hemisphere) spatial reasoning capacities may be incomplete. Griffith and Davidson (1966) also suggested that, although verbal-spatial disparities following hemispherectomy may diminish with time, such disparities remain more easily detectable in the more intelligent patients. Accordingly, Table 3-II presents test scores of the most intelligent patient (PK) among the ten with right hemispherectomy, and of the most intelligent (BL) among the fourteen with left hemispherectomy.

In addition to providing evidence bearing on earlier diverse findings, presentation of the scores for these two young adults (Table 3-II) permits comparisons with performances on the same tests by four older adults with right and one with left hemispherectomy. Since our neuropsychological battery includes several tests that were standardized in studies of normal adults with two intact hemispheres, Table 3-II also provides evidence of the extent to which language, verbal reasoning, and visual ideational and other non-

TABLE 3-II

RIGHT AND LEFT HEMISPHERECTOMY FOR INFANTILE HEMIPLEGIA

	Right	Left
	IH$_1$ (PK)	IH$_2$ (BL)
Postop Interval	4 yrs	16 yrs
Age/Education (years)	24/13	21/12
	(WAIS)	
Information	17/11	22/13
Comprehension	14/8	27/19
Arithmetic	10/9	10/9
Similarities	15/11	17/12
Digit Span	9/7	9/7
Vocabulary	. . . .	59/13
Digit Symbol	38/7	45/8
Picture Completion	9/7	17/12
Block Design	28/9	36/11
Picture Arrangement	22/9	24/10
Object Assembly	20/7	26/8
Verbal IQ	96	113
Performance IQ	85	98
Full Scale IQ	90	107
Peabody Picture Vocab	109	125
Visual Memory	6	7
Copying Designs	10	10
Colored Matrices	31	32
Visual Organization	23	27½
SDMT Written	40	36
SDMT Oral	47	55
Porteus Maze	. . . .	. . . .
DSS (Face-Hand)	left sensory	normal

language functions may develop in a single remaining left or right hemisphere.

PK was one of Dr. Paul Bucy's patients, and thanks to his kindness, Professor John Wiley and I examined her on November 11, 1968. Her reported medical history (#3 in Ignelzi and Bucy, 1968) lists encephalitis at the age of ten months, resulting in left hemiparesis, and mental and neurological retardation; and the development of seizures and frequent episodes of destructive behavior, neither of which were controlled by a variety of medications. At the age of twenty, she underwent a right hemidecortication, performed by Dr. Bucy. Comparisons of preoperative and postoperative findings, including the elimination of seizures and of mental aberrations in PK and three similar patients, were described in a report on early postoperative findings (Ignelzi and Bucy, 1968).

Dr. Oscar Sugar kindly arranged for our examination of BL. Following delivery by Cesaerian section, right hemiparesis was noted at the age of five months. Seizures developed at the age of four years, and despite anticonvulsant drugs, increased to ten to twelve per day. Preoperative language studies indicated that although verbal comprehension was apparently normal, speech was distorted and difficult to understand. At the age of 5.5 years, Dr. Sugar performed a left hemispherectomy with, as Table 3-II shows, the most salutary results. The absence of a right facial paralysis immediately after left hemispherectomy, as recorded by Dr. Sugar, is especially noteworthy. Speech, which had been almost unintelligible, rapidly improved and became normal. In addition to the cessation of seizures without the use of medication, Table 3-II reflects the subsequent development of normal or above normal language, verbal reasoning, visual ideational, and other non-language capacities.

If the transfer of functions from BL's left hemisphere (injured at birth and removed 5.5 years later) to the right hemisphere was "incomplete" (Griffith and Davidson), and/or the lateralization of different functions can *not* "really be reversed with complete impunity" (Teuber, 1967); or if the limitations on residual functions after right or left hemispherectomy "bear particularly heavily upon language as opposed to non-language functions" (McFie, 1961), language and verbal reasoning capacities sixteen years after removal (and 21 years after birth injury) of the left hemisphere should be less well developed than nonlanguage functions.

Special orofacial and language examinations of both BL and PK by Professor Wiley and the neuropsychological test battery, however, failed to reveal any suggestion of even a slight defect in speech, auditory comprehension, reading, writing, or orofacial functions.

If conclusions were based only on Wechsler tests, we may note that in contrast to the findings of Griffith and Davidson and of McFie, BL's Verbal IQ (113) was fifteen points higher than his Performance IQ (98), placing him in the 80th percentile or higher than four of five adults with two intact hemispheres in verbal intelligence. It is also interesting to observe that BL's Verbal IQ (113), Performance IQ (98), and Full Scale IQ (107) sixteen years after *left* hemispherectomy for birth injury are strikingly comparable to those of Griffith and Davidson's first patient (Verbal IQ 121, Performance IQ 91, Full Scale IQ 109) fifteen years after *right* hemispherectomy.

Comparisons of language and nonlanguage test scores of BL with left and PK with right hemispherectomy also reveal consistently higher scores by BL in almost all nonlanguage as well as language tests. (The only measure showing a higher score by PK was the written form of the Symbol Digit Substitution Test (Smith, 1967) in which writing with the left hand handicapped BL by blocking the standard. However, this did not occur in the WAIS Digit Symbol subtest, and comparisons of the *oral* form of the Symbol-Digit test reflected the pattern of superior capacities shown by BL in other measures.)

Comparisons of PK's Verbal[96] and Performance[85] IQ's, however, suggest that nonlanguage functions have not developed as much as language functions four years after right hemispherectomy. (This might suggest that the development of nonlanguage functions was selectively attenuated in cases with right hemispherectomy. However, Performance IQ's were higher than Verbal IQ's in only 3—one aphasic and 2 severely retarded—of 13 cases with left hemispherectomy; and in one of 8 with right hemispherectomy.)

The tests in the neuropsychologic battery were selected or constructed to differentiate impairment in test modalities (i.e. those involved in perceptions of and responses to the presented tasks) from impairment of the "higher" mental functions the tests were designed and are assumed to measure. Although slightly subnormal scores in the Benton Visual Retention and Hooper Visual Organization tests also suggest less development of the specific nonlanguage visual perceptual functions involved, correct responses to thirty-one of the thirty-six problems in the Raven Coloured Progressive Matrices tests indicated normal capacities for nonverbal analagous reasoning, or the ability to abstract in "visual systems of thought."

Time is one of the most important factors in evaluating the effects of brain lesions (Smith, 1962), and Meyers (1958) has emphasized the importance of lifetime studies in efforts to evaluate initial and later effects of hemispherectomy. We may therefore note that PK's preoperative, two-year postoperative, and four-year postoperative performances revealed continuing postoperative increases in Performance IQ's (75 versus 80 and 85) compared to an initial postoperative increase followed by little change in Verbal IQ's (85 versus 95 and 96). Follow-up studies of these and other patients with hemispherectomy for tumor as well as for IH are therefore of special interest with respect to possible changes in the organization or levels of cerebral functions with time.

The pattern of higher Verbal than Performance IQ's following left hemispherectomy was also demonstrated by EK, one of Dr. Joseph Ransohoff's cases with birth injury and surgery at the age of 7.8 years. In addition to cessation of seizures, a Verbal IQ of 98, Performance IQ of 77, Full Scale IQ 88, Peabody Picture Vocabulary of 107 when tested at the age of 15.6 years, normal responses in Double Simultaneous (face-hand) stimulations were shown by only one other patient (BL) among the twenty-three tested.

Thus, consistent with the findings of Basser, Carlson *et al.*, and Wilson, our neuropsychological and language tests revealed no evidence of dysphasia in twenty-three of twenty-four cases with left[14] or right[10] hemispherectomy for IH, and no evidence of significant differences in effects of right or left hemispherectomy on language and nonlanguage tests. In contrast to the findings in Verbal-Performance IQ comparisons, higher Performance IQ's in three of thirteen patients with left and one of nine cases with right hemispherectomy might suggest that effects of removals of either hemisphere are more marked on nonlanguage capacities. Indeed, one of the most striking findings in studies of twenty-four patients thus far was that with only one exception (an aphasic hospitalized for continuing psychotic episodes, examined 3 years after left hemispherectomy), correct grammatical speech had developed in all patients, including four whose intelligence test scores were below the lowest limits.

The consistent findings of subsequent development or improvement of language functions after right or left hemispherectomy for IH in almost all reported studies suggest that, in the reorganization of functions in the drastically reduced neuroanatomical economy resulting from removal of either hemisphere, *there may be a developmental hierarchy in which the development of language functions takes precedence over nonlanguage and verbal reasoning functions.* Language was described by Nissen (1951) as "a stupendously complicated symbolic system, not even approximately achieved by any other organism." The suggested priority and independence of language in the development of cerebral functions is indicated by two patients with right and two with left hemispherectomy whose verbal and nonverbal reasoning capacities were below the lowest limits of standardized intelligence tests for children or adults. In addition to similar cases reported in earlier studies of hemispherectomy for IH, priorities for the selective development of speech and verbal comprehension (but *not* of reading and writing) are also evident in the severely mentally retarded. Thus, the findings indicate that the *acquisition* of (or the development, organization, and integration of the complex processes involved in) speaking and understanding speech are "no more learned than , say ability to walk is learned" (Chomsky, 1967).

Clearly, then, the biological substrata of language functions, and I would add, for nonlanguage visual ideational functions that are manifested in normal adults, are duplicated in each hemisphere. In those reported cases in which normal language and other capacities fail to develop after left or right hemispherectomy for IH, such failures may reflect limitations on the residual hemisphere superimposed by insults either concomitant with or subsequent to the initial obvious lesion resulting in infantile hemiplegia. (In the case of PK, for example, although left hemiparesis clearly reflected involvement of the right hemisphere, the underlying encephalitis almost assuredly affected both hemispheres in contrast to the birth injury of BL, which was restricted to the left hemisphere. The usual development of normal language before or after hemispherectomy for IH has been described as evidence of the *interhemispheric* "transfer" of functions, and as reflecting the "functional plasticity" of the immature brain. However, the gradual disappearance of persisting dysphasia *following* left or right hemispherectomy may also reflect *intrahemispheric* "plasticity." As McFie (1961) noted, the high proportion of abnormal EEG's over the residual hemisphere, usually associated with severe impairment in verbal and nonverbal reasoning, suggested the presence of preoperative bilateral lesions. The high proportion of persisting dysplasia in McFie's cases shortly after hemispherectomy thus suggests that the structures that normally mediate language functions in the residual hemisphere had been compromised before surgery.

Although chronic dysphasia in unoperated adults with a history of early right hemiplegia is relatively rare, the development of normal language following early speech difficulties has been interpreted as evidence that language functions had shifted to the presumably intact right hemisphere. However, the proportion of dysphasics in Wilson's (1970) later follow-up studies of fifty cases (including the 34 studied by McFie) was markedly lower than that indicated in the earlier study by McFie (1961). The apparent recovery from early aphasia might therefore be interpreted as evidence that, *in the presence of damage to structures in the remaining hemisphere in which language normally develops in cases without bilateral lesions, other intact structures in the immature brain provided the biological substrata necessary for the development of normal language.*

PATHOLOGICAL OCULAR DOMINANCE

In addition to the obvious alteration of handedness in IH according to involvement of either hemisphere, the markedly higher than normal incidence of sinistrality among nonhemiplegic populations with early brain insult (e.g. epileptics, cerebral palsied, mentally retarded) reflects "pathological lefthandedness" (Hecaen and Ajuraguerra, 1964; Smith, 1968).

Ferrier (1878) suggested that preferred use of the right or left eye might reflect differences in the role of the two hemispheres in visual ideation. On the face of it, Ferrier's notion is more logical than the demonstrated but still unexplained relationships between handedness and hemispheric specialization in language. Yet possible relationships between eyedness, hemispheric specialization in visual ideational functions, and differential effects of lateralized brain lesions on eyedness and nonlanguage functions have largely been overlooked.

Prompted by Ferrier's suggestion, ocular dominance tests were added to our neuropsychological test battery in 1965. Although data on premorbid eyedness in clinical populations are usually unavailable, Christiaens, Bize, and Maurin (1962) reported that in normal right-handed men and women, the incidence of left-eyedness is 15 percent and 21 percent, respectively. It is therefore interesting to note that in 110 right-handed stroke patients with chronic aphasia, sighting dominance tests showed an incidence of *18* or *23 percent* left-eyedness in *seventy-eight* men, and *9* or *28 percent* in *thirty-two* women.

Comparisons of the nature and degree of language disturbances revealed no significant differences between right-eyed and left-eyed aphasics. However, comparisons of nonlanguage tests revealed markedly lower scores by the left-eyed group in all measures. Although we cannot determine whether the higher incidence of left-eyedness in this population precedes or reflects the effects of often diffuse and extensive cerebrovascular lesions, the findings in experimental and clinical studies of hemispherectomy suggest bases for such a determination.

Since handedness and possibly eyedness reflect differences in hemispheric functions unique to man, generalizations of the results of hemispherectomy in other twin-brained species are obviously qualified. However, Kruper, Boyle, and Patton (1967) reported preoperative random eye preference in eight monkeys systematically shifted to preference for the eye homolateral to the ablated right or left hemisphere. Although adequate data for eyedness following hemispherectomy for tumor in adults are lacking, Dr. Burklund has reported that immediately following removals of the left hemisphere in six cases and the right hemisphere in six others, the pupil on the paretic side was 1.5 to 2 times larger than the other pupil in all twelve cases.

It is therefore interesting to note that in postoperative studies of ten cases of right hemispherectomy for IH, nine were right-eyed, the single exception being a child with bupthalmus of the right eye; and of thirteen with left hemispherectomy, nine were left-eyed. Although these limited data warrant no conclusions, they suggest that in addition to injury to the peripheral structures involved in vision, marked differences in visual acuity between the two eyes, hereditary, and other possible postnatal factors (e.g. left or right homonymous hemianopsia and hemiplegia), like "pathological left-handedness," eye preference may reflect lateralized lesions in the young or mature brain.

THEORETICAL IMPLICATIONS

In view of the numerous sources of ambiguity inherent in studies of hemispherectomy and the small samples in the present study, the above findings warrant few firm conclusions. Almost a century ago, Goltz (1888) wrote, "The research into the functions of the brain is a very old question. Many have tried and many have erred." As Dr. Burkland has said, it is important to keep an open mind. But, it is often difficult, since we have all been more or less indoctrinated by teachers and textbooks.

The accumulating findings in studies of effects of focal lesions and of hemispherectomy at different stages in the development of the brain suggest different patterns in the maturation of normal hemispheric functions which have been described elsewhere. However, two consistent findings merit brief consideration.

Studies of hemispherectomy for IH have demonstrated that although two hemispheres are necessary for normal sensory and motor functions, only one intact hemisphere—either the left or right—will suffice for the development of normal language, verbal, and nonverbal reasoning capacities. In fact, as noted above, verbal reasoning capacities developed to appreciably higher levels than those of normal adults in BL after left hemispherectomy and in Griffith's first patient with a right hemispherectomy for IH. Has nature, then, been overly extravagant in providing us at birth with two equal brains, each capable of the development of "higher" mental processes?

In a little noted but remarkable essay, however, Berry Campbell (1960) called attention to "The Factor of Safety in The Nervous System." He quoted Meltzer's elegant observation on the large safety factor in the duplication of the kidney, and of other paired organs. Studies of hemispherectomy for IH thus suggest that at birth, the presence of two intact hemispheres constitutes a similar safety factor to that of the two kidneys—but, with one important difference. The two kidneys in man provide a reserve or safety factor for compensation of normal functional decrements with advancing age, or for loss of function in one kidney because of disease throughout life. The safety factor in two cerebral hemispheres, however, is increasingly reduced in most—but not all people—by the progressive specialization of the left hemisphere in speech, reading, writing, and verbal reasoning functions; and of the right hemisphere in visual ideational and other nonlanguage functions. The "critical period," or the age at which either hemisphere can no longer fully compensate for loss of functions of one has been reported to occur sometime between the first and fifteenth birthday. Hopefully, future studies will provide more specific and definite findings.

The second recurring finding has especially important theoretical implications. Krynauw and others cited above have reported the marked improvement of speech after left or right hemispherectomy for IH in several cases. This improvement was associated with the rapid return of preoperatively abnormal EEG's over the intact hemisphere to normal levels. Thus, Krynauw and others have pointed out that in cases of IH, the effects of lateralized lesions may radiate to the opposite hemisphere and disrupt its functions.

The disappearance of dysarthria in Dr. Burklund's case #9 after left hemispherectomy, and the striking improvement in recovery of motor functions of the left leg in his patient #1 immediately after right hemispherectomy may, as Dr. Burklund has suggested, also be due to removal of inhibitory influences of the tumor in the left or right cerebral hemisphere on the remaining ipsilateral caudal structures.

Whether or not the inhibited mechanisms are in the opposite hemisphere or in the remaining ipsilateral caudal structures following hemispherectomy, these findings indicate that partial or total loss of specific cerebral functions may be due to either *destruction*—or *inhibition*—of their underlying neuroanatomical substrata. Since the potentials for restitution of the specific functions would obviously differ, differentiations of the nature of impairment in functions and of the specific structures involved are of conceivable theoretical as well as practical importance.

In closing, it is interesting to observe that in Lashley's attempts to generalize the findings of experimental animal studies to human brain functions, he gradually recognized that his earlier concept of equipotentiality was in error and modified his views. It is therefore not surprising that later in his career, Lashley (1941) urged the coalescence of neurology and psychology. The recent emergence of clinical neuropsychology as a discrete field of specialization, and the increasing collaboration of neurosurgeons, neurologists and neuropsychologists reflects the growing recognition that the problems of brain-behavior relationships overlap the borders of different disciplines.

ACKNOWLEDGMENTS

This investigation was supported by PHS Grant No. MH 16470-01 from the National Institute of Mental Health. The kind interest of Drs. P. Bucy, C. Burklund, G. Fischer, W. Gardner, M. Girgis, R. Goodall, A. Greenberg, E. Hendrick, E. Laskowski, M. Perlstein (deceased), J. Ransohoff, D. Richardson, E. Todd, and P. Vogel and often extensive cooperation in arranging examinations and providing clinical data for their patients is gratefully acknowledged. Special thanks are also due to Prof. John Wiley for independent studies of language functions; Dr. J. Bogen for assistance in locating and examining four patients; to Dr. J. Arbit, I. Mensh, and J. Wishner for providing previous test data; and especially to Dr. C. Netley, who administered the neuropsychological test battery to Dr. Hendrick's patients.

REFERENCES

1. Austin, G. M., and Grant, F. C.: Physiologic observations following total hemispherectomy in man. *Surgery, 38:*239-258, 1955.
2. Basser, L. S.: Hemiplegia of early onset and the faculty of speech with special reference to the effects of hemispherectomy. *Brain, 85:*427-460, 1962.
3. Bennett, A. H., and Godlee, R. J.: Case of cerebral tumor. *Brit Med J, 1:*988-989, 1885.
4. Bogen, J. E.: The other side of the brain. *Bull Los Angeles Neurol Soc, 34:*73-105, part I (a), 135-161, part II (b), 1969.
5. Bramwell, B.: On "crossed" aphasias. *Lancet, 1:*1473-1379, 1899.
6. Broca, P.: Sur la faculte du langage articule. *Bull Soc D'Anthropologie (Paris), 6:*493-494, 1865.
7. Bruell, J. H., and Albee, G. W.: Higher intellectual functions in a patient with hemispherectomy for tumor. *J Consult Psychol, 26:*90-98, 1962.

8. Cairns, H., and Davidson, M. A.: Hemispherectomy in the treatment of infantile hemiplegia. *Lancet, 2:*411-415, 1951.

9. Campbell, B.: The factor of safety in the nervous system. *Bull Los Angeles Neurol Soc, 25:*109-117, 1960.

10. Carlson, J., Netley, C., Hendrick, E. B., and Prichard, J. S.: A reexamination of intellectual disabilities in hemispherectomized patients. *Trans Amer Neurol Ass, 93:*198-201, 1968.

11. Chomsky, N.: In Millikan, C. H., and Darley, F. L. (Eds.) : *The General Properties of Language in Brain Mechanisms Underlying Speech and Language.* New York, Grune and Stratton, 1967, pp. 73-88.

12. Christiaens, L., Bize, P. R., and Maurin, P.: Les gaucheurs au travail. In *VIIth Journees Nationales de Medicine du Travail.* Paris, Masson and Cie, 1962, p. 5-6.

13. Critchley, M.: Disorders of higher nervous. In Vinken, P. J., and Bruyn, G. W. (Eds.): *Handbook of Clinical Neurology.* New York, John Wiley and Sons, 1969, vol. 3, pp. 1-10.

14. Dandy, W. E.: Physiological studies following extirpation of the right cerebral hemisphere in man. *Johns Hopkins Hosp Bull, 53:*31-51, 1933.

15. Dandy, W. E.: Removal of right cerebral hemisphere for certain tumors with hemiplegia. Preliminary report. *JAMA, 90:*823-825, 1928.

16. Falconer, M. A., and Wilson, P. J. E.: Complications related to delayed hemorrhage after hemispherectomy. *J Neurosurg, 30:*413-426, 1969.

17. Feld, M.: De L'hemiplegie cerebrale infantile aux encephalapothie catricielles. Place et signification des hemispherectomies, *Vth Int Neurol Congress, 4:*387-391, 1953.

18. Ferrier, D.: *The Localization of Cerebral Disease.* London, Smith, Elder, and Company, 1878.

19. Flourens, P.: *Recherches Experimentale sur les Proprietes et des Fonctions du Systeme Nerveux dans les Animaus Vertebres.* Paris, Chez Crevot, 1824.

20. French, L. A., Johnson, D. R., Brown, I. A. and Von Verben, F. B.: Cerebral hemispherectomy for control of intractable convulsive seizures. *J Neurosurg, 12:*154-164, 1955.

21. Gardner, W. J., Karnosh, L. J., McClure, C. C., and Gardner, A. K.: Residual function following hemispherectomy for tumor and for infantile hemiplegia. *Brain, 78:*487-502, 1955.

22. Goltz, F.: On the functions of the hemispheres. *Pflugers Archiv fur die gesamte Physiologie, 42:*419-467, 1888. (Translated by Gerhardt von Bonin in *Some Papers on the Cerebral Cortex.* Springfield, Thomas, 1960, pp. 118-158.)

23. Griffith, H., and Davidson, M.: Long-term changes in intellect and behaviour after hemispherectomy. *J Neurol Neurosurg Psychiat, 29:*571-576, 1966.

24. Gros, C., and Vlahovitch, B.: Etude de la sensibilite dans les hemispherectomies. *Congre Neurologique International, 4:*320-322, 1953.

25. Hebb, D. O.: Intelligence in man after large removals of cerebral tissue: Defects following right temporal lobectomy. *J Gen Psychol, 21:*437-446, 1939.

26. Hecaen, H., and Ajuriaguerra, J. de: *Left-handedness.* New York, Grune and Stratton, 1964.

27. Hillier, W. F.: Total left cerebral hemispherectomy for malignant glioma. *Neurology, 4:*718-721, 1954.

28. Ignelzi, R. J. and Bucy, P. C.: Cerebral hemidecortication in the treatment of infantile cerebral hemiatrophy. *J Nerv Ment Dis, 147:*14-30, 1968.

29. Jackson, H.: Case of large cerebral tumor without optic neuritis and with left hemiplegia and imperception. *Roy Lond Opthalmic Hosp Rep, 8:*434, 1876.

30. Kennard, M. A., and Fulton, J. F.: Age and reorganization of the central nervous system. *J Mount Sinai Hosp, 9:*594-605, 1942.

31. Kennedy, F.: Stock-brainedness, the causation factor in the so-called "crossed aphasias." *Amer J Med Sci, 6:*849-859, 1916.

32. Kruper, D. C., Boyle, B., and Patton, R. A.: Eye preference in hemicerebrectomized monkeys. *Psychol Sci, 7:*105-106, 1967.

33. Krynauw, R. A.: Infantile hemiplegia treated by removing one cerebral hemisphere. *J Neurol Neurosurg Psychiat, 13:*243-267, 1950.

34. Lashley, K. S.: Coalescence of neurology and psychology. *Proc Amer Philosoph Soc, 84:*461-470, 1941.

35. Liepman, H. K.: Die linke hemisphere und das handeln. *Med Wchnschr, 52:*2322-2326, 1905.

36. Lenneberg, E. H.: *Biological Foundations of Language.* New York, John Wiley and Sons, 1967.

37. Lereboullet, J.: Removal of left cerebral hemisphere. *Paris Med, 1:*358-360, 1936.

38. Lhermitte, J.: L'ablation complete de l'hemisphere droit dans les cas de tumeur cerebrale localizee compliquee d'hemiplegie: La decerebration supra-thalamique unilaterale chez l'homme. *Encephale, 23.1:*314-323, 1928.

39. McFie, J.: The effects of hemispherectomy on intellectual functioning in cases of infantile hemiplegia. *J Neurol Neurosurg Psychiat,* 1961.

40. McHenry, L. C., *Garrison's History of Neurology.* Springfield, Thomas, 1969.

41. McKenzie, K. G.: The present status of a patient who had the right cerebral hemisphere removed. *JAMA, 111:*168, 1938.

42. Mensh, I. N., Schwartz, H. G., Matarazzo, R. G., and Matarazzo, J. D.: Psychological functioning following cerebral hemispherectomy in man. *Arch Neurol Psychiat, 67:*787-796, 1952.

43. Meyers, R.: Recent advances in the neurosurgery of cerebral palsy. In Illingworth, R. S. (Ed.): *Recent Advances in Cerebral Palsy.* London, Churchill, 1958, pp. 330-386.

44. Monakow, C. V.: Localization of brain functions. *J Fur Psychologie und Neurologie, 17:*185-200, 1911.

45. Nissen, H. W.: In Stevens, S. S. (Ed.): *Handbook of Experimental Psychology.* New York, John Wiley and Sons, 1951, pp. 367-386.

46. Obrador, S. A.: Hemisferectomia en el tratamiento de las convlsiones de la hemiplegia infantil por hemiatrofia cerebral. *Arq Neuro-psiquiat (S Paulo), 9:*191-197, 1951.

47. Patterson, A., and Zangwill, O. L.: Disorders of visual space perception associated with lesions of the right hemisphere. *Brain, 67:*331-358, 1944.

48. Patterson, A., and Zangwill, O. L.: A case of topographical disorientation associated with unilateral cerebral lesion. *Brain, 68:*188-212, 1945.

49. Pool, J. L.: Answer to question "Would you recommend hemispherectomy for treatment of a cerebral glioma?" *Clin Neurosurg,* 1968, p. 286.

50. Roberts, L.: Aphasia, apraxia, and agnosia in abnormal states of cerebral dominance. In Vinken, P. J., and Bruyn, G. W. (Eds.): *Handbook of Clinical Neurology.* New York, John Wiley, 1969, vol. 4, pp. 312-326.

51. Rowe, S. N.: Mental changes following the removal of the right cerebral hemisphere for brain tumor. *Amer J Psychiat, 94:*604-612, 1937.

52. Smith, A.: Ambiguities in concepts and studies of "brain damage" and "organicity." *J Nerv Ment Dis, 135:*311-326, 1962.

53. Smith, A.: Speech and other functions after left (Dominant) hemispherectomy. *J Neurol Neurosurg Psychiat, 29:*467-471, 1966.

54. Smith, A.: Neuropsychological aspects of learning disorders. In *Learning Disorders,* Seattle, Washington, Special Child Publications, 1968, vol. 3, pp. 83-91.

55. Smith, A.: Nondominant hemispherectomy, *Neurology, 19:*442-445, 1969.

56. Smith, A.: Objective indices of severity of chronic aphasia in stroke patients. *J Speech Hearing Dis,* 1971 (in press).

57. Smith, A., and Burklund, C. W.: Dominant hemispherectomy. *Science, 153:*1280-1282, 1966.

58. Smith, A., and Burkland, C. W. B.: Nondominant hemispherectomy: Neuropsychologic implications for human brain functions. *APA, 1967 Convention Prog.,* pp. 103-104.

59. Sperry, R. W., Gazzaniga, M. S., and Bogen, J. E.: Interhemispheric relationships. In Vinken, P. J., and Bruyn, G. W. (Eds.) : *Handbook of Clinical Neurology.* New York, John Wiley and Sons, 1969, vol. 4, pp. 273-290.

60. Strong, O. S., and Elwyn, A.: *Human Neuroanatomy.* Baltimore, Williams and Wilkins, 1943.

61. Subirana, A.: Handedness and cerebral dominance. In Vinken, P. J., and Bruyn, G. W. (Eds.) : *Handbook of Clinical Neurology.* New York, John Wiley and Sons, 1969, Vol. 4, pp. 248-272.

62. Terman, L. M., and Merrill, M. A.: *Measuring Intelligence.* Boston, Houghton Mifflin, 1936.

63. Teuber, H. L.: Lacunae and research approaches to them. In Millikan, C. H., and Darley, F. L. (Eds.) : *Brain Mechanisms Underlying Speech and Language.* New York, Grune and Stratton, 1967, pp. 204-216.

64. Vulpian, A.: Lecons sur la physiologie generale et comparee du systeme nerveux. *Paris Balliere, 6:*920, 1866.

65. Weisenburg, T. H., and McBride, K. E.: *Aphasia: A Clinical and Psychological Study.* New York Commonwealth Fund, 1935, p. 322.

66. Weisenburg, T. H., Roe, A., and McBride, K. E.: *Adult Intelligence.* New York Commonwealth Fund, 1936.

67. White, H. H.: Cerebral hemispherectomy in the treatment of infantile hemiplegia, *Confin Neurol, 21:*1-50, 1961.

68. Wiley, J., Speech and language functions before and after left (dominant) hemispherectomy. *A. S. H. A. Convention,* 1968.

69. Williams, D. J., and Scott, J. W.: The functional responses of the sympathetic nervous system of man following hemidecortication. *J Neurol Psychiat, 2:*313-322, 1939.

70. Wilson, P. J. E.: Cerebral hemispherectomy for infantile hemiplegia. *Brain, 93:*147-180, 1970.

71. Zangwill, O. L.: *Cerebral Dominance and Its Relation to Psychological Function.* Edinburgh, Oliver and Boyd, 1960.

72. Zangwill, O. L.: Speech and the minor hemisphere. *Acta Neurologica et Psychiatrica Belgica, 67:*1013-1020, 1967.

73. Zollinger, R.: Removal of left cerebral hemisphere. *Arch Neurol Psychia, 34:*1055-1064, 1935.

Chapter 4

Effects of Psychotropic Drugs on Computer Analyzed Resting and Sleep EEG Following Hemispherectomy in Man*

BERND SALATU AND TURAN M. ITIL

INTRODUCTION

SEVERAL investigators have demonstrated that in spite of the surgical removal of a human cerebral hemisphere, scalp recorded electrical potentials can still be recorded on that side of the head (Marshall and Walker, 1950; Cobb and Pampiglione, 1952; Ueki, 1966; and Lorenz *et al.*, 1968). It has been assumed that these potentials spread from the remaining hemisphere by conduction through the skull, scalp, and fluid (Obrador and Larramendi, 1950; Cobb and Sears, 1960). However, in a recent study, by means of quantitative analysis, we demonstrated that the EEG in the hemispherectomized side is not just a smaller version of the activity originating in the unoperated side (Itil and Saletu, 1971). The occurrence of certain frequency potentials more often in the operated than in the unoperated hemisphere during resting and sleep recordings suggests the existence of indigenous bioelectrical phenomena in the operated hemisphere, most likely originating in the thalamus, hypothalamus, and brain stem. Based on these findings, we were interested in investigating the mode of action of psychotropic drugs on a hemispherectomized patient using digital computer analyzed resting and sleep EEGs.

MATERIAL AND METHOD

Case History

We studied a twenty-two-year old white male patient who had been ill for nineteen years. At the age of three years his parents noticed that he had frequent headaches, vomiting, and dizziness, followed by prolonged periods of sleep. The first definite seizure activity began at the age of six years with a right adversive Jacksonian seizure. The patient was admitted to the hospital where an EEG suggested a left frontal-parietal focus, while a pneumoencephalogram was normal. Despite anticonvulsive treatment, the patient experienced approximately three seizures a month. Two years later (1956) he was again admitted to the hospital with an EEG showing moderately slow dysrhythmia and transient paroxysms without a focal tendency. In 1959 the patient was admitted for the first time to a psy-

*Supported in part by USPHS grant MH-11381 and the Psychiatric Research Foundation of Missouri.

69

chiatric hospital, as a result of aggressive and combative behavior. A physical examination revealed a right hemiparesis with right central facial paralysis and dysphasia. The pneumoencephalogram exhibited a slight dilation of the left anterior horn, suggesting cortical atrophy in this region. In 1967 the patient was again admitted to the hospital as a result of frequent outbursts of aggressive destructive behavior, numerous Jacksonian seizures, and three to four grand mal attacks per month. A pneumoencephalogram and a cerebral arteriogram revealed mild atrophy of the left cerebral hemisphere. The EEG showed delta and theta waves in the left cerebral leads, with higher amplitude and phase reversal in the left temporal region, indicating some brain damage to the left cerebral hemisphere. On August 18, 1967, a left hemispherectomy was performed leaving the thalamus and a part of the basal ganglia. The pathological findings revealed an old infarct of the insula, putamen, caudate nucleus, frontal and parietal lobes, and hippocampalgyrus. Postoperatively the patient had a dense right hemiplegia, hemihypesthesia, aphasia, and a right homonymous hemianopsia. The hemiplegia and aphasia improved with physical and speech therapy, so that the patient was able to return home for a trial visit on October 25, 1967, experiencing no further seizures.

The present admission (1968) resulted from the patient again becoming agitated, attacking his mother. Physical examination at this time showed no changes.

Methods of Investigation

During a one-month investigation period, the patient was kept on Dilantin® medication (300 mg daily). At this time, we made a series of all-night sleep recordings (7-8 hours duration) following one adaptation night. Preceding the sleep recordings, we also took a resting EEG of ten to fifteen minutes. A monopolar recording (indifferent electrode on the ear) was carried out from the frontal, central, temporal, and occipital areas of both the hemispherectomized and unoperated sides. Six channels (two central, two temporal, and two occipital) were recorded on tape (Ampex SP-300), and one channel was analyzed on-line using period analysis programs (Burch *et al.,* 1964; Shapiro and Fink, 1966) with a digital computer system (IBM 1620/1710). This method permits analysis of each EEG sample (10-second, 20-second, 30-second or 60-second samples) based on nineteen measurements (14 different frequency bands for zero cross and first derivative measurements, zero cross and first derivative average frequencies, average frequency deviation of zero cross analysis, average absolute amplitude and amplitude variability).

In the sleep investigations, EMG, EKG, and rapid eye movement (from both sides) were recorded simultaneously with the EEG. The sleep stages were determined using the digital computer "sleep print" method (Itil and Shapiro, 1968; Itil *et al.,* 1969). With this method each thirty-second EEG epoch is continuously and automatically classified into one of the three-stage (slow wave spindle sleep, low voltage fast sleep, neither), five-stage

(Dement and Kleitman, 1957), and nine-stage sleep classifications (Itil and Shapiro, 1968), based on the seven zero cross measurements of the period analysis. Using other computer programs, it was also possible to obtain the percentage of time spent in each sleep stage of the three systems of sleep classification, as well as to classify each artefact-free epoch of the sleep record by its distance from the resting (awake) record in terms of the resting (wakening) EEG variability measure (Itil, 1969). The length of the REM periods were evaluated visually based on a low voltage fast EEG pattern, the occurrence of the rapid eye movement, and the disappearance of muscle potential. It was also determined whether each REM sample had predominantly single or burst REM activity.

Thioridazine and LSD-25 were selected for the psychopharmacological investigations. The first compound is a major tranquilizer, effective in controlling psychotic symptoms, while the latter is a hallucinogenic drug, which produces experimental psychosis. In this study, thioridazine was given orally both in a single dose of 100 mg and in 300 mg daily chronic administration. LSD-25 was administered parenterally in a dosage of 70 mcg.

RESULTS

Investigations with Thioridazine

Resting EEG

The mean values of EEG period analysis measurements demonstrated that there were statistically significant (two sample t-test) differences between the right and left hemisphere in the central, temporal, and occipital recordings, before as well as after 100 mg thioridazine orally. Before drug administration central and temporal recordings showed more 0-12 cps activity (zero cross measurements) and superimposed very high frequency beta waves over 40 cps (first derivative measurements) in the operated than the unoperated side (Fig 4-1). The unoperated side exhibited more 16-40 cps (zero cross measurements) and superimposed 0-40 cps (first derivative measurements) activity. In the occipital recordings all the EEG measurements in the two hemispheres were similar with the exception of alpha activity and beta waves: Eight to sixteen cps activity was greater in the unoperated side, and 26-40 cps activity was greater in the operated side. The amplitude was greater in all regions on the unoperated side.

The thioridazine-induced changes were different in the two hemispheres. The operated central region showed a greater decrease in average frequency and 26-40 cps activity and a greater increase in 5-16 cps waves (zero cross measurements) than the unoperated side (Fig. 4-2). In contrast, the unoperated side exhibited a greater decrease in 0-5 cps waves and a greater increase in 16-26 cps activity (zero cross measurements) than the operated

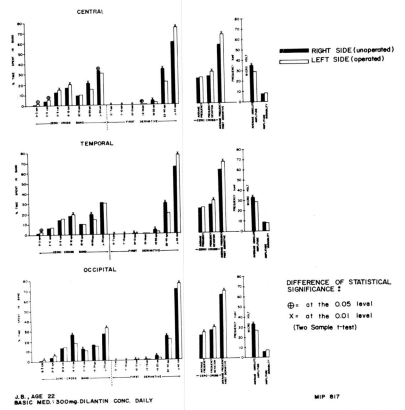

Figure 4-1. Mean values of computer period analysis measurements of a hemispherectomized patient during awakening (second placebo week). Nineteen EEG variables of the period analysis are shown in the abscissa. The ordinate on the left shows the percentage of time spent in each band, while that on the right indicates frequency in cycles per second and amplitude in microvolts. In the central and temporal regions, 0-3, 3-5, 5-8, and 8-12 cps activities of the zero cross measurements and the over 40 cps activity and average frequency of the first derivative measurements are greater in the operated than in the unoperated side. In contrast, 16-26 cps and 26-40 cps activity of the zero cross measurements and 10-13, 13-16, 16-22, and 22-40 cps bands of the first derivative measurements are greater in the unoperated than in the operated side. The differences were often at a level of statistical significance. In the occipital area, the opposite was true of only 8-12 and over 26 cps bands in the zero cross measurements.

side. During thioridazine treatment, the average absolute amplitude decreased significantly in the unoperated side while it significantly increased in the operated side. (P < .01, t-test).

Sleep EEG

All-night sleep recordings were carried out before and during, as well as following, chronic oral treatment with thioridazine (300 mg daily). It was ob-

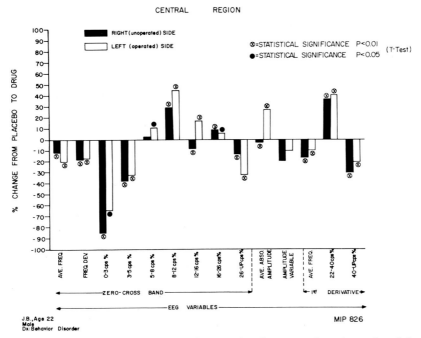

Figure 4-2. Thioridazine-induced EEG changes in the central region of a left hemispherectomized patient. (100 mg mellaril orally, based on computer period analysis.) 14 EEG variables of the period analysis are shown in the abscissa. The percentage change from placebo to drug is represented in the ordinate. The operated side shows a greater decrease in average frequency and 26-40 cps activity and a greater increase in 5-16 cps waves than the unoperated side. The unoperated side exhibits a greater decrease in 0-5 cps and a greater increase in 16-26 cps waves than the operated side. The average absolute amplitude decreases in the unoperated side, while it increases in the operated side.

served that chronic thioridazine medication, as compared with placebo, increased the length of the deep sleep stages (Fig. 4-3). REM periods seemed to decrease after discontinuation of thioridazine treatment (Fig. 4-4.) Because of technical difficulties, the differences between the right and left hemispheres of the sleep recordings during thioridazine medication could not be analyzed.

Investigation with LSD-25

Sleep Prints

The onset of deep sleep stages after 70 mcg LSD-25 I.M. was delayed for a period of four to five hours (Fig. 4-3) . Analysis of the length of sleep stages, based on the five-level sleep stage classification of sleep prints (artefact free samples primarily at the end of the night) , showed that after LSD-

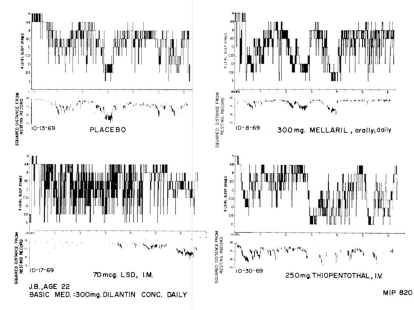

Figure 4-3. Drug effect on the sleep print and squared distance from the resting record of a left hemispherectomized patient. (Based on computer period analysis of the right occipital EEG.) Time (6 hours) is represented in the abscissa; in the ordinate the nine sleep stages (A = awakening, E = deepest sleep) and the squared distance from the resting record are shown. Chronic thioridazine medication, as compared with placebo, increases the length of deep sleep stages. 70 mcg LSD i.m. delays the onset of deeper sleep for a period of four to five hours.

25 administration the occipital region of the unoperated side spent more time in awakening and light sleep stages. In the central area the unoperated side exhibited more awakening and stage three sleep, whereas the operated side spent more time in sleep stages one and two (Fig. 4-5).

Computer EEG Measurements

Several EEG measurements showed interesting findings after I.M. administration of 70 mcg LSD—a hallucinogenic compound—which decreases alpha activity and increases fast activity. Eight to 12 cps activity decreased to a significantly greater degree in the operated than in the unoperated side, suggesting that LSD-25 has primarily an effect on the subcortical function system (Fig. 4-6). As is known, subcortical structures are predominantly responsible for the origin of the 8-12 cps activity. Obviously, because of the interaction of the sleep tendency with LSD-25, 16-26 cps waves decreased on both sides, but less on the operated than on the unoperated side. The significant differences between the two hemispheres in these frequency

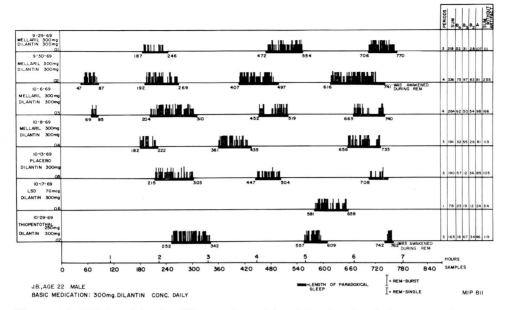

Figure 4-4. REM activity in different drug-nights following hemispherectomy in man. The amount, onset, and end of REM periods in different nights, as well as the number of thirty second samples spent in paradoxical sleep with single REM (B_4), REM burst (B_3), and non-REM (B_2) activity are shown. During chronic thioridazine medication the patient has 3-4 REM cycles per night and many REM bursts. After discontinuation of thioridazine, REM activity decreases, and in the LSD night only one delayed REM period can be seen.

bands, which were observed during the resting recording, were still present six to seven hours after LSD administration, but at this time they were reversed. This may be related again to the interaction of the sleep process with LSD-25, but in any case, it indicates that the differences between the right and left hemispheres are not due to either the spreading of activity or artefact, but to real functional differences. Before and after LSD administration, 22-40 cps activity (first derivative measurement) was greater in the unoperated than operated side (Fig. 4-7). However, in comparison to the pre-LSD record, a marked increase of 22-40 cps activity was observed after LSD, and this increase was greater in the operated side. The very high frequency superimposed beta activity (over 40 cps in the first derivative measurement) was prevalent in the operated side both before and after LSD administration. Again, LSD-induced changes were predominant in the operated side.

REM Activity

REM sleep (paradoxical sleep) occurred with a considerable amount of latency (late onset) after LSD-25 administration as compared with all-night

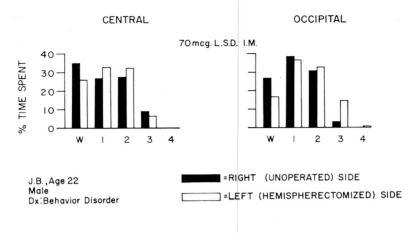

Figure 4-5. Length of sleep stages of two hemispheres (5 stage classification) after drug administration based on digital computer sleep print method. Sleep stages (W = awakening, 4 = deepest sleep) are shown in the abscissa and in the ordinate percentage of time spent in different sleep stages. In the occipital region the unoperated side spent more time in sleep stages W and 1, whereas the operated side spent more time in sleep stages 2 and 3. In the central region more awakening stages can again be seen on the unoperated side, while the operated side exhibits more stage 1 and 2.

sleep without LSD-25 (Fig. 4-4). Only one period of rapid eye movement was observed (6th hour of sleep), and during that period more single REM activity occurred than burst REM activity.

DISCUSSION

This study demonstrated that thioridazine, a major tranquilizer, increased alpha activity and theta waves, and decreased very fast activity in the EEG of a left hemispherectomized patient. On the other hand, LSD-25, a hallucinogenic compound, decreased alpha activity and increased 22-40 cps fast activity. That thioridazine produces a slowing in the EEG activity, has previously been described by several authors (Hollister and Barthel, 1959; Ulett *et al.*, 1964; Itil 1968). The desynchronization and acceleration effect of LSD on the EEG is known as well (Gastaut *et al.*, 1953; Bradley and Elkes, 1957; Itil *et al.*, 1969).

Since subcortical activity can be detected from the operated side and predominantly cortical activity can be detected from the unoperated hemisphere of a hemispherectomized patient (Itil and Saletu, 1971; Saletu *et al.* in press), it was tried in this study to determine whether LSD-25 and thioridazine act predominantly on subcortical or on cortical structures. After thioridazine, 8-13 cps, 12-16 cps, and 5-8 cps activity showed a greater increase in the operated hemisphere than in the unoperated hemisphere, suggesting

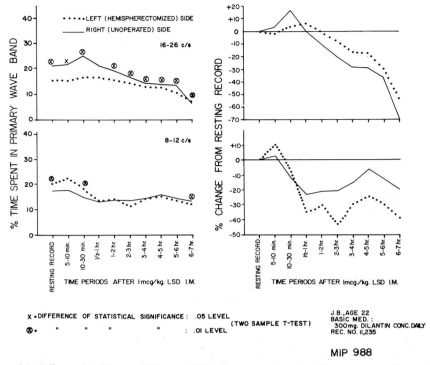

Figure 4-6. Effect of LSD on different EEG frequency bands. The abscissa shows different time periods, while in the left ordinate, percentage time spent in the 16-26 and 8-12 cps band, and in the right ordinate the percentage change from the resting record in these bands, are shown. 8-12 cps activity decreases more and 16-26 cps decreases less in the operated than in the unoperated side.

that the drug has an effect primarily on the subcortical substrates, which have previously been correlated with these activities (Jung *et al.*, 1950; Okuma *et al.*, 1954; Andersen and Andersson, 1968). The increases in alpha activity and amplitude and the decrease in average frequency, as well as frequency and amplitude variability, indicate the inhibitory influence of thioridazine on the reticular activating system of the brain stem and thalamocortical integration system. That thioridazine apparently acts on the ascending reticular activating system and through the thalamic and hypothalamic nuclei on the cortex was suggested by Prat Homs and Rom Font (1965), when they observed a synchronization of cerebral bioelectrical activity in thioridazine-treated catatonics.

After LSD-25, 8-12 cps activity decreased and 22-40 cps activity increased—this more in the operated than in the unoperated side. Again, the fact that the decrease of the alpha and increase of fast activity was greater in the operated than in the unoperated side indicates that the predominant

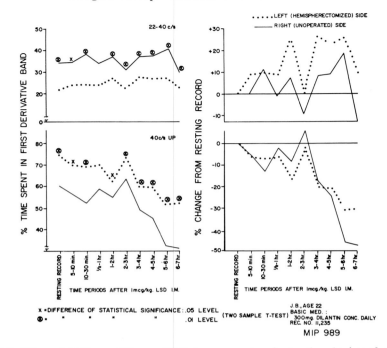

Figure 4-7. Effect of LSD on different EEG frequency bands. In the abscissa the different time periods are shown. Percentage of time spent in the 22-40 cps and 40 up cps band of the first derivative are shown in the left ordinate, while the right ordinate shows the percentage change from the resting record in these bands. 22-40 cps activity is always dominant on the unoperated side, and over 40 cps waves are dominant on the operated side. However, LSD-induced changes can be seen better in the operated than in the unoperated side.

effect of LSD is not on the cortex but on the subcortical structures, most likely exerting a stimulatory effect on the reticular activating system of the brain stem.

Chronic administration of thioridazine induced a greater amount of deep sleep and REM activity as compared with the placebo night. In contrast, LSD-25 delayed the onset of sleep for a period of four to five hours and decreased REM activity. That LSD-25 markedly inhibits the sleep cycles has previously been found in man (Itil, 1968) as well as in animals. Hobson (1964) observed that 2 mcg per kg LSD-25 interfered with sleep generally and reduced LVF sleep selectively in eight cats with chronically implanted electrodes.

SUMMARY

The mode of action of two psychotropic drugs on a left hemispherectomized patient was studied using digital computer analyzed resting and sleep

EEGs. After administration of thioridazine, a major tranquilizer, 5-16 cps activity showed a greater increase in the operated than in the unoperated hemisphere, suggesting that the drug primarily has an effect on subcortical substrates. In contrast, LSD-25, a hallucinogenic compound, decreased 8-15 cps and increased 22-40 cps activity. Since these changes were greater in the operated than in the unoperated side, it was concluded that the predominant effect of LSD is not on the cortex but on subcortical structures, most likely stimulating the reticular activating system of the brain stem. Thioridazine generally increased the length of deep sleep stages and REM activity; LSD-25 delayed the onset of deeper sleep stages for a period of four to five hours and decreased REM activity as well.

ACKNOWLEDGMENT

We would like to thank Dr. A. Marrazzi and Dr. S. Woodruff for their cooperation with our investigations involving their patient and Mr. W. Hsu for statistical analysis. Dr. Sidney Goldring performed the hemispherectomy at Barnes Hospital.

REFERENCES

1. Andersen, P., and Andersson, S. A.: *Physiological Basis of the Alpha Rhythm.* Appleton-Century-Croft, New York, 1968.
2. Bradley, P. B., and Elkes, J.: The effects of some drugs on the electrical activity of the brain. *Brain, 80:*77-115, 1957.
3. Burch, N. D., Nettleton, W. J., Sweeney, J., and Edwards, R. J.: Period analysis of the electroencephalogram on a general purpose digital computer. *Ann NY Acad Sci, 115:*827, 1964.
4. Cobb, W. A., and Pampiglione, G.: The electroencephalogram in relation to human cerebral hemispherectomy. *Rev Neurol (Paris), 87:*465, 1952.
5. Cobb, W., and Sears, T. A.: A study of the transmission of potentials after hemispherectomy. *Electroenceph Clin Neurophysiol, 12:*371-383, 1960.
6. Dement, W. C., and Kleitman, N.: Cyclic variations in EEG during sleep and their relation to eye movements, body motility, and dreaming. *Electroenceph Clin Neurophysiol, 9:*673-690, 1957.
7. Gastaut, H., Ferrer, S., Castells, C., Lesevre, N., and Luschnat, K.: Action de la Diethylamide de l'acide d-lysergique (LSD-25) sur les fonctions psychiques et l'electroencephalogramme. *Confin Neurol, 13:*102-120, 1953.
8. Hobson, J. A.: The effect of LSD on the sleep cycle of the cat. *Electroenceph Clin Neurophysiol, 17:*52-56, 1964.
9. Hollister, L. E., and Barthel, C. A.: Changes in the electroencephalogram during chronic administration of tranquilizing drugs. *Electroenceph Clin Neurophysiol, 11:*792-795, 1959.
10. Itil, T. M., and Saletu, B.: Digital computer analyzed—resting and sleep EEG's (sleep prints) after hemispherectomy in man. Electoenceph. Clin. Neurophysiol *30:*457-461, 1971.
11. Itil, T. M., and Shapiro, D.: Computer classifications of all-night sleep EEG (sleep prints). In Gastaut, H., Lugaresi, E., Ceroni, G. B., and Coccagna, G. (Eds.): *The abnormalities of sleep in man.* Aulo Gaggi, Bologna, 1968, pp. 45-53.

12. Itil, T. M.: Electroencephalography and pharmacochpsychiatry. In: Freyhan, F. A., Petrilowitsch, N. and Pichot (Eds.) : Clinical Psychopharmacology, Modern Problems of Pharmacopsychiatry. S. Karger, Basel/New York. 1968, pp. 163-194.

13. Itil, T. M., Keskiner, A., and Holden, J. M. C.: The use of LSD and Ditran in the treatment of therapy resistant schizophrenics. *Dis Nerv Syst, 30:*93-103, 1969.

14. Itil, T. M.: Effects of psychotropic drugs on computer "sleep prints" in man. In Cerletti, A., and Bove, F. J. (Eds.) : *The present status of psychotropic drugs.* Excerpta Medica, Amsterdam, 1969, pp. 167-169.

15. Itil, T. M.: Automatic classification of sleep stages and the discrimination of vigilance changes using digital computer methods. *Agressologie, 10:* Numero special: 603-610, 1969.

16. Itil, T. M., Shapiro, D. M., Fink, M., and Kassebaum, D.: Digital computer classifications of EEG sleep stages. *Electroenceph Clin Neurophysiol, 27:*76-83, 1969.

17. Jung, I. R., Riechert, T., and Meyer-Mickeleit, R. W.: Uber intracerebrale Hirnpotentialableitungen bei hirnchirurgischen Eingriffen. *Dtsch Z Nervenheilk, 162:* 52-60, 1950.

18. Lorenz, R., Grutzner, A., and Vogelsang, H.: Elektroencephalographische Befund bie hemisphärektomierten Patienten. *Dtsch Z Nervenheilk, 193:*18-40, 1968.

19. Marshall, C., and Walker, A. E.: The electroencephalographic changes after hemispherectomy in man. *Electroenceph Clin Neurophysiol, 2:*147-156, 1950.

20. Obrador, S., and Larramendi, M. H.: Some observations on the brain rhythms after surgical removal of a cerebral hemisphere. *Electroenceph Clin Neurophysiol, 2:* 143-146, 1950.

21. Okuma, T., Schimazono, Y., Fukuda, T., and Narabayashi, H.: Cortical and subcortical recordings in non-anesthetized and anesthetized periods in man. *Electroenceph Clin Neurophysiol, 6:*269-286, 1954.

22. Prat Homs, J., and Rom Font, J.: Revision del concepto de catatonia, su posible interpretacion fisiologica y su tratamiento con la thioridazine. *Actas Luso Esp Neurol Psiquiat, 24:*28-43, 1965.

23. Saletu, B., Itil, T. M., and Saletu, M.: Evoked responses after hemispherectomy. *Confin Neurol* (in press) .

24. Shapiro, D. M., and Fink, M.: *Quantitative analysis of the electroencephalogram by digital computer methods.* St. Louis, Psychiatric Research Foundation of Missouri, Publication No. 66-1, 1966.

25. Ulett, G. A., Bowers, C. A., Heusler, A. F., Quick, R., Word, T., and Word. V.: A study of the behavior and EEG patterns of patient receiving tranquilizers with and without the addition of chlordiazepoxide. *J Neuropsychiat, 5:*558-565, 1964.

26. Ueki, P.: Hemispherectomy in the human with special reference to the preservation of function. In Tokizane, T., and Schade, J. P. (Eds.) : *Correlative neurosciences —Part B: Clinical studies.* Amsterdam, Elsevier, 1966, pp. 285-338.

PART II

CEREBRAL BLOOD FLOW

Chapter 5

The Process of Atheroma

D. HYWEL DAVIES

A THEROMA is the substance which is deposited in the walls of arteries during the development of atherosclerosis. The word derives from the Greek "athare," meaning porridge; formerly the name was applied to cysts on the scalp, with contents of the consistence of porridge. Atherosclerosis occurs spontaneously in various species besides man, such as the dog, the eagle, the gorilla, and even the two-toed sloth.[1] It may affect arteries supplying any territory of the body, with corresponding effects.

Sometimes it is present in all arteries, sometimes in only some. Thus, we may see diffuse atherosclerosis affecting virtually every artery in the body. On other occasions we may see severe coronary disease with no evidence of disease elsewhere. Such selectivity makes it difficult to generalize about the nature of the disease process, for it may be multifactorial in its origin. So I shall take as my point of reference atherosclerotic disease of the coronary arteries, for this is my most familiar territory. I think it is reasonable to assume that there are certain features which are common to both coronary and cerebral arterial disease, though of course it does not follow that all conclusions must apply equally to both territories. It is worthwhile taking a look at the topic again, for certain "conclusions" which are nothing more than assumptions have been repeated until they have become standard thinking. Perhaps this is not so terrible, but when nationwide action is advocated on the basis of these statements, particularly when they are propounded confidently by men with loud voices, it is time to pause and take stock. Let us then examine a few of the basic questions concerned with atherosclerosis, with especial reference to the coronary circulation.

The presence of atheroma in the inner lining of a blood-vessel represents the presence of disease, whether or not this is clinically important. We assume that the absence of atheroma represents normality, and this is seen uniformly at birth and sporadically later. In a normal blood-vessel from a boy aged four months the intima consists of a single layer of endothelial cells lining the lumen, and there is an internal elastic lamina which is seen as a wavy line. The media consists of smooth muscle fibers, the external elastic lamina of layers of elastic fibers. Vasa vasorum from the adventitia supply the media.

"Normal" arteries like this are sometimes found late in life, and the view that atheroma formation is a necessary accompaniment of aging is thus not tenable. (One could argue in fact that in order to become old one needs good coronaries.) It is nevertheless a very common accompaniment of age-ing, as we all know, and the coronary artery from a man of forty-five shows the typical luminal occlusion of severe atheroma. Clearly some people are especially prone to the development of atheroma, and others are not. The factors concerned in this, hereditary, metabolic, or environmental, are of course the subject of intensive study.

A commonly held view is that atheromatous coronary disease is rampant-ly increasing in our Western societies and that it is afflicting younger age groups. The disease has been called, somewhat histrionically, an *epidemic* and has been the subject of major national and international advisory dicta. Not all will agree with the points of view so expressed, as we shall see. No-one will disagree, however, that coronary disease is common, and that we see it present its fully-developed picture often in the fourth decade of life. It is therefore appropriate to ask when the disease begins, and to establish some concept of an "incubation period." For this I draw from Osborn's monograph entitled "The incubation period of coronary thrombosis."[2]

Osborn illustrates clearly that intimal arterial lesions may occur in young children, his example being taken from a five-month-old baby who died from tonsillitis. The deposit in the intima is mucin and is again seen in a child of thirteen months who died from gastroenteritis. Another of his cases is a man aged twenty-two years who died from a ruptured liver: The lumen of the coronary artery is greatly compromised "as a result of mucoid in-filtration and fibrous thickening of the intima. Some lipid laden foam-cells are seen in the deep parts near the media, and secondary vascularization has developed." A further case is that of a woman of thirty-nine years who died of pontine hemorrhage, showing almost complete occlusion of the coronary artery by mucoid infiltration and fibrous proliferation, with proliferation of smooth muscle fibres in the lower part of the section. Secondary vasculariza-tion has prevented necrosis. Another woman, aged seventy-five years, died from coronary disease. Great bundles of smooth muscle fibers are present in the region of the pin-point lumen, with various condensations of elastic fibers.

In none of these lesions are there any lipids, and this point is made strongly by Osborn; the lesions shown are essentially of mucoid, fibrous, elastic, and smooth muscle composition in varying degree. The nature of these lesions in early life is intriguing, and it is worth noting that the sec-tions shown above from children were all from subjects who had suffered dehydration and collapse. The intimal deposits, furthermore, tend to occur in two main sites in the vessel: opposite the mouth of a branch and around the mouth of a branch, suggesting that mechanical factors play a part in their development. Lipid infiltration, beginning with foam cells, would appear to be a secondary phenomenon. According to Adams and Tuqan (1961) ,[3] degenerating elastic fibers provide a source of lipids. The muscle of the media proliferates radially and later may be seen in whorled bundles not unlike leiomyomata. So eventually we see a "complex mixture of mucus, collagen, proliferating and degenerating elastic fibers and smooth muscle fibers occurring singly or in tumour-like masses."

It is clear, then, that stenosing lesions can exist in the coronary arteries in infancy. What relationship, if any, these bear to adult atheroma is not clear, for the series of Osborn is small and selected. What the data tell us is that the lumen of the coronary arteries can in certain circumstances be compromised at an early age and by a process in which lipids appear to play no part. Likewise in later life coronary occlusive lesions may be seen without the presence of lipid.

Let us look now at the evidence in young adults. In 1948 Yater *et al.*[4] described their findings in a large number of soldiers who died from coronary disease, among these being two hundred who were under thirty years of age. Since they died, these could of course not be looked on as typical of the community as a whole, and it was necessary to examine the coronary arteries of young people who had died from other causes. The information was forthcoming in 1953 and was based on American soldiers who were killed in Korea.[5] The coronary arteries of three hundred of these were examined, the average age of the soldiers being 22.1 years. Disease of the coronary arteries was present in three quarters of the men, ranging from slight thickening of the wall to complete blockage.

The findings were confirmed in 1960, when a group of American Air Force doctors[6] examined the hearts of 206 young and healthy flyers who were killed in flying accidents. One hundred and thirty-one were under the age of thirty. Two thirds showed significant disease of the coronary arteries.

We see, thus, that disease does not exist in the coronary arteries at birth, that in certain infants who die at the age of a few months mucoid and fibrous intimal lesions are seen, that these can become infiltrated with lipids, and that fully developed atheromatous lesions of the coronary arteries are frequently seen in young American males as early as the third decade in life. These are isolated observations, and before we link them together into the same elephant that the blind men are feeling, we must have evidence that the lesions of infancy which Osborn has described are the precursors of the lesions seen in the older people. Only then can we define the "incubation period" of coronary arterial disease with confidence.

Be that as it may, the data about young Americans is hard, and since we can be sure that fully-fledged atheroma takes time to develop, something must be happening to the arteries of many youngsters in their teens and possibly earlier. What the factors are which determine this we do not know, but it has been linked with our way of life, and I would therefore like to examine critically some of the evidence which bears on this.

First, the question of *lipids*.

It is exceptional to find lipids deposited in the coronary arteries below the age of five, and it then becomes commoner until between the ages of sixteen and twenty over half the subjects examined are affected.[2] Lipids first appear in foam cells which are seen in close relation to the intima, and they are not seen where the arterial wall is normal. It seems therefore that the arterial wall must be "conditioned" in order to receive them. It is not certain where the foam cells come from, and there are three possibilities. (a) They are macrophages which have entered from the blood in the lumen. (b) They may come from the lining endothelial cells themselves. (c) They may come from other cells of the intima. The most likely source is (b),[2] and the foam cells then migrate into the deeper parts of the wall, where they are seen to contain cholesterol crystals. Fresh collagen bundles are laid down to separate the collections of foam cells from the lumen, and in this process there is compromise of the lumen. This, according to Osborn, constitutes the essential nature of the lipid process, i.e. a superficial fibrous layer and a deep lipid layer. In his view there is no evidence that the lipid layer is in any way derived from thrombus in the lumen. Necrosis, calcification, and hemorrhage are later complications giving use to the complex final picture. Finally, fibrous bands may be seen occasionally which are independent of lipids. Whether or not disturbance of lipid metabolism is a major causative factor remains, however, to be established.

The whole subject is bedevilled by the emotionalism which enters any consideration of diet and health. Vilhalmur Stefansson said, "There is probably no field of human thought in which sentiment and prejudice take the place of sound judgement and logical thinking so completely as dietetics." I would be foolish to deny that lipids *may* play an important part in the development of atheroma, but this is far from proved, and the state of our knowledge certainly does not justify a social program such as that advocated by such august bodies as the American Heart Association, involving the advocacy of a low low-fat cholesterol diet for all—particularly when the lesions are fully developed. As Dr. William Evans used to say, "When you look at coronary disease in the post-mortem room, you can realize that nothing out of a bottle can reverse that."

The advocacy of the low low-fat cholesterol diet for atherosclerosis is based on several pieces of "evidence," which are widely quoted by the vociferous proponents of the antilipid school.

(1) That feeding high-cholesterol diets to some animals can lead to the development of atheroma-like lesions of the aorta. Whilst true, this bears

no major relevance to the problem of coronary disease in man, for even in man there is no necessary relationship between aortic and coronary atheroma.

(2) That atheromatous disease is common and increasing in our society, and that we must do *something* about it or we are lost—an amusing conclusion when we consider that in a neighbouring room an antipopulation meeting might at the same time be concluding that we are lost if we do do something about it.

Now the conclusion that the coronary problem is on the increase has been widely accepted, but in my view does not bear critical examination. The relationship of coronary disease to sudden death was mentioned by Leonardo da Vinci in the sixteenth century. In 1793 John Hunter died after a stormy meeting of the governors of St. George's Hospital, and necropsy (performed by his friend Dr. Price) showed severe coronary disease; he had had angina pectoris for about twenty years. However, the clinical diagnosis of coronary disease remained unusual until the third decade of this century, following Herrick's papers in 1912, 1918, and 1919 on the clinical aspects of angina pectoris coronary arterial occlusion. Actually, Parkes Weber in 1896 described a patient with angina pectoris who died with obliteration of the right coronary artery from an organizing thrombus.

We may wonder at this time why such descriptions as Parkes Weber's merit mention, unless it be that the condition was uncommon then. However, the association between occlusive coronary arterial disease and angina pectoris simply did not exist in the minds of most physicians at that time— Sir Clifford Allbutt, for example, maintained until 1925 that angina pectoris had nothing to do with coronary disease, but was due to a "lesion of a knot of exalted sensibility to tension at the base of the aorta." Sir William Osler by 1910 was asking the question, "Has angina pectoris increased in the community? Has the high pressure life of modern days made the disease more common?"

With the growing awareness, therefore, of coronary disease in the 1920's and subsequently, it is not surprising that from this time it begins to figure more commonly in necropsy records—it would be surprising if it did not. Under what guise, therefore, was it masquerading before that time? The answer is to be seen in the next slide, from Robb-Smith,[10] showing that before 1920 much degenerative heart disease was being registered as "Other Heart Disease," and between 1925 and 1940 as "Myocardial Degeneration." As "Coronary and Arteriosclerotic Heart Disease" increased, so did "Myocardial Degeneration" decrease to the same extent. The total death rate from degenerative heart disease remained the same.

Such differences in registration procedures, together with the changing age distribution of the population, can account for the apparent increase in frequency of the disease in the community. We do not have to go off on wild-goose chases to find a reason for something that does not exist.

Another piece of evidence quoted by the lipid enthusiasts is that during the Second World War in Europe the crude death rate for circulatory diseases fell abruptly. However, the statistics are laden with such diagnoses as "apoplexy," "chronic myocarditis," "endocarditis," etc. Further, the Norwegian data,[7] much quoted, are made more difficult to assess by the fact that the Norwegian statistical office changed their categorizations of disease in 1940. The difficulties of accurate recording in the circumstances that prevailed at that time need no emphasis. To conclude further that because dietary fats were restricted at that time then they are responsible for coronary disease seems more than odd.

Another fruitful source of occupation and income for a large number of people is the comparison of mortality statistics from various countries. A look at the World Health Organization's statistics show that the risk of dying from coronary disease in various parts of the world is as follows (from *World Health Statistics Annual,* vol. 1, 1966) :

	M	F	
Finland	530	85	
United States	465	112	
Scotland	430	110	
Norway	226	34	*Age 50–54*
Switzerland	154	48	Per 10^5
France	91	17	
Japan	63	37	

Now in order for such comparisons shall be meaningful, and especially before conclusions are drawn from them, it would seem to me to be an elementary precaution to ensure that the habits of death registration should be comparable. But this is clearly not the case, as the following examples serve to show.

In France, Moine (1952)[8] noted that in 1947 nearly a fifth of all declarations for death registration were not accompanied by a death certificate and that in some departments the majority lacked this. Moreover, the French doctors have a particular bias towards diagnosing "maladie du coeur, cause inconnu" and senility. Before we conclude that garlic and wine are responsible for low coronary rates, we had best beware, though many of us will continue to act as though this were so.

In Japan, in 1952, only 43 percent of sick people were treated by physicians, the remainder being cared for by acupuncturists, judo-orthopoedists, or folk-medicine practitioners. (Survey of Japanese Ministry of Health,

1954.) Further, the age structure of the Japanese is different from that of, for instance, the United States, for 80 percent of the people in Japan are under forty-five years of age, compared with 60-70 percent here.

In Ceylon, according to De Fonseka (1960),[9] 75 percent of death certificates are completed by lay persons without medical knowledge.

In Britain, one of the most sophisticated of countries in this regard, things are not all they might be. I recall in the middle 1950's glancing at the counterfoils (stubs) of the death certificates made out by our local general practitioner. I was interested to observe that about one half of the patients dying in his practice succumbed from aortic stenosis—a relatively rare condition of which one would have expected him to see only one or two cases per annum.

Such, then, are the problems of drawing conclusions from inaccurate data and of trying to make a silk purse out of a sow's ear. On experimental as well as epidemologic grounds, the case against lipids is simply not proven.

Accordingly, we have focused our attention on patients with coronary disease which has been demonstrated by angiography of the coronary arteries, in an attempt to discern whether or not there was any demonstrable abnormality of lipid profile that we could relate to their propensity to have the disease. Time does not permit of the presentation of details of this work, but briefly we have found that especially in our young patients with coronary disease lipid abnormalities are as frequently absent as present, and that a number of very old people have lipid abnormalities (e.g. Frederickson Type IV hyperlipidemia) without there having any compromise of longevity.

The growing awareness of the weakness of the antilipid case is presumably one reason for the increasing feeling in some circles that carbohydrates are the villains, particularly perhaps fructose. However, many of these conclusions are based on tenuous evidence and cannot yet be accepted.

My own view is that gluttony and sloth are likely to take their toll of the arteries (though this is probably the result of my own nonconformist Welsh upbringing, where there was still a certain moral stigma about indulgence). I think the human body has enough resource to convert fats to carbohydrates to proteins at will and that it is the total intake of food that counts if food counts at all. To smear your bread with margarine instead of butter and cutting the fat off the ham seems to me to be as ridiculous a way of safeguarding against atherosclerosis as stepping on alternate cracks between the paving-stones of a sidewalk.

Then there is stress, smoking, physical activity, hypertension, and the way you have chosen your parents to say nothing of the effect of blood-clotting in the causation of atheroma and its complications. Each of these is a lengthy topic in its own right.

May I conclude with a thought, expressed first by Moynihan, I believe, that famine and want have in the past been part of the lot of mankind and that the people who used their limited calories most economically were those most likely to survive. These are probably the same people who in times of plenty become fat and have a tendency to diabetes—and arterial disease. Shortage may therefore have tended to select out those people most prone to arterial disease.

I would like to express my indebtedness to the works, mentioned below, of Dr. Osborn and Professor Robb-Smith for at least some of the conclusions expressed.

REFERENCES

1. Ratcliffe, H. L.: Environmental factors and coronary disease. *Circulation, 27:*481, 1963.
2. Osborn, G. R.: *The Incubation Period of Coronary Thrombosis.* London, Butterworths, 1963.
3. Adams, C. W. M., and Tuqan, N. A.: Elastic degeneration as source of lipids in the early lesion of atherosclerosis. *J Path Bact, 82:*131, 1961.
4. Yater, W. M.: Coronary artery disease in men 18 to 39 years of age. *Amer Heart J, 36:* 334, 481, 683, 1948
5. Enos, W. F., Beyer, J. C. and Holmes, R. H.: Pathogensis of coronary disease in American soldiers killed in Korea. *JAMA, 158:*912, 1955.
6. Rigal, R. D., Lovell, F. W., and Townsend, F. M.: Pathologic findings in the cardiovascular systems of military flying personnel. *Amer J Cardiol, 6:*19, 1960.
7. Strøm, A., and Jensen, R. A.: Mortality from circulatory diseases in Norway 1940-45. *Lancet, 1:*126, 1951.
8. Moine, M.: Eur l'augmentation de quelques causes de deces. *Bull Inst Nat Hyg (Paris), 7:*729, 1952.
9. De Fonseka, T. E. J.: Difficulties in the classification of diseases and certification of deaths. *J Ceylon Pub Health Ass, 1:*7, 1960.
10. Robb-Smith, A. H. T.: *The Enigma of Coronary Heart Disease.* London, Lloyd-Luke, 1967.

Chapter 6

New Methods for Regional Cerebral Blood Flow Measurement and Their Significance

MARVIN E. JAFFE AND LAWRENCE C. McHENRY, Jr.

INTRODUCTION

T HE ERA of quantitative measurement of cerebral blood flow in man opened with the work of Seymour Kety and Carl Schmidt in the wards and laboratories of the University of Pennsylvania and Philadelphia General Hospital in 1945.[1] To contribute to this book with Dr. Kety, twenty-five years later in order to review what is current in this field, is a great honor and responsibility. It is in this historical perspective that our work has continued at the Philadelphia General Hospital with a full cognizance of our debt to the past, as well as our eye to the future. In order to understand fully the value of the newer methods, one must first be familiar with the older one.

The Kety-Schmidt method is based on the Fick principle. The technique requires measurement of the concentration of an inert tracer substance in both the arterial blood arriving at the brain and the venous blood leaving the brain via the jugular vein. The original technique utilized saturation of the brain with nitrous oxide and determination of arteriovenous differences for nitrous oxide using the Van Slyke apparatus. Technical modifications in the procedure have been made by various investigators. Among the most significant are the substitution of a radioactive, inert gas, Krypton-85, as a tracer[2] instead of nitrous oxide and in making measurements during the desaturation period,[3] while the brain is being cleared of tracer rather than during the saturation phase, increasing the experimental accuracy.[4] The preferred method of performing Fick principle cerebral blood flow studies at this time is the Krypton-85 desaturation method.[5]

Dr. Kety's method has resulted in the accumulation of a great deal of important, quantitative data concerning cerebral blood flow and metabolism in a variety of disease states, as well as in the healthy normal. Information extends from childhood to old age. Responses to a variety of physical and pharmacological agents have been detailed in recent reviews.[6,7]

There is, however, one major limitation in interpreting information gained by this technique. The "tissue sample" or venous blood, drawn from

*This work has been supported by USPHS Grant No. NB-06520, and the Strasburger Foundation.

91

the jugular bulb, is a mixture of venous blood draining from many brain areas. There may be variable admixture from right and left and from supratentorial and infratentorial structures, depending on the variable anatomy of the venous drainage in each individual.

It is likely that areas of slower flow are not fully labeled by the tracer during the period of saturation and that areas of more rapid flow may be overrepresented.[8] Autoradiographic studies in animals reveal many different rates of blood flow in the brain and a marked difference between gray and white matter. During sensory stimulation, regional changes in blood flow occur in the receptor areas.[9] These regional variations are not reflected by the original techniques.

There are two aspects to neurological disease, one concerned with diffuse abnormalities in brain function, as seen in intoxications, infections, metabolic disturbances, etc. and the other associated with disturbances in function related to discrete brain lesions, such as occur in vascular disease and tumors. There are also two approaches to the study of brain blood flow and metabolism. The newer regional method is complementary to the original method, which does not reveal focal flow disturbances in the larger mass of more normally functioning brain tissue.

XENON INJECTION METHOD OF rCBF MEASUREMENT

The first studies of local blood flow in man were performed over surgically- exposed cortex using O_2 recorders or radioisotopes.[10,11] The promise of these early studies encouraged the application of this method to measure blood flow in man through the intact skull. The first reports of the successful application of this approach were by Glass and Harper[12] and Lassen and colleagues[13] in 1963, both of whom reported on the use of carotid injection of a radioactive gas dissolved in saline with external detection.

Since then, there has been increasing interest in the application of the technique of regional cerebral blood flow measurement.[14,15,16,17] Instrumentation has been improved by the use of smaller crystal detectors in order to localize more accurately the area of observation and by the application of rapid data handling devices. I will review the technique in detail since it is of some help in understanding the applications and limitations of the method and where the need for further refinement exists.

Studies of rCBF are usually performed in conjunction with cerebral angiography. After common carotid artery puncture, under fluoroscopic guidance, a small catheter is passed into the internal carotid artery. In this way, the isotopic activity is limited to the distribution of the internal carotid artery, and extracranial tissues do not receive the tracer, except in minute amounts.

The arrival and subsequent clearance of the isotope is monitored by a bank of scintillation detectors containing small thallium-activated NaI crystals. In our laboratory, they are 0.5 inches in diameter and 0.5 inches thick. The probes, containing the crystals and photomultiplier circuits, are housed in a collimator block, and each one sees the washout of the isotope from a core of brain tissue approximately 1.5 inches in diameter. The location of the probe and the distribution of the branches of the internal carotid artery determine the area of brain in which regional flow is measured. Usually, most of the probes are over the distribution of the middle cerebral artery, the remaining being over the anterior or posterior cerebral artery territories.

The clearance of isotope from each brain region may be recorded separately on multiple channel magnetic tape or multichannel scalers. Each clearance curve is then reproduced individually through a digital scaler and plotted on a chart recorder or analyzed automatically without drawing it. The computer program most commonly used is based on that developed by Sveinsdottir for Lassen.[18]

The data may be analyzed in several ways. The methods in most frequent use are:

(1) The ten-minute flow index or stochastic method. The cerebral blood flow is calculated by the height divided by area formula, after multiplying by the tissue/blood solubility coefficient to xenon.

$$rCBF_{10} = \frac{H_{10}}{A_{10}} . \chi \lambda \ 100 \ ml / 100 \ gm / minute$$

where H_{10} = the initial height of the curve less the height at ten minutes.

A_{10} = the area under the curve for ten minutes.

λ = the tissue blood solubility coefficient.

The mathematical derivation is given by Zierler.[19]

(2) Initial slope index (ISI) or two-minute flow index. It has been noted that the initial portion of the cerebral clearance curve declines almost monoexponentially when plotted on semilogarithmic paper. If one takes the logarithmic slope during the first minute as percent of a decade and multiplies it by two, the result is an estimate of flow which is remarkably close in many cases to the 10-minute flow value. The method has the advantage of rapidity, since the initial slope can be taken directly from an oscilloscope screen using a bank of logarithmic rate meters displaying simultaneously on the screen.[20,21]

(3) Compartmental analysis: The most elegant use of regional cerebral blood flow studies is in separating gray matter flow from white matter flow. Reivich[22] has shown that normal brain blood flow fits a bimodal Gaussian distribution which is closely predicted by a two

exponential model. By graphic methods of curve peeling or by computer methods of curve fitting, two exponential values can be derived from nearly any cerebral blood flow washout curve. Values are obtained for the zero time intercepts and also the half times for each component. From these, one may calculate the relative weights of a rapidly clearing component and a more slowly clearing compartment equated with the gray and white matter under each detector. The absolute flow through each of the compartments may be derived, as well as the mean flow in each region.[23,24]

(4) Visual analysis: There are interesting qualitative features in the clearance curves in addition to the quantitative data revealed by mathematical analysis. In the initial portion of the curve, one may often see peaks or areas of rapid shunting. The most frequent site where normal peaks are seen is over the carotid siphon. This is a very brief peak, lasting five to six seconds. It may occasionally be found over the sylvian fissure also. Abnormal, brief arterial peaks are seen over arteriovenous malformations and very vascular tumors. These may be recognized by their abnormal location away from the carotid artery, and the nature of the lesion can be confirmed angiographically. Less rapidly clearing peaks, called tissue peaks or super-fast components, may be seen over areas of hyperemia, so-called "luxury perfusion," in diseased tissue. They are usually associated with angiographically recognizable blushes or early filling veins. These peaks represent abnormal perfusion at a precapillary or capillary level and are probably associated with hyperoxia in the involved vascular territories.

The importance of peaks and shunts is whether such phenomena are beneficial by increasing flow, providing more oxygen and glucose and removing metabolic products of tissue destruction in the area involved. On the other hand, they may represent a low pressure bypass by means of which blood is diverted away from ischemic areas, resulting in a deleterious clinical effect. It is fairly certain that the rapid shunts, represented by the arterial peaks of arteriovenous malformation, are not associated with high rates of tissue flow.[25] The blood flow to the head as a whole is high, but the metabolically exchanging flow at tissue level is severely reduced. The progressive mental deterioration sometimes seen with AVM may be this sort of tissue starvation in the midst of plenty.

There are several shortcomings to the regional cerebral blood flow method as currently performed by us and in most centers. First is the requirement for carotid puncture and internal carotid artery catheterization. Although this is a safe procedure in experienced hands, there is a definite incidence of serious complications, as well as the relative discomfort to the patient. In patients with severely stenosed or occluded arteries, the study cannot be done. Repeated studies at intervals of days or weeks are rarely performed because of the reluctance to perform repeated carotid puncture.[5]

Second, results of the rCBF study are delayed and are not readily available to the clinician. This is due to a time lag in processing data for computer analysis. This problem can be solved by on-line computer analysis.[26]

Third, although regional cerebral blood flow data is obtained, regional metabolic data is not.

OTHER METHODS OF rCBF MEASUREMENT

Several other methods for measuring regional cerebral blood flow are being developed. Although none has yet achieved the clinical usefulness or wide applicability of the Xe-133 injection method, they may resolve some of the limitations.

(1) Inhalation of Xe-133 has the advantage of avoiding carotid puncture. There is, however, contamination of the extracerebral tissues with isotope, rendering the calculation and interpretation of results most difficult. A deconvolution computer program has been developed by Obrist which may solve these problems.[27] If successful, this atraumatic procedure will make this study technically easy and safe for a multitude of applications, including serial studies at relatively close intervals.

(2) Implanted H_2 electrodes or microscintillation detectors[28] permit tissue clearance to be measured directly. They require the chronic implantation of electrodes and are, therefore, limited to neurosurgical applications.

(3) The use of radioactive ^{15}O permits the simultaneous measurement of regional cerebral blood flow and regional cerebral oxygen metabolism.[29,30] The limitations are, again, those of carotid artery injection. In addition, the fifteen-minute half-life of the isotope requires a cyclotron in the immediate vicinity to keep isotope available. Although limited to very specialized centers, it promises to yield otherwise unobtainable data. It is probably the most important new technique since the Kety-Schmidt method.

(4) The use of positron-emitting isotopes with coincidence counting well permit greater regionalization of the data and will decrease the scatter effect which is a serious problem with a low energy isotope such as xenon.[31]

(5) Gamma camera methods, using either diffusible or nondiffusible isotopes, suffer from a lack of resolution. They may give some qualitative impressions of circulation time, but do not have the inherent resolution of crystal detectors.

RESULTS OF rCBF MEASUREMENTS

Normal values for rCBF have been reported in only a few cases. Such series have been reported from Sweden,[32] England,[33] and from our laboratory[34] (Table 6-I). The results are very similar in each laboratory. The values shown are mean hemisphere flow values. That is, an average value was taken for all the detectors over the hemisphere. The normal values obtained by this method are very similar to those of the Kety-Schmidt technique.

TABLE 6-I

REGIONAL CEREBRAL BLOOD FLOW VALUES IN NORMAL INDIVIDUALS

	Sweden	*England*	*PGH*
Number	7	10	5
ApCO$_2$ (mmHg)	38.6	45	39
Gray Flow	79.7 ± 10.7	86.6 ± 17.1	77.0 ± 5.6
White Flow	20.9 ± 2.6	21.7 ± 3.7	21.9 ± 1.2
% Weight Gray	49.2 ± 3.9	45.5 ± 4.8	54.0 ± 6
rCBF	*	50.9 ± 9.3	51.6 ± 3.2
rCBF$_{10}$	49.8 ± 5.4	*	54.4 ± 2.7

Flow values are in cc/100 gm/min $\pm$ standard deviation.
rCBF is weighted compartmental value.
rCBF$_{10}$ is the ten-minute height/area value.
*Not reported.

In two further studies, one done by Lassen and Hoedt-Rasmussen[35] and the other done in our laboratory,[34] cerebral blood flow studies were repeated in the same patient by two different methods. Lassen compared the krypton saturation modification of the Kety-Schmidt technique[36] with intra-arterial xenon injection. We compared the krypton desaturation modification[3] with intra-arterial xenon injection. The mean values were extremely close by both methods. There is, however, a tendency toward a greater discrepancy between the two methods in patients with focal brain disease.

Besides its reproducibility between laboratories, the technique is reproducible in serial studies on the same patient. Several such studies by ourselves[34] and others[32,33] show a standard error of the difference of 3 percent to 8 percent between serial injection carried out thirty to sixty minutes apart in normals and in a variety of abnormal conditions.

Also of importance is the problem of normal interregional differences between brain areas. In our studies, we have found no significant interregional differences between brain areas when the rCBF$_{10}$ or ten-minute stochastic values are used[37] (Fig. 6-1). There is a relatively slower gray flow in the temporal lobe. Wilkinson *et al.* have reported similar findings.[33] The perfusion of gray matter was significantly decreased in the temporal region and was elevated in the precentral region. Differences in weight of gray matter are due to the geometrical relationships between the detectors and the head; a greater weight or percent gray is seen in tangential areas and lesser amounts over the center of the hemisphere where more white matter lies under the detector.

NORMAL VALUES

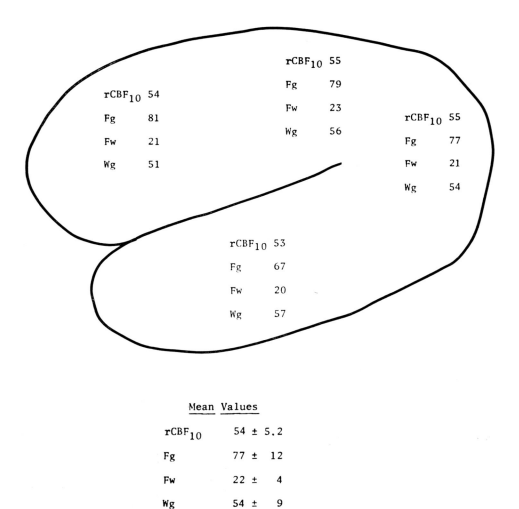

$rCBF_{10}$ 55
Fg 79
Fw 23
Wg 56

$rCBF_{10}$ 54
Fg 81
Fw 21
Wg 51

$rCBF_{10}$ 55
Fg 77
Fw 21
Wg 54

$rCBF_{10}$ 53
Fg 67
Fw 20
Wg 57

Mean Values

$rCBF_{10}$	54 ± 5.2
Fg	77 ± 12
Fw	22 ± 4
Wg	54 ± 9

Figure 6-1. The normal values for four brain areas and the hemispheric mean are shown. There is no significant difference between the ten-minute stochastic values ($rCBF_{10}$) or the white matter flow component (Fw). The gray matter flow (Fg) is reduced in the temporal lobe. All flow values are in cc/100 gm/min.

The physiological responses of the cerebral circulation are well-known.[6,7] The current major themes are the increase in CBF associated with hypercapnia[38] and the stability of CBF despite relatively wide variations in arterial blood pressure.[39] However, the regional method allows one to determine focal abnormalities of flow in the resting state, as well as local abnormalities of responsiveness during the stresses induced by changes in blood gases or blood pressure. The regional effects of vasodilating agents can also be assessed (Fig. 6-2).

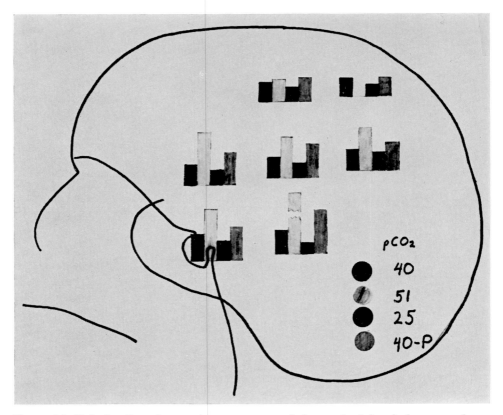

Figure 6-2. Relative flow changes in seven areas of the cerebral hemisphere are shown in a patient with severe stenosis of the anterior cerebral artery. The two upper sets of bars are in an area of compromised vascular supply. The lower five are over presumably normal middle cerebral artery territory. Raising the arterial pCO_2 from 40 to 51 mmHg (Bars 1 and 2) results in a marked increase in flow in the normal regions and no increase in flow in the anterior cerebral artery distribution. One area did not receive enough isotope to measure flow. The third bar shows the effect of hyperventilation, reducing the $ApCO_2$ to 25. The last bar demonstrates that intravenous papaverine was able to cause a flow increase in the normal vessels, but did not cause a blood flow increase in the anterior cerebral artery area.

REGIONAL CEREBRAL CIRCULATION IN STROKE

Having satisfied ourselves that the method was safe, accurate, reproducible, and compared favorably with the long-validated Kety-Schmidt technique, we next established a set of criteria by which we could evaluate stroke patients. We wanted to know:

(1) If cerebral blood flow was normal or abnormal?
(2) If abnormal, was it increased or decreased?
(3) If the derangement was focal or global?
(4) If there was any abnormality in autoregulation or CO_2 responsiveness?
(5) The effect of vasodilators?

The values used in establishing normalcy were based on our own results, shown in the previous Table. First, the $rCBF_{10}$ or regional value in each area is compared to the normal to determine if there is a local absolute increase (values over 66) or decrease (less than 49 cc/100 gm/min) in flow. The most important step is to compare each individual probe value with the hemispheric mean value. Since the coefficient of variation between areas in the normal study was approximately 10 percent, we took twice this, a 20 percent difference from the hemispheric mean, to represent a focal relative increase or decrease in flow.

In order to decide if a significant change had occurred between studies, either after administration of a drug, CO_2, induced hypertension, or other stress, data were applied from our serial study. We found a coefficient of variation between serial studies of 3.8 percent for hemispheric mean values and 10.1 percent for individual probe values in patients with a variety of neurological diseases. Therefore, we require a change of over 7 percent in the hemispheric mean or 20 percent in a single probe value before a change is considered significant.

In addition, all cases are evaluated independently by the neuroradiologist who defines angiographically abnormal areas by the criteria of significant focal stenosis or occlusion of vessels, areas of avascularity or hyperemia, early filling veins, patterns of collateral circulation and alterations in hemispheric or regional circulation times.

These are rigorous criteria for significant change, more rigorous than those used by most other investigators. We chose to use our own laboratory criteria because of the lack of uniformity of such criteria in the literature.

Most of our data is on patients with cerebral vascular disease. The patterns of abnormality in cerebral blood flow in stroke include:

(1) general depression of flow
(2) focal depression of flow

(3) focal hyperemia

(4) vasoparalysis

The type of pattern seen bears a relationship to the time after the stroke that the patient is studied, the site or sites of the vascular lesion and resultant patterns of collateral circulation, the presence of associated factors such as hypertention, hypercapnia, or the use of vasodilator drugs, along with the status of the intrinsic cerebral autoregulatory reflexes and cardiac function.[40]

Recent clinical reports have attempted to subdivide stroke cases into those with evident focal vascular occlusion or stenosis at the time of the study,[41] and those without evidence of arterial occlusion.[42] The nature of the study eliminates from consideration patients with severe stenotic or occlusive disease in the extracranial circulation since selective internal carotid catheterization cannot be carried out.

A review of the findings from various centers[41,42,43,44,45] indicates that focal hyperemia (luxury perfusion) is seen most frequently in the first few days after the stroke and most often in patients *without* demonstrable arterial occlusions. This is not to say that a transient arterial occlusion may not have occurred with subsequent return of flow because of lysis of the thrombus or dissolution of an embolus. It indicates that both a diseased brain area and an adequate perfusion pressure are necessary to cause hyperemic foci. The vasodilatation is probably the combined result of tissue acidosis and loss of autoregulation.[46]

Focal decreases in flow are much more frequent than hyperemic foci. They may be seen during the acute or chronic phases of the illness and in the presence or absence of demonstrable focal vascular stenoses. In acute disease such foci most likely represent the actual areas of ischemia, but in chronic disease they are probably areas of cerebral scarring with resultant decreased metabolism resulting from neuronal loss.

Global decreases in hemispheric CBF occur most frequently in large lesions, especially in the presence of depressed level of consciousness or with clinical evidence of diffuse cerebral involvement or multiple lesions. The cerebral oxygen consumption is also decreased in these patients.[6]

The observation of changes in the cerebral vascular responses to physiological stimuli will yield further information on the nature of the vascular abnormality in stroke. A variety of responses have been found to occur to similar stimuli in different patients and in the same patient at different times. It is impossible to predict what the response in an individual case wll be from the angiogram or from the clinical presentation. This is why rCBF measurements are particularly valuable. For instance, the usual response to an increase in arterial pCO_2 is vasodilatation with increase in CBF which is normally related to the absolute change in pCO_2. Most patients also show an increase in blood pressure when breathing CO_2, but relatively little attention has been paid to this as an additional factor in the resulting vasomotor response.

Fieschi has reported a normal interregional variability in CO_2 responsiveness with a ratio between the most reacting and least reacting regions of as high as 2.4 in young subjects.[47] This means that relatively large variations between regions after CO_2 administration must be accepted as falling into the normal range, and the criteria for interregional variability may have to be expanded for CO_2 administration. Such a large interregional variation in normal persons has yet to be confirmed by others.

However, certain changes seen after CO_2 administration must be accepted as being clearly abnormal. For example, an overall failure of blood flow increase (seen in 37% of Fieschi's cases) or focal flow decreases during hypercapnia (steal phenomenon). Similarly, an increase in flow during hypocapnia, induced by forced hyperventilation, is also a paradoxical response and clearly abnormal. It has been called the inverse steal phenomenon. These paradoxical responses are probably the result of maximal dilatation in an ischemic area resulting from local tissue acidosis. As hypercapnia dilates the normal vessels, blood is diverted away from the area of ischemia for no further vasodilatation can occur in this area. Hypocapnia, on the other hand, causes the normal vessels to constrict, increasing resistance to flow through them, resulting in shunting through the involved area where resistance to flow is low.

Local edema in the area of infarction may potentiate this reaction by further increasing capillary resistance. Cerebral blood volume increases during hypercapnia.[48] The associated hypertension may also increase the edema in the diseased areas.[49] Although a great deal of emphasis has been laid on the possible diversion of blood away from ischemic foci during CO_2 administration, it must be remembered that in the majority of cases this does not occur. The areas of ischemia usually react by increasing blood flow during CO_2 administration. It is not known whether this is due entirely to vasodilatation from hypercarbia. Loss of autoregulation and the associated hypertension and increased cardiac output, caused by CO_2, also play a part.[50]

Vasoparalysis is demonstrated by observing blood flow changes in response to changes in blood pressure. Normally, the cerebral vessels compensate for changes in blood pressure by dilating or constricting to maintain CBF constant over a wide range of blood pressure. However, in vasoparalyzed areas the vessels behave like passive tubes. Blood flow increases as the pressure increases and falls as pressure decreases. Under unusual circumstances, clinical changes can be shown to parallel changes in blood pressure.[51]

Usually, loss of response to hypercapnia is associated with loss of autoregulation to changes in blood pressure also, but occasionally these responses can be dissociated. One of two responses may occur: (a) the vessels may lose autoregulation, but continue to react to hypercapnia, or (b) they may be able to constrict in response to increased blood pressure or hypocapnia but fail to dilate to hypercapnia.

The first instance may represent a tissue acidosis, which resets the responsiveness to blood pressure changes to a higher level although maximal vasodilatation has not yet occurred. The second type of dissociation is not so easily explained. Increased edema and elevated intracranial pressure resulting from vasodilatation may increase local vascular resistance to flow sufficiently in the diseased areas to decrease flow.[52] This response, on the other hand, may be an artifact of the method.

The paradoxical nature of some of these responses is apparent. Since this review is concerned with measurement of alterations in cerebral blood flow in man, I shall not enter into a discussion of the work which is being done to resolve some of these problems in animal models. There are several hypotheses[41,42] regarding the site of CO_2 action, the importance of extracellular pH in regulating CBF, alterations in sodium exchange across blood vessel membranes, effect of cerebral edema, etc., all of which probably contribute to some extent in the pathophysiology of the cerebral circulation in cerebral vascular disease. On the basis of too few cases (and sometimes strictly on a theoretical basis), therapeutic recommendations have been made suggesting hyperventilation to induce hypocapnia or vasoconstrictor treatment with aminophylline as a possible treatment for stroke. Although clinical trials of these therapies should be made, a blanket recommendation for therapy is not warranted.

PHARMACOLOGICAL STUDIES OF rCBF IN STROKE

Vasodilator drugs have been generally ignored in recent quantitative studies of rCBF in cerebrovascular disease. The inference has been made that since carbon dioxide seemed to cause steals, and vasoconstrictors reversed them, any type of vasodilator is contraindicated in the treatment of stroke. We have begun a series of studies to test the effects of vasodilators in stroke.

Both papaverine[53] and hexobendine have been evaluated in our laboratory. Papaverine has repeatedly been shown to cause cerebral vasodilatation.[6] The regional effects of parenteral papaverine in patients with cerebral infarction have not been previously documented. In a series of six patients with focal vascular disease, demonstrated angiographically, we found increases in mean hemispheric flow and regional blood flow in both angiographically normal and abnormal areas. In only one normal area was a steal phenomenon noted.

In a second series of patients, a new cerebral vasodilator, hexobendine,[54] was used (Fig. 6-3). Again, increases were seen in both angiographically involved and noninvolved areas. In this series no steals were produced, but they will probably be seen as more patients are studied.

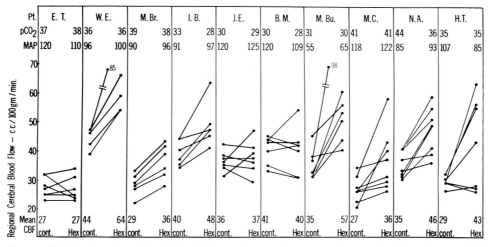

Figure 6-3. Regional cerebral blood flow values ($rCBF_{10}$) before and after the administration of intravenous hexobendine are shown in ten patients with cerebrovascular disease. The arterial pCO_2 and mean arterial blood pressure (MAP) values are above the regional blood flow results and the hemispheric mean CBF values below for each patient. Three patterns of response take place: (a) all areas may increase (W.E., M.Br., and I.B.), (b) all areas show no significant response (E.T., J.E. and B.M.), and (c) only certain areas increase (M.Bu., M.C., N.A. and H.T.)

As with CO_2 several patterns of response to vasodilators are seen. All areas may increase; all areas may fail to react, or only certain areas may increase. The factors controlling this peculiar selectivity of response are presently unknown.

SUMMARY

The currently available methods of regional cerebral blood flow measurement have reopened a large number of questions on the interpretation of the pathophysiology of cerebral vascular disease and cerebral vascular reactivity in other disease states. Considering the relatively poor spatial resolution of the crystal detector systems and the contributions from neighboring areas because of scatter, it is surprising that focal flow changes are found or can be produced so often in patients with no angiographic evidence of focal vascular occlusions. Such data tends to support a cortical involvement by ischemia in such cases. An alternative hypothesis is that the cortical function is depressed in a retrograde manner after deep lesions affecting critical cortical pathways, but such a hypothesis is not supported by the results of functional CBF tests. These seem to bear out the presence of an abnormality of vascular reaction relatively superficially in the cortex.

Carrying such reasoning one step further, one may also hypothesize that the majority of such episodes are thromboembolic in nature. The failure to demonstrate focal significant stenoses in many patients, the presence of hyperemia in the area of involvement, and the lack of clinical evidence of hypotension all speak against the theory of hemodynamic vascular crises in the etiology of such cases of nonhemorrhagic stroke.

Another corollary to the studies so far done in stroke patients is that one cannot generalize in regard to effective therapy. If one assumes that increasing CBF through ischemic foci is beneficial and that diverting blood away is not, it would seem that although some patients may benefit from hypercapnia, others require hypocapnia; some need vasodilators, but some would require vasoconstrictors; some should have their blood pressure raised; probably none should have it lowered, and some patients should not be treated pharmacologically at all. The performance of controlled clinical trials of all of these treatments is necessary in order to decide if any actually shorten morbidity, reduce mortality, or lead to an improved quality of survival. But such clinical trials will be meaningless unless parallel cerebral circulation studies are done to determine if the treatment being used is increasing or decreasing rCBF in that particular patient.

It appears that it would be clinically valuable to test the cerebral vascular reactivity of each stroke patient to determine which treatment, if any, may be useful. Repeated testing may be necessary to assess changes in reactivity associated with the time course of the illness and changes in treatment initiated as indicated. Such testing is not feasible with the current method of intra-arterial injection, but may be practical when a valid inhalation method is available.

REFERENCES

1. Kety, S. S., and Schmidt, C. F.: Determination of cerebral blood flow in man by use of nitrous oxide in low concentrations. *Amer J Physiol, 143:*53, 1945.
2. Lassen, N. A., and Munck, O.: Cerebral blood flow in man determined by use of radioactive krypton. *Acta Physiol Scand, 33:*30, 1955.
3. McHenry, L. C., Jr.: Quantitative cerebral blood flow determinations, application of krypton-85 desaturation technique in man. *Neurology, 14:*785, 1964.
4. Ingvar, D. H., and Lassen, N. A.: Methods for cerebral blood flow measurements in man, *Brit J Anaesth, 37:*216, 1965.
5. Harper, A. M.: Measurement of cerebral blood flow in man. *Scot Med J, 12:*349, 1967.
6. Lassen, N. A.: Cerebral blood flow and oxygen consumption in man. *Physiol Rev, 39:*183, 1959.

7. Sokoloff, L.: Action of drugs on cerebral circulation. *Pharmacol Rev, 11*:1, 1959.

8. McHenry, L. C., Jr.: Cerebral blood flow. *New Eng J Med, 274*:82, 1966.

9. Sokoloff, L.: Local cerebral circulation at rest and during altered cerebral activity induced by anesthesia or visual stimulation, In Kety, S. S., and Elkes, J.: *Regional Neurochemistry*. New York, Pergamon, 1961, p. 107.

10. Meyer, J. S., and Hunter, J.: Polarographic study of cortical blood flow in man. *J Neurosurg, 14*:382, 1957.

11. Ingvar, D. H., and Lassen, N. A.: Quantitative determination of regional cerebral blood flow in man. *Lancet, 2*:806, 1961.

12. Glass, H. I., and Harper, A. M.: Measurement of regional blood flow in cerebral cortex of man through intact skull. *Brit Med J, 1*:593, 1963.

13. Lassen, N. A. *et al.*: Regional cerebral blood flow in man determined by krypton. *Neurology, 13*:719, 1963.

14. Hoedt-Rasmussen, K.: *Regional Cerebral Blood Flow*. Copenhagen, Munusgaard, 1967.

15. Ingvar, D. H., and Lassen, N. A. (Eds.) : Regional cerebral blood flow: An international symposium. *Acta Neurol Scand*, Suppl. 14, 1965.

16. Ingvar, D. H., Lassen, N. A., Siesjo, B. K., and Skinhoj, E. (Eds.) : Cerebral blood flow and cerebrospinal fluid: III international symposium. *Scand J Clin Lab Invest*, Suppl. 102, 1968.

17. Brock, M., Fieschi, C., Ingvar, D. H., Lassen, N. A., and Schurmann, K. (Eds.) : *Cerebral Blood Flow*. Berlin; Springer-Verlag, 1969.

18. Hoedt-Rasmussen, K., Sveinsdottir, E., and Lassen, N. A.: Regional cerebral blood flow in man determined by intra-arterial injection of radioactive inert gas. *Circ Res, 18*:237, 1966.

19. Zierler, K. L.: Equations for measuring blood flow by external monitoring of radioisotopes, *Circ Res, 16*:309, 1965.

20. Paulson, O. B., Cronquist, S., Risberg, J. and Jeppesen, F. I.: Regional cerebral blood flow: A comparison of 8 detector and 16 detector instrumentation, *J Nucl Med, 10*:164, 1969.

21. Hutten, H., and Brock, M.: The two minute flow index (TMFI) . In Brock *et al.* (Eds.) : *Cerebral Blood Flow*. Berlin, Springer-Verlag, 1969, p. 19.

22. Reivich, M., Slater, R., and Sano, N.: Further studies on exponential models of cerebral clearance curves. In Brock *et al.* (Eds.) : *Cerebral Blood Flow*. Berlin, Springer-Verlag, 1969, p. 8.

23. Sveinsdotter, E.: Clearance curves of krypton-85 and xenon-133 considered as sum of compartments each having monoexponential outwash function, description of computer program for simple case of only two compartments. *Acta Neurol Scand*, Vol. 69, Suppl. 14, 1965.

24. Hoedt-Rasmussen, K., and Skinhoj, E.: In vivo measurements of the relative weight of gray and white matter in the human brain. *Neurology, 16*:515, 1966.

25. Haeggendal, E. *et al.*: Pre- and Post-operative measurement of regional cerebral blood flow in three cases of intracranial arterio-venous aneurysm. *J Neurosurg, 22*:1, 1965.

26. Hill, R., Clifton, J., Gallager, T., and Potchen, E. J.: Regional cerebral blood flow in man: II Data acquisition and analysis. *Arch Neurol, 20*:384, 1969.

27. Obrist, W. D. *et al.*: Determination of regional cerebral blood flow by inhalation of 133-xenon, *Circ Res, 20*:124, 1967.

28. Sem-Jacobson, C. W., Styri, O. B., and Mohn, E.: Simultaneous focal intracerebral

blood flow measurements in man around 18 chronically implanted electrodes. In Brock *et al.* (Eds.) : *Cerebral Blood Flow.* Berlin, Springer-Verlag, 1969, p. 44.

29. Ter-Pogossian, M. M., Eichling, J. O., Davis, D. O., and Welch, M. J.: The simultaneous measure in vivo of regional cerebral blood flow and regional cerebral oxygen utilization by means of oxyhemoglobin labelled with radioactive oxygen[15]. In Brock *et al.* (Eds.) : *Cerebral Blood Flow.* Berlin, Springer-Verlag, 1969, p. 66.

30. Ter-Pogossian, M. M., Eichling, J. O., Davis, D. O., Welch, M. J., and Metzger, J. M.: The determination of regional cerebral blood flow by means of water labeled with radioactive oxygen[15]. *Radiology, 93:*31, 1969.

31. Potchen, E. J., and Welch, M.: 13N$_2$O coincidence counting for rCBF measurements. *Scand J Lab Clin Invest, XI (Suppl. 102):* J, 1968.

32. Ingvar, D. H. *et al.*: Normal values of regional cerebral blood flow in man, including flow and weight estimates of grey and white matter. *Acta Neurol Scand,* Suppl. 14, p. 72, 1965.

33. Wilkinson, I. M. S. *et al.*: Regional blood flow in the normal cerebral hemisphere. *J Neurol Neurosurg Psychiat, 32:*367, 1969.

34. McHenry, L. C., Jr., Jaffe, M. E., and Goldberg, H. I.: Regional cerebral blood flow measurement with small probes, I. Evaluation of the method. *Neurology, 19:* 1198, 1969.

35. Lassen, N. A., and Hoedt-Rasmussen, K.: Human cerebral blood flow measured by two inert gas techniques. *Circ Res, 19:*681, 1966.

36. Lassen, N. A. and Munck, O.: Cerebral blood flow in man determined by radioactive krypton. *Acta Physiol Scand, 33:*30, 1955.

37. Jaffe, M. E., Goldberg, H. I., McHenry, L. C., Jr., and Kawamura, J.: Interregional differences in cerebral blood flow in stroke. *Excerpta Medica ICS, 193:*232, 1969.

38. Reivich, M.: Arterial pCO$_2$ and cerebral hemodynamics. *Amer J Physiol, 206:*25, 1964.

39. Lassen, N. A.: Autoregulation of cerebral blood flow. *Circ Res, 14 and 15 (Suppl I):* I-201-204, 1964.

40. Jaffe, M. E., McHenry, L. C., Jr., and Goldberg, H. I.: Regional cerebral blood flow measurement with small probes: II application of the method. *Neurology, 20:* 225, 1970.

41. Paulson, O. B.: Regional cerebral blood flow in apoplexy due to occlusion of the middle cerebral artery. *Neurology, 20:*63, 1970.

42. Paulson, O. B., Lassen, N. A. and Skinhoj, E.: Regional cerebral blood flow in apoplexy without arterial occlusion. *Neurology, 20:*125, 1970.

43. Hoedt-Rasmussen, K. *et al.*: Regional cerebral blood flow in acute apoplexy: The "luxury perfusion syndrome" of brain tissue. *Arch Neurol, 17:*271, 1967.

44. Jaffe, M. E., Goldberg, H. I., and McHenry, L. C., Jr.: Regional cerebral blood flow in middle cerebral artery occlusion and stenosis. *Circulation,* Supp VI, p. 106, 1968.

45. Fieschi, C. *et al.*: Derangement of the regional cerebral blood flow and of its regulatory mechanisms in acute cerebrovascular lesions. *Neurology 18:*1166, 1968.

46. Lassen, N. A.: The luxury perfusion syndrome. *Lancet, II:*1113, 1966.

47. Fieschi, C. *et al.*: Impairment of the regional vasomotor response of cerebral vessels to hypercarbia in vascular diseases. *Europ Neurol, 2:*13, 1969.

48. White, J. C., Verlot, M., Selverstone, B. and Beecher, H. K.: Changes in brain volume during anesthesia: The effects of anoxia and hypercapnia. *Arch Surg, 44:* 1, 1942.

49. Schutta, H. S., Kassell, N. F., and Langfitt, T. W.: Brain swelling produced by injury and aggravated by arterial hypertension. *Brain, 91:*261, 1968.

50. Cooper, E. S., West, J. W., Jaffe, M. E., Goldberg, H. I., Kawamura, J., and McHenry, L. C., Jr.: The relation between cardiac function, cerebral blood flow, and cerebral angiography in stroke patients. *Stroke* (in press).

51. Wise, G. R.: Vasopressor-drug therapy for complications of cerebral arteriography. *New Eng J Med, 282:*610, 1970.

52. Lassen, N. A. and Paulson, O. B.: Partial cerebral vasoparalysis in patients with apoplexy: Dissociation between carbon dioxide responsiveness and autoregulation. In Brock, M. *et al.* (Eds.): *Cerebral Blood Flow.* Berlin, Springer-Verlag, 1969, p. 117.

53. McHenry, L. C., Jr., Jaffe, M. E., Kawamura, J., and Goldberg, H. I.: The effect of papaverine on regional blood flow in focal vascular disease of the brain. *New Eng J Med* (in press).

54. Meyer, J. S., Kondo, A., Szewezykowski, J., Nomura, F., and Teraura, T.: The effect of a new drug (hexobendine) on cerebral hemodynamics and oxygen consumption in monkeys. *J Neurol Sci, 10:*25, 1970.

PART III

DEVELOPMENTAL AND METHODOLOGICAL
APPROACHES TO DRUG STUDY

Chapter 7

Methodological Considerations in Developmental Studies

MARCEL KINSBOURNE

EXPERIMENTAL groups are selected, relevant behaviors measured, and these measures may then be repeated after some treatment has been applied. We will consider problems of specificity in subject selection and of appropriateness in choice of behavioral index, in the context both of the evolution of behavior in the young and its dissolution in the old. Selection of an experimental group has the aim of assembling subjects as homogeneous as possible as regards the behavior to be studied. Criteria for selecting an experimental group may specify age, etiology, psychometric characteristic, or performance. One may use children or old people; victims of a particular disease entity; subjects of a given intelligence quotient or a given discrepancy of scores between tests of different aspects of intelligence; or persons who diverge from the norm to a critical extent as regards some particular behavior or skill.

Etiology is the least useful way to assemble a group with some communality in behavior. Etiologies overlap in their effects on brain, and a given etiology may be diverse in its cerebral effects. Because the nature of a behavioral anomaly depends primarily on the location of the central nervous lesion, groups defined without reference to localization, for the presence of global entities such as brain damage, chronic brain syndrome, and organicity, although they perform inferiorly in many tasks, show no specific behavioral anomalies interpretable in terms of brain mechanism.

Chronological age is more relevant in that it covaries with behavior. Children progress through definable cognitive states as their brains mature (Piaget, 1947). But when children of a given age show a diversity of performance, this reflects on relative cerebral maturation only if they are drawn from a homogeneous background. The potential generated by brain maturation supports performance only to the extent permitted by the environment, and in the culturally heterogeneous American society, initial test failure of "disadvantaged" children is ambiguous in implication. To sort out the cognitively handicapped from the undermotivated underachiever, one has to persist with a trial of teaching, then retest. The teaching will familiarize the children with the nature of the demands of the task and foster the competitive attitude which leads subjects to perform at the limits of their

111

capacities when formally tested. If these goals are realized, the underachievers will advance at a rate not open to children who are cognitively immature.

The phonics aptitude test (Kinsbourne and Lohrbauer, in preparation) requires subjects to break down the sound of words into their several phonemic elements (an essential step in learning to read by phonics). A sample of middle class entering first graders scored far better on this measure than did a comparable lower class sample, and only for the former group was the result predictive of subsequent reading achievement. Retest four months later revealed disproportionate gains for the lower class group, and their scores were now significantly related to reading performance. It appears that the first test of the lower class group elicited near random performance from these children who were quite unused to performance testing. After several months in school, they had begun to adopt the competitive and individualistic middle class approach. Now their performance more accurately represented their innate capabilities and thus was predictive of reading achievement.

One need not wait for months to observe the transforming effect of familiarization on performance. Deficit in figure copying (constructional apraxia) reflects cerebral disease. Yet normal lower class persons often perform alarmingly poorly on these tests at first encounter. But in contradistinction to the organically impaired, they can easily be taught the task in question. After familiarization any residual performance deficit becomes of diagnostic significance.

A similar cultural problem confounds the comparison of older persons with younger controls in that at a given socioeconomic level the older people as a group often have had less prolonged and thorough early education, so that in effect a cultural imbalance obtains.

The definition of groups in the area of aging is particularly treacherous. Nothing is easier than to show that the aged, like the brain damaged, or any other group of suboptimal cerebral competence, perform inferiorly to controls, both in horizontal and in longitudinal comparisons. But does the cumulative cognitive deficit during aging reflect more than the cumulative intervention of diseases, with an overall pattern of deficit reflecting the relative prevalence of the major disease entities and their usual loci of maximum impact on central nervous function? Sudden drops in performance presage death (Lieberman, 1969). In view of this the form of the gradual cognitive decrement revealed by group data (Fig. 7-1) could be the result of multiple individual sharp decrements distributed in time (Fig. 7-2). Should one construct a "backward dying curve" (Fig. 7-3) in which performance is plotted backwards from the time of death, the form of the "age decrement" in performance might undergo drastic change, and the study of aging might become an exercise in the effect of brain damage preceding death on behavior.

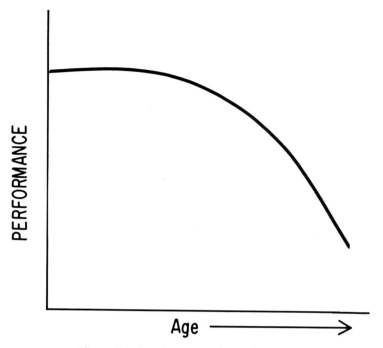

Figure 7-1. Age decrement in performance.

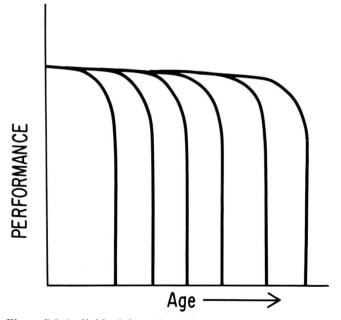

Figure 7-2. Individual drops in performance preceding death.

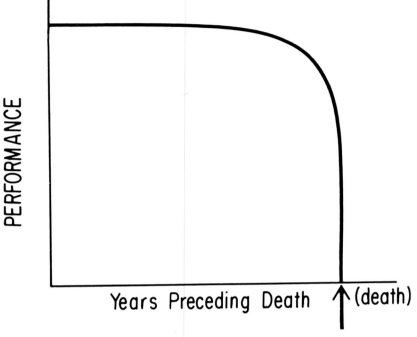

Figure 7-3. Backward dying curve.

Elderly persons do also have in common experiences contingent on having long been alive. Do these include cognitive and maturational changes which might impair test performance, such as overlearned behavior difficult to extinguish, caution reflected as an undue reluctance to participate in speeded, albeit imperfect performance, and a failure to rise to the challenge of a difficult task because of a socially induced low self esteem? An early effort to demonstrate an over-learning effect (Ruch, 1934) could not be confirmed (Korchin and Basowitz, 1957), and no evidence exists that the notorious caution of old people is other than justified by a correct appraisal of their own dwindling capability.

In studying the old, one studies a miscellaneously brain-damaged population. Such studies can not be expected to reveal more communality of behavior than can attach to such diverse case material. The capabilities of old people as a group, however stage-managed the test situation, always fall short of those of young healthy controls, and the intragroup variance is greater. The more appropriate inquiry is into the relative strengths and weaknesses in the performance spectrum of the old, as compared to the relative capabilities of the young, while admitting the inexorable nature of the absolute deficits incurred as time passes.

Young and old subject groups are confronted with tachistoscopic displays of randomly scattered black discs and rings of equal diameter, but varying in thickness (Kinsbourne and Butts, in preparation). Subjects are asked to enumerate the discs only, while ignoring the rings. The higher the count, the longer the latency of response. But also the more numerous the irrelevant rings and the thicker (i.e. the more like discs) they are, the longer the latency. A trade off is established, "enumeration time" versus "discrimination time." The old are, of course, slower both at enumerating and at discriminating. But relatively speaking, discrimination is the function that has suffered disproportionately.

Looking for such discrepancies permits one to delineate a cognitive profile characteristic of old people, with obvious vocational implications. We may also ask of a treatment not only does it restore the prior (young) level of performance (it never will), but also, more modestly, does it correct the age-dependent imbalance between different cognitive processes?

Psychometric criteria often define a group, usually in combination with an age criterion. For children "equal mental age" comparisons are in style. The old are constantly matched with the young on a measure such as a vocabulary test. Such matching would be logical if older mentally dull children were in important cognitive respects like younger bright ones, or if mentally bright old people were like duller young adults. The evidence does not support this monotonic theory of evolution and dissolution of mind. When one matches different age groups on a particular psychometric criterion, one finds them unmatched on most other performance measures. Which group does better on the additional measure depends on the nature of the arbitrarily chosen test on which initial matching was performed. Such results are artifacts of the matching procedure.

The logic of these considerations directs us to regard as most appropriate for the definition of experimental groups the subjects' skill at the particular performance that is the focus of the investigation, better still, the efficiency of the underlying process or processes.

Cognitive functioning may be broadly divided into selection and processing. The observer selects from the environment and from memory, that subset of information necessary for the continual decision making that underlies adaptive behavior. He processes that information up to the point at which his decision criterion is satisfied; then he acts or withholds action, whichever is deemed appropriate. Inappropriate decision making, which is the kernel of cognitive deficit, will result either when the observer is lacking in processing ability or when he applies suboptimal selection strategies to the task, by attending to an inappropriate input subset or by attending for too short a time (before reliable decisions can be made) or for too long a time (beyond that at which all decision-relevant information has been extracted.) It becomes clear that the identical performance deficit can arise on account of inadequacies either in selection or in processing. When one selects groups on a performance criterion, this distinction should not be overlooked. It may be illustrated with an instance bearing on children's ability to discriminate spoken words.

Wepman has introduced a test in which children are asked to judge spoken word pairs as being the same or different. The pairs may indeed be the same word spoken twice or two words differing in one initial or terminal phoneme. Failure on this task is attributed to defective auditory discrimination (Wepman, 1961). The only restriction on this verdict is the need for the child to have mastered the concept of "sameness-difference," which, at the age at which this test is performed, is generally true of normal children. A failure of auditory discrimination would be categorized as failure of processing.

We observed that in the Wepman Test children mostly err in judging different words to be the "same" rather than the reverse and do so particularly when the objective difference arises in the terminal phoneme (Kinsbourne and Levy, in preparation). Might the excess of terminal over initial phoneme errors represent a selection rather than a processing deficit? Perhaps children were failing to incorporate the comparison of the terminal phonemes into the information on which they based their judgements.

This turned out to be the case. When we added to the test one further requirement—each time to repeat the second word of the pair *after* making the judgement, the excess of terminal over initial phoneme errors disappeared, and performance improved to that extent. The instruction to repeat modified the children's listening strategies, and the terminal phoneme information, previously ignored, which they now attended to on account of "set to repeat," they also incorporated in their sameness-difference judgements. The errors that still remain can now more reasonably be attributed to discrimination difficulty.

Now suppose some treatment improves children's word-matching performance? Have we improved childrens' ability in auditory discrimination, or have we modified their listening habits? The former type of explanation is too readily offered. The experiment illustrates how the two mechanisms can be sorted out.

Faulty selection strategies are pervasive in childhood. Children ignore dimensions of visual input such as orientation, which they are demonstrably capable of discriminating (Kinsbourne and Hartley, 1968). The way to improve performance deficit based on ignoring a relevant dimension is to exclude all other dimensions from the test situation. The children who commit copious reversal errors in reading and writing have no particular difficulty in remembering and reproducing various orientations when form is held constant (Kinsbourne and Rosof, in preparation). Children who have difficulty learning to discriminate mirror image forms ([ ]) simultaneously exposed, have less difficulty when these are exposed successively (one at a time). Successive exposure eliminates the irrelevant dimension of relative position and permits children to attend to the only remaining one, that of orientation itself (Kinsbourne, in preparation). As with animals, so with children it is possible to demonstrate response hierarchies. Children are more apt to base hypotheses on dimensions high in hierarchy, such as position, intensity, color, than on one that is low, such as orientation. What changes in maturation is the extent to which the individual persists with his initial hypothesis in the face of disconfirming feedback and the size of the set of hypotheses he is able to entertain successively before abandoning the task. When a treatment has resulted in improved discrimination learning, has discrimination been strengthened, or has selective attention been guided to the dimension appropriate for handling the problem? (Hochberg, 1968.)

The objective evaluation of a treatment hinges on measuring in isolation the process that is presumptively affected. It is pointless to apply a potentially important method, for instance, hyperbaric oxygenation, to an indiscriminately wide population that is characterized by dementia, and quote as evidence of benefit a decrease in psychometric signs of organicity after treatment (Jacobs, *et al.* 1969). Organicity in psychometric data is an empirically defined set of findings, reflecting no identifiable cerebral process, and is the resultant of countless uncontrolled variables. Ultimately, such looseness in behavioral index is self-defeating and can cause potentially useful treatments to fall into disrepute. It is still more discouraging to find as radical a treatment as shunting of the cerebrospinal fluid circulation in the presumed entity of normal pressure hydrocephalus (Adams *et al.,* 1965) validated as regards its effect on cognition and memory by purely anecdotal evidence. The choice of appropriate indices of relevant cerebral process is critical in cases like this.

A patient with normal pressure hydrocephalus tested by us showed no improvement at all in his postoperative WAIS Score, but he improved dramatically on measures of visual recognition span, visual enumeration span, and paired associate learning. The relevant processes were not ones caught in Wechsler's arbitrarily selective psychometric net. An adequate double-blind study both of hyperbaria and of shunting of normal pressure hydrocephalus remains to be made. In general, the temptation is to specify as target for treatment some overwide man-made category such as "perception" or "memory" or "social adaptation" and sample these for change by means of empirically assembled test batteries. Any real effect of treatments is then obscured by the sheer mass of additional test scores relevant to quite other cerebral processes.

Of a test for disordered performance we should know what it measures, and it should measure what we want to know. These two stipulations are not necessarily identical. Take the treatment of hyperkinesis. Hyperkinetic children are overactive, overresponsive to external change, and distractible from the main task. The hypothesized causal sequence of drug treatment is hyperactivity ⎯⎯⎯⎯⎯→ inattention ⎯⎯⎯⎯⎯→ school failure. Improving attention is the drug's proximate effect; reversing school failure the ultimate effect. If we then only measure school performance, we do not know how the drug worked, by its effect on activity level or in some other way. If we only measure activity level, we do not know what effect changes in that level have actually had on the real life situation. Both the proximate and ultimate effects of a drug have to be studied in the course of its evaluation (Fig. 7-4).

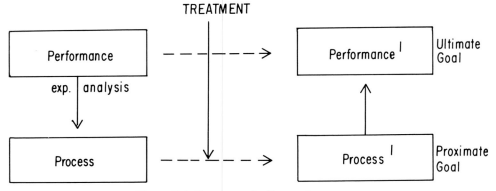

Figure 7-4. Process underlies performance.

Similarly with remedial methods a child undergoes "perceptual training" with a view to optimizing reading ability. After training, proximate effects relate to perception—is it now sharpened? Ultimate effects relate to reading; is it now improved? Unless we can answer both questions, we can not understand the effect of the treatment.

A second attribute of a test might be suggested—that it is standardized, that norms are available. Is this necessarily so?

If we wish to measure the extent to which a deviant population is impaired as compared to normals, we must of course have normal data to compare to the results. For instance, it is futile to see in any failure to copy a cube or a star, evidence of brain damage when the majority of a normal but ill educated group will similarly fail (Kinsbourne, unpublished) ; or to see without qualification in a child's writing reversals evidence of minimal cerebral dysfunction when all normal children are at some time or other guilty of that error. But that by no means implies a need for the elaborate standardization procedures that characterize the development of a test of general intellect, like Wechsler scales. It merely states that a normal control group is needed.

The use of commercially available standardized test material is a double-edged sword. Rarely will the designer of the test have had in mind a purpose identical to that for which the investigator needs this instrument. Thus in investigating brain damage, one is looking for impairment of process. One would hardly choose the curious miscellaneous clutter of questions that constitute the WAIS for such a purpose. The WAIS is more a test of content than of process. It turns out that persons with the greatest fund of knowledge will usually have acquired that knowledge by dint of superior process. But the exceptions to this are so numerous as to invalidate these tests as experimental tools.

A second more insidious danger is in the interpretation of the results. It should be noted that failure on a given item by an old person may mean something quite different from failure by a younger man. The factorial loading of the WAIS performance of the elderly differs materially from that which prevails with the young (Cohen, 1957). But with the old at least we know what that loading is; we have no such information about the brain damaged, the psychotic, the institutionalized mentally retarded. Wechsler did not include such groups in his standardization sample. Therefore, when used on such groups, the WAIS and WISC are nonstandardized tests; the results are obscure and even obscured by what we know about these tests in their more usual context.

Another example applies to Raven's Progressive Matrices. This test is highly loaded on the factor of general intelligence, "g" (Klonoff, 1951); reasoning power is the performance-limiting factor for normals and perhaps for left cerebral hemisphere damaged subjects also. But when right hemisphere damaged subjects do badly on this test, it is for quite other reasons. They are spatially disoriented, and this failure to grasp spatial relationships deprives their reasoning faculty of its raw material. A spatial factor becomes performance limiting. In right hemisphere damaged patients, the Raven's Progressive Matrices test something quite different from that which they test in normals (Warrington, James and Kinsbourne, 1966).

Standardized tests have a solitary advantage when used on deviant case material. They make for excellent background documentation to give others a fair idea of the type of patient one is working with. But he who wishes to measure a process almost always finds himself having to design a test specifically suited to his purpose.

The measuring of effects of treatments on reading backwardness is a prime instance of the substitution of measures of performance for those of process. Teachers' ratings and reading achievement test data before and after treatment are of course of practical interest, but if there is an improvement, they do not betray whether that effect was specific to reading or general to the child's adaption to the school situation nor do they specify on which of the many interacting processes that constitute reading and writing capacity the treatment exerted its influence. Analytical measures of reading ability are essential. They will enable children to be classified in terms of the particular process affected, rather than thrown together into miscellaneous groups of readers backward for whatever cause. Potentially rational remedial measures can then be tried out without fear that even if effective on a subset of subjects, this effect will not appear in the group statistic. Not until a good range of analytical reading tests is available can we approach the fundamental question in remediation, as applied to reading; teach to strength or teach to weakness?

An analytical reading test should simulate the processes involved in reading as closely as possible, short of using the actual graphic symbols of the written language, which would contaminate the measure through a mixture of an unknown amount of prior experience. Thus, we analyze the early reading process into nine constituent operations and simulate each one by use of arbitrary stimulus material (Kinsbourne and Rosof, in preparation). The analysis consists of a three-by-three matrix (Fig. 7-4) and must be regarded as based on a minimal model of this complex skill:

	Form	*Orientation*	*Sequence*
Discrimination	×	×	×
Retention	×	×	×
Association	×	×	×

In the design of presumptively process-specific measures, the variable of task difficulty is crucial, and yet it is rarely taken into consideration. There is general awareness of the fact that ceiling and floor effects must be avoided. But potentially much more misleading is the situation in which a group of efficient performers and a group of less efficient ones are compared on a task, and quantitative conclusions are drawn. These difficulties arise from the fact that the degree to which a subject applies himself to a task is not unrelated to his notion of how well he is doing and his expectations as to how well he might do.

When a task is made somewhat more difficult, the quantitative performance decrement may be deceptively small on account of a "challenge" effect. The subject invests more effort so as to meet the challenge. On the other hand, an overwhelming incidence of failure may evoke disengagement from the task. The subject "gives up" and does even his limited capacity far less than justice. Whether a given level of difficulty is interpreted as challenging or as basis for disengagement depends greatly on the subject's life history. While normal, young, white, middle class adults are prone to view difficulty as a challenge, the reverse is true of many groups, notably the aged and the mentally retarded who react with defeatism against the background of multiple failure experiences. This may lead to gross overestimation of the individual's intellectual deficit (Zigler, 1967).

It has long been argued that old people are peculiarly unfitted to work under "paced" conditions (Canestrari, 1965; Eisdorfer, 1968) though agreement is lacking as to the explanation for this. The implication is that if only one gives the elderly enough time, they will finish the job. Yet attractive as are the moral overtones of this position, the results of actually giving the old that extra time do not necessarily fulfill these optimistic expectations (Heron and Chown, 1967). Is it really pacing per se that makes a task harder for the old? Or is it that the paced task is in general more difficult and old people do badly with difficult tasks whatever the origin of that difficulty; is their performance in fact unsafe at any speed?

Existing demonstrations of pacing effects on age-related performance confound rate of presentation with task difficulty. The paced learning task affords the subject less overall learning time. We decided to investigate the effect of pacing presentation of paired associates, holding total learning time constant (Kinsbourne and Berryhill, in preparation). Young control subjects do equally well at each of the three rates chosen, so long as total time is held constant (Cooper and Pantlee, 1968). We find the old to behave likewise; if anything, they do least well on the slowest presentation rate. When overall task difficulty (total time available for learning) is held constant, the rate of presentation ceases to be a relevant variable.

In tests of problem-solving ability the demoralizing effects of task difficulty may be avoided by use of materials graduated in difficulty, with a predetermined criterion for when testing is to be stopped, related to the degree of success at various stages of the test. A similar method may be applied to tests of information transmitting capacity (Kinsbourne, 1970). Consider a measure of learning ability, using the paired associate paradigm.

A set of *n* paired associates is customarily presented serially 1-n, and the presentation is repeated till a performance or time criterion is met. In order to obtain an estimate of learning ability, rather than immediate memory span, the number of pairs presented is greater than can be recalled at the first run through. Thus the subject is initially given an overload of information to remember; the poorer a learner he is, the greater the overload. Now if the amount of overload is itself a variable relevant to the difficulty of a learning task, then good and poor learners are being unequally treated if the same number of pairs is serially presented to each. This is true irrespective of the mechanism of this variable. That mechanism will probably be maturational; the subject is intimidated by the amount he is supposed to master. There may however also be cognitive factors. At the second run through the subject responds incorrectly to some of the stimuli. He then has the further complicating task of remembering in subsequent reappearances of that stimulus which was the corrected response and which was his error. It follows that any method presenting materials for learning that reduces the incidence of these two factors should make a more suitable vehicle for the clinical assessment of learning ability.

One way of minimizing wrong responses is by presenting the right response very quickly after the stimulus comes on. Only if the subject is very sure will he answer so quickly as to anticipate the displayed response, and he will then usually be right. This "errorless" technique is in fact very effective in enhancing the amount children learn in a given time (Kinsbourne, 1970). But another method, the "cumulative" shares the advantage and is preferable as regards motivation (Kinsbourne, 1970).

In the cumulative paradigm of paired associate learning, pairs are phased in in stages with rehearsal of all previous items after introduction of each new pair, thus:

$$p_1$$
$$p_2 \; p_1$$
$$p_3 \; p_2 \; p_1, \text{ etc.}$$

with sequence randomized within rows.

This method has two advantages; the full set of pairs for learning is not initially revealed. Indeed, if a criterion of number of errors is set for discontinuance of testing, then the child may never know what the full set would have been, and he will lack a proper appreciation of the degree of his failure. At the same time, because the early loading on memory is minimized, there will be fewer wrong responses subsequently to discriminate from the corrections. The paradigm in fact yields far better learning per unit time than does the standard method, and we are now using it as a vehicle for presenting material in an analytical reading test battery (Kinsbourne and Rosof, in preparation).

So far we have discussed the type of measures appropriate for cognitive evaluation at various stages of development. Further problems are faced when these are repeated to evaluate the effects, if any, of some in intervening treatment. These are the following: the effect of the observer's expectations both on treatment and on evaluation; the problem of whether to teach to the skill to be measured or to seek to trace back and first attack its simpler origins; the question of specificity of the effect and of the generality of that specific effect.

To contrast treatment with no treatment is obviously unsound, on account of the halo effect of action. It is preferable to contrast multiple treatments, as should it be the case that both treater and treated have equally high expectations of both, or are unaware as to which is happening. The evaluation should be similarly in the dark; the double-blind method of running dry trials is now very familiar. Unfortunately double blind is not always practicable, as for instance when a drug has an evident side effect. It is hardly possible blindly to evaluate 5-hydroxytryptophan in the treatment of Down's Syndrome when the agent patently increases muscle tone (Bazelon, 1967). The danger of being misled in such cases is not only that the evaluator be misled in his measurement, but also that his expectations communicate themselves to the subjects, who perform accordingly—the so-called Rosenthal (1968) effect.

Does one teach to a skill or to its presumed antecedents? Certainly one trains not a complete skill as a whole but its elements, prior to their combination; no one would suggest starting an illiterate child age eight in the third grade and then reiterating this grade for remedial purposes. But the more fundamental question is, should one go back further to some earlier acquired but still supposedly related skill? Does one learn reading by "perceptual training" or on the trampoline?

Systematic studies of the matter are lacking. The appropriate paradigm is to teach in two ways, holding total teaching time constant: teach to the skill; teach to its "antecedent"; compare results. Pending such studies there is no reason at present to doubt that the most reliable and effective way of teaching any skill is to teach it rather than something else.

Then there is the matter of specificity of the mechanism of the treatment. This fundamental problem can only be discussed in its various specific contexts. Suffice it to note that in areas in which multiple methods of remediation coexist and no one is self-evidently the best, it is likely that all are nonspecific in their mechanism and relatively ineffective.

How general is the result? The surest way to success is to test, train on that very test, and test again. Actually in skill learning this is precisely what should be and is done. In concept learning the point is crucial. Can the subject generalize the concept beyond the particular context in which he acquired it? The training of conservation in young children (Wallach, 1963) is open to such suspicion of nontransferability. Whenever any individual is taught something that at his age or with his level of intelligence he would not have been expected to master, the question must be faced; is that of use to him? It can not be assumed that he will utilize the principle it embodies in as general a way as would someone at a later developmental stage.

It is hard to imagine anything more difficult than to define an experimental group in terms of valid criteria, analyze the performance under scrutiny into its underlying processes, and correctly ascertain the effect of a treatment both on the target process and on the resulting performance, and correctly evaluate the generality of one's findings.

REFERENCES

1. Adams, R. D., Fisher, C. M. Hawkins, S., Ojemann, R. G., and Sweet, W. H.: Symptomatic occult hydrocephalus with "normal" cerebrospinal fluid pressure: A treatable syndrome. *New Eng J Med, 273:*117-126, 1965.
2. Bazelon, M.: Reversal of hypotonia in infants with Down's Syndrome by administration of 5-hydroxytryptophan. *Lancet,* pp. 1130-1133, 1967.
3. Canestrari, R. E.: Age changes in acquisition: Theoretical and methodological issues. Annual Meeting Gerontological Society, Los Angeles, 1965.
4. Cohen, J.: The factorial structure of the WAIS between early adulthood and old age. *J Consult Psychol, 21:*283-290, 1957.
5. Cooper, E. H., and Pantle, A. J.: The total time hypothesis in verbal learning. *Psychol Bull, 4:*221-234, 1968.
6. Eisdorfer, C.: Arousal and performance: Experiments in verbal learning and a tentative theory. In Talland: *Human Behavior and Aging: Recent Advances in Research and Theory.* New York, Academic Press, 1968, pp. 189-216.
7. Heron, A., and Chown, S.: *Age and Function.* London, Churchill, 1967.
8. Hochberg, J.: In the mind's eye. In Haber, R. N. (Ed.) : *Contemporary Theory and Research in Visual Perception.* 1968.
9. Jacobs, E. A., Winter, P. M., Albis, H. S., and Small, S. M.: Hyperoxygenation effect on cognitive functioning in the aged. *New Eng J Med, 281:*753-757, 1969.
10. Kinsbourne, M.: Optimal learning conditions for fast and slow learners. American Association on Mental Deficiency, Washington, 1970.
11. Klonoff, H.: *An Exploratory Study and Analysis of the Wechsler-Bellevue Intelligence Scale and the Raven's Progressive Matrices.* Unpublished Master's Thesis, University of Toronto, 1951.
12. Korchin, S. J., and Basowitz, H.: Age differences in verbal learning. *J Abnorm Soc Psychol, 54:*64-69, 1957.
13. Piaget, J.: *The Psychology of Intelligence.* Routledge and Kenan Paul, Ltd. Broadway House, 1947.
14. Rosenthal, R., and Jacobson, L.: *Pygmalion in the Classroom.* New York, Holt, Rinehart and Winston, 1968.
15. Wallach, M. A.: Research in children's thinking. In National Society for the Study of Education: 62nd Yearbook, *Child Psychology.* Chicago University Press, 1963.
16. Warrington, E., James, M., and Kinsbourne, M.: Drawing disability in relation to laterality of cerebral lesion. *Brain, 89:*53-82, 1966.
17. Wepman, J. M.: The interrelationship of learning, speech and reading. *The Reading Teacher, 14:*245-247, 1961.
18. Zigler, E.: Familial mental retardation: A continuing dilemma. *Science, 155:*292-298, 1967.

Chapter 8

EEG Ontogenesis in Normal Children

DAVID R. METCALF* AND KENT JORDAN

T HIS PRESENTATION represents an overview report on some of the results of a recently completed long-term study of EEG development in a group of normal children. The purpose of this chapter is to detail some ontogenic features of the EEG as revealed in this study. We have chosen for our focus those aspects of EEG development which are most subject to misinterpretation, in particular misinterpretation of normal EEGs as being abnormal. The subjects of this study, as will be noted later, were from volunteer families. Families were enrolled in the program† *before* the study-child was conceived, or shortly thereafter. Mothers were intensively followed during pregnancy. Each child was seen several times a year for a large variety of investigations of which repeat EEGs were only one (BMR, x-rays, physical anthropometry, psychological evaluation, physical examination, interval history, etc.) . Thus, within any practical limit, these are known to be "normal" children. Any intervening disturbance (illness, injury, behavioral disturbance, etc.) was documented; there were antecedent and subsequent studies with reference to such disturbances. Thus, for the EEG, the effects of an injury on one child's EEG could be properly documented. This report, therefore, deals with normal EEG development in a long-term, longitudinal study of normal infants and children studied from the neonatal period until the age of ten to fifteen years. Individual variability during the course of development can be delineated; the group size (N = 80) makes cross-sectional statements, as well, valid.

The electroencephalogram (EEG) is a widely used diagnostic tool in neurology, psychiatry, and neurosurgery where it is used for the nontraumatic study of actual or potential organic brain disturbance. It has had many applications in the clinical research of brain electrophysiology. At the present time the use of the EEG with adults is well established on both empiric and theoretic grounds as a useful medical diagnostic and research tool. On the contrary, the diagnostic usefulness of the EEG with infants and children is severely limited by factors relating to the relative complexity and

*Dr. Metcalf is currently supported by NIMH Research Scientist Development Award No. 5-K2-MH-40, 275-02.

†Child Research Council, Department for the Study of Human Growth, University of Colorado Medical Center, Denver, Colorado.

variability of their EEGs. Children's EEGs show much interindividual and intraindividual variability in contrast to the relative stability and predictability of adult's EEGs.

Electroencephalography in infants and children has sometimes been regarded with suspicion, if not disrepute, because of the contradictions between EEG diagnosis on the one hand and clinical diagnosis and ultimate outcome on the other. Conflicting EEG results are seen in EEGs separated by brief time intervals; conflicting interpretations are seen in different laboratories. These conflicts and lack of predictability between the EEG and current clinical status, prognosis and clinical outcome are in part because of the general lack of adequate normative standards for infant's and children's EEGs. A blatantly abnormal EEG in association with highly suggestive clinical findings can be of clear diagnostic value. The problem arises when a moderately abnormal or "borderline" or "nonspecifically" abnormal EEG is coupled with equivocal clinical findings. There exist few standards to help differentiate in children between certain normal but unusual EEG patterns and abnormal EEG patterns of similar appearance in children. To further add to the dilemma, abnormal EEG findings in the child often disappear after a period of time; the mechanisms for this "normalization" are not understood, the meaning, significance and prognosis of such normalizing with respect to clinical findings is not known nor is the general developmental course of such evenescent patterns understood. Thus, there is a need for increased knowledge about the normal EEG in infancy and childhood, particularly with reference to aspects of the EEG that are critical for clinical diagnosis. Not to be neglected is the parallel, related, but slightly separate need for such standards for research and scientific purposes.

Despite the current state of our ignorance, there is a broad, deep, and important literature on children's electroencephalograms; that interest in normal EEGs of children is very old, having its inception with the first human clinical EEGs done by the "father of electroencephalography," Hans Berger, in the early 1930's. The major goal of this presentation is to describe a few aspects of EEG development in a group of normal children who were followed intensively from birth through adolescence.* This intensive study (including repeated neurological examinations, physical examinations, reports of illness, nutritional histories, school reports, etc.) insures that we are working with children who fall well within the range of normal variation along many parameters, i.e. they are "clinically normal." Illnesses, injuries, and other aspects of life history could be directly related to EEG findings, past, current, and future in this long-term, anterospective, longitudinal

---

*These data were all obtained in the EEG program which was part of the general research program of the Child Research Council, Department for the Study of Human Growth at the University of Colorado Medical Center in Denver, Colorado.

study. Thus, occurrence of EEG variability, findings of deviations from the expected norm, as well as the pathway of most common and expectable EEG development are all observable. Hypothetical clinical correlations and their predicted sequelae can be tested. Where questions as to significance of a specific EEG finding occurred, it was always possible to correlate such EEG disturbances against concurrent clinical status as well as search for future consequences of such EEG disturbances in this unique EEG series.

The general unavailability of normal standards for infants and children, particularly on a longitudinal, individual developmental basis, leads not only to difficulty in understanding any single EEG, but more serious difficulty in using children's EEGs diagnostically. This difficulty is further compounded when the EEG is part of a diagnostic battery in studying children with possible minimal brain dysfunction. In these instances there is little expectation of finding more than a minimal brain physiological disturbance (in contrast to the situation with epilepsy, brain tumor, or cerebral trauma). Lack of full knowledge of expected EEG development in infants and children can lead to misinterpretation of single EEGs. Misdiagnosis can and often does lead to improper medical treatment including ill-advised use of medications. This longitudinal study, therefore makes it possible to delineate many "normal" deviations (temporary or enduring) from expectable developmental trends.

A knowledge of normal EEG development and its expected variability is at least equally important for investigators of human development. The course of EEG development is not smooth, straightforward, or cleanly predictable. Varying rates of EEG development, specific periods of increased or decreased variability, age periods during which EEG deviation is particularly prevalent all have a bearing on any study of neurological development, personality development, behavioral development, learning in relationship to development, etc. Through this avenue, the relationship of brain maturation and development to broad issues in biopsychological development comes into contact with questions about critical developmental periods, "developmental lags," etc. Exploration of these issues rests heavily on clear and accurate knowledge of normal brain physiological development and can be clarified by this type of broadly based, longitudinal EEG study.

Implied in the foregoing is the fact that the EEG changes throughout the life cycle from earliest times (including prematurity) to old age. These changes are particularly rapid during the first two years. Development continues at a decelerating rate through adolescence after which there is a trend toward relative "plateauing" of development. The marked developmental changes in the EEG from birth to adolescence have led behavioral scientists to seek relationships between brain maturation (as seen with the EEG) and other areas of development, whether they be at the physical, physiological, or psychological levels. We have noted, for instance, that the EEG changes associated with adolescence are correlated with the very earliest sign of adolescence (epiphyseal closure—presumably under hormonal control), and therefore precedes adolescence as typified by secondary sex changes, psychological changes, and physical growth changes.

EEGs at all ages are quite different for all levels of consciousness (awake, drowsy, sleep, and intermediate categories). In general, a full clinical EEG includes awake and sleep recording because of the different types of pathology and different developmental indices found in different levels of consciousness. The variability of infant's and children's EEGs makes it particularly necessary to study each level of consciousness and to understand what is acceptable under each circumstance.

We choose here to focus primarily on some aspects of the sleep EEG without minimizing the importance of the awake EEG. In general, the sleep EEG (especially quiet, NREM sleep) shows greater variability at any single age than does the awake EEG. There is also a significant developmental change with age, particularly after three years. Variability and complexity of sleep electroencephalograms render them difficult and confusing to evaluate, but the greater variability also is an asset when these EEGs are used for developmental research. The variability of the sleep EEG, the variable rates of development in individual children, and related confusing factors have resulted in less knowledge about expected variability, expected patterns, and range or normality to be expected at any age or under particular circumstances. Consequently, there is less knowledge among EEG clinicians about sleep EEGs in children than about awake EEGs. Lastly, it is a fact that certain attributes of normal sleep patterns in children often resemble abnormal patterns seen in adults. Thus, in summary, the complexity, general insufficient knowledge of the data, and similarity of sleep EEG findings to certain common abnormal patterns all make it an important area for further clarification. This report will focus on the development of spindles and K-complexes as well as variations in spindle and K-complex morphology. Through this means an attempt will be made to construct a hierarchy in terms of closeness to and distance from "midline normality" as well as construct a developmental-ontogenic picture of the sleep EEG in infancy and childhood.

This is not a study of abnormal EEGs in an abnormal population or EEG correlates against clinical abnormality. This is a study of essentially normal EEGs and normal EEG variability within a clinically normal population. This population has been intensively studied for many years, and the possibile clinical outcome or clinical correlates of intercurrent diseases, intercurrent EEG disturbances, learning disturbances, physical growth alterations, etc. have been carefully explored. On the basis of these data it is hoped that this report will help the clinician evaluate the single EEG with respect to a given clinical problem.

As part of this thinking, the general concept of normality, particularly as applied to developing children needs careful understanding. Normality may be conceptualized as an approach to some ideal state. The concept of normality may also carry implications for the capacity for adaptation or for range of adaptability available to the individual. Normality also carries implications of an ethological nature in terms of fulfilling survival needs or having survival value for an individual in terms of concepts about "species survival." Normality may also carry statistical connotations, i.e. events which occur very rarely would be by definition "abnormal" whereas common events would be "normal." In general, we tend to combine the statistical and adaptive concepts in our judgments about normality. Thus, although it might be statistically normal for an individual to have a severe upper respiratory infection, this would be also considered as a biological or adaptive abnormality.

A knowledge of human development and an appreciation of concepts of normality within this concept implies, therefore, an understanding and appreciation of theories of "critical developmental period." Thus, within the schema of human development it is assumed that there are times (ages, points in development, etc.) when developing physiology, social demands, status of hormonal systems, etc. are so interrelated and perhaps developing at such a pace that physiological and/or psychological systems may be particularly vulnerable to disturbance or vulnerable in such a way that induced deviation may have unusually enduring or serious sequelae.

EEG ontogenesis procedes in a relatively unbroken line from the intrauterine situation, through the perinatal period and on into infancy and childhood. The ontogenic course of the awake and sleep EEG in prematurely-born infants has been thoroughly documented by Dreyfus-Brisac and her co-workers, by Parmalee, Monod, and others. The strong relationship between EEG morphology and gestational age in prematures is now well known. In brief, the sleep EEG of young prematures of about thirty-two weeks can be said to show three principal types of activity. Large amounts of time (up to 70% of sleep) are spent in Stage I eye movement sleep, commonly called Stage I-REM or merely REM sleep (rapid eye movement). This is a situation where the EEG is relatively low in amplitude, polyrhythmic, and continuous; there are numerous jerky, rolling eye movements (rapid eye movements), and the infant shows irregular pulse, irregular respiration and much facial activity, spontaneous smiling, finger, hand and fist movements, and squirming and twisting of arms, legs and body.

An outstanding attribute of the EEG of prematurity is the tracé alternant EEG which, after thirty to thirty-two gestational weeks, is primarily associated with "quiet sleep." Quiet sleep is that stage of sleep during which there are no rapid eye movements (NREM), and respirations are quite regular in contrast to previously noted REM sleep or "active sleep." The tracé alternant EEG consists of relatively flat or isoelectric periods of eight to ten or fifteen seconds duration interspersed by brief bursts of slow and polysharp activity lasting from one to five seconds. These bursts may appear simultaneously in all scalp regions, but are generally randomly distributed and more evident in parietal-occipital regions than elsewhere. The morphology of the bursts is mixed and usually of moderate to high amplitude, sometimes reaching $100\mu v$. As the premature infant becomes older (in terms of postconceptional age), the flat interburst intervals become of shorter duration and gradually become "filled in" by polyrhythmic but generally slow (1-4 Hz) EEG activity. The intermittent slow and sharp bursts tend to become lower amplitude, less clearly evident against the EEG background, and gradually become encompassed within the developing EEG rhythms as they "fill in" the isoelectric interburst periods. By the time a premature infant approaches the approximate point of "full term," i.e. forty gestational weeks, the tracé alternant recording has almost completely disappeared although some remnants of this discontinuous quality of the record remains. The intermittent and relatively discontinuous record after forty gestational weeks is not evident in early quiet sleep, but remains evident in very deep, quiet sleep.

It is particularly important not to mistake the tracé alternant recording for abnormality particularly in premature infants, but also in full-term infants as will be discussed subsequently. The sharp and slow bursts in the premature infant can resemble atypical polyspike and slow "epileptiform" discharges. When these bursts appear against the background of an alternating record and are seen randomly in all scalp regions, they are most likely to represent the normal recording for this age. On the other hand, persistence of clear tracé alternant recording or persistence of clear polysharp and slow bursts around the time of expected term is quite uncommon and raises the suspicion that a cortical-subcortical disturbance exists. One must remember that alternating EEGs in pathological situations can be brought about by extremely deep anesthesia, cortical undercutting (as a sequela of prefrontal lobotomy), or as one finding in severe idiopathic panencephalitic-like disturbances such as "hypsarrhythmia." The electrographic diagnosis of seizures in prematures and neonates often depends on the witnessing of clinical seizure manifestations in association with electrographic disturbance.

In full-term neonates, there is always a visible remnant of sharp and slow bursts alternating with lower amplitude recording very similar to that seen in premature infants. This is most evident in deep quiet sleep (regular respirations, no eye movements, no body activity except for intermittent spontaneous startles, and no facial activity), particularly five to ten minutes after this stage of sleep has commenced. During deep quiet sleep the tracé alternant recording, to a progressively lesser degree, persists until age four to five weeks in full-term infants, but is rarely seen after six weeks. Thus, an alternating recording particularly with intermittent polysharp and slow bursts after seven or eight weeks in full-term infants is again an unusual and suspicious finding whereas previous to this time it would be within normal limits.

Of a somewhat nonelectroencephalographic nature but worthy of mention is the "switch-over" from an infantile type of sleep mechanism to a more mature type of sleep mechanism which takes place at about age three months in full-term infants (the ontogenesis for premature infants is unknown at this time). Before age three months, infants routinely fall asleep directly into active, eye movement sleep after which they drift into quiet or high voltage slow wave sleep (with spindles after age 5-7 weeks). After about age three months, infants fall asleep almost directly into spindle sleep, i.e. Stage II sleep preceded by a very rough and poorly formed high voltage, moderately regular slow wave type of EEG, which is the precursor of hypersynchronous drowsy patterns to be seen later. Additionally, before age three months large amounts of indeterminate or undifferentiated states are seen. By this we mean, in particular, the simultaneous presence of Stage I eye movement EEG in association with physiological patterns belonging to nonbehavioral sleep situations, such as sucking, drowsiness, crying, and fussing (Emde and Metcalf, Metcalf and Emde).

After age three months rapid eye movements and the low amplitude irregular "active" EEG is almost exclusively associated with the behavioral state of sleep. We do not yet know whether a prolongation of this "switchover point" to age four or five months could be termed pathological, but we would be quite interested to explore the clinical correlates of such an event. Parenthetically, it should be noted that after significant trauma, such as circumcision (Emde *et al.*), infants will fall directly into quiet sleep and show much longer episodes of quiet sleep than are otherwise seen; this alteration of sleep control lasts at least ten hours and possibly a little longer.

First, well-defined EEG sleep spindles begin to make their appearance in full-term infants between four and six weeks of age. Sleep spindle bursts are rarely seen before age four weeks in full-term infants and also on rare occasions may not develop before age seven or eight weeks. The terms "well-defined" or "clearly defined" refer to sleep spindles which are vertex dominant or exclusively recorded at the vertex, fairly well fixed in a narrow frequency band around 12-14 Hz and appear only during high voltage slow wave (HVS) sleep. The presence of spindling during the early stages of HVS sleep is one of the primary defining criteria for the presence of Stage

II sleep. The ontogenesis of sleep spindles before the well-defined spindles appear occupies approximately one week. Before the development of well-defined sleep spindle bursts, spindles of lower amplitude and poorly fixed frequency control are also seen in the vertex region. These have been termed by us "Grade I" spindles, the well-defined spindles being termed "Grade II." Rudimentary spindles can be seen at almost all ages in full-term infants before Grade I spindles develop. Rudimentary spindles have been demonstrated by us with computer analysis to be an almost continuous, 16-18 Hz vertex dominant rhythm of extremely low ($5\mu v$-$8\mu v$) amplitude. When Grade I spindles first develop, 12-14 Hz spindles are seen to coexist with the faster 16-18 Hz rudimentary spindles; the latter disappear as Grade II spindles develop. Rudimentary spindles are often not visible because of high frequency cut-off of the EEG amplifiers, pens that are too dull and other limiting technical factors. The general definition and description of sleep spindles is adequate for EEGs of humans of all ages whereas this would not be the case for any of the rhythms of the awake EEG. Despite this unusual stability of spindles throughout life, there are some noteworthy changes in spindle characteristics during infancy and childhood (Metcalf, Lenard) .

After Grade II spindles develop, they are seen to be vertex dominant, well controlled in the 12-14 Hz range, and generally of $30\mu v$-$50\mu v$ amplitude. At about age two to three months, it is not uncommon for spindle episodes to be extremely long, occasionally of eight to ten seconds duration and sometimes $40\mu v$-$50\mu v$ amplitude. By age three to five months, spindle bursts tend to be one to three seconds duration and occur with a frequency of about one to three bursts every ten seconds. Thus, a diagnosis of "extreme spindles" is difficult to make under age four months when spindles may be very high amplitude and of extremely long duration in normal children. During the first six months, spindle morphology remains smoothly contoured, and the number of spindle bursts per unit time gradually increases until about eighteen months when we may see four to five short spindle bursts per ten seconds of EEG.

At about five to six months of age, spindles become very sharply contoured, usually comb-like with positively directed sharp components when recording front to back or vertex to ear. Also at this time, but less often, spindles may be saw-toothed and sharp. Comb-like spindles usually persist until about 1-1.5 years; persistence after 2.5-3 years is regarded as an unusual persistence of an immature pattern without known clinical correlates. After age 1-1.5 years, comb-like and sharp spindles are seen less often, and the most common type of spindling is smoothly contoured, regular, fixed in frequency, and tending toward good symmetry between the hemispheres but without phase-synchrony between the hemispheres. It is quite common, however, for hemispherical voltage asymmetry of a complete or incomplete variety to be seen in EEGs of children through age four years although less so after age three years. This asymmetry tends to be shifting, that is, the higher amplitude spindling appears at random in one or the other hemisphere rather than being a persistent asymmetry. Because development of the sleep EEG from birth to three years appears to be fairly smooth and regular, one might assume that this regularity of development continues thereafter. This is not the case. Between age three and nine years, there is a great increase in variability of spindle morphology as well as variability along a number of other EEG parameters.

It should be noted that the well-known drowsy hypersynchrony consisting of 3-5 Hz high amplitude synchronous activity in all scalp regions during behavioral drowsiness and preceding sleep begins to take form between three and six months with some variability between children. Certainly, drowsy hypersynchrony no longer should be confused with abnormal slow wave bursts. However one must always be on guard not to mistake small interspersed sharp waves or fast activity in the midst of drowsy hypersynchrony for isolated sharp discharges which may make such a record appear to contain a spike and slow "epileptiform" disturbance. Similarly, hypersynchronous patterns are seen after arousal from sleep. These hypersynchronous patterns before and after sleep may last anywhere from one to five minutes.

The EEG of Stage II sleep becomes differentiated from deeper sleep at about age three to four months. This change first makes it possible to differentiate Stage II sleep from what might be called a combined Stage III-IV sleep. The Stage III-IV sleep is characterized by being higher amplitude, slower, and a little less regular than the EEG of Stage II sleep; also spindle activity is less evident during Stage III-IV sleep. After age four to five months, it is possible to distinguish all four "classical" stages of sleep, i.e. Stage I, Stage II, Stage III, and Stage IV. These differentiations become quite clear from six months on.

The next major change in the EEG takes place between ages five and six months with the development of spontaneous K-complexes (Metcalf *et al.*). K-complexes, which are typical biphasic and triphasic medium to high amplitude, 500 msec discharges occurring in posterior vertex scalp regions during spindle sleep and deeper stages of sleep, develop rapidly after age six months from poorly differentiated forms to well differentiated forms by age three years. After age three to four years there is increased variability of K-complex morphology although K-complexes continue to develop toward the ultimate mature forms seen during midadolescence, late adolescence, and early adulthood. In order to study K-complex development more carefully and objectively, we have evaluated K-complexes in our normal group in accord with different parameters as follows:

(1) Vertex focus: referring to the presence or absence of vertex dominance of the K-complex.

(2) Individuation: referring to the degree to which a K-complex is readily differentiated from background EEG activity and fulfills the traditional criteria for waveform and triphasic pattern.

(3) Repetition: the amount of rapid repetition of individual K-complexes without intervening EEG activity.

(4) Spread: the occurrence of K-complexes, which although vertex dominant, are also recorded at distant scalp regions such as fronto-temporal and temporal-occipital.

(5) Sharp K-complexes: referring to sharpness of the initial high voltage component.

We find that each of these parameters has its own developmental pattern with the most immature K-complexes showing poor vertex dominance because they are almost inextricably intermingled with ongoing high amplitude slow EEG activity and also showing a significant amount of "spread" because the K-complexes appear in lateral and lateral-posterior scalp regions 100-300 msec after appearing at the vertex. The most prominent aspect of gradual development of K-complexes consists of a gradual sharpening and regularizing of the various K-complex components so that ultimately the total pattern becomes relatively invariant and well differentiated from ongoing random activity, becomes well limited to the vertex region, and tends to occur as single isolated discharges rather than groups of intermingled discharges. Ultimately, in the well-organized EEG of late adolescence and young adulthood, it is most common for K-complexes not to repeat themselves more than once per second or once in every two or three seconds, thus permitting the development of "slow" components of the K-complex, each K-complex showing the full triphasic morphology limited to the vertex region. Previous to age two years, the initial high voltage component of the K-complex is rounded and of relatively long duration at the peak. At somewhat older ages, these initial components become more sharp and also higher voltage, often reaching $300\mu v$-$400\mu v$. Sharp K-complexes become somewhat reduced in voltage after age seven years, but the sharpness persists during adolescence and contributes to the distinctness of K-complexes during adolescence. This sharpness gradually abates during adulthood leaving the smooth rounded K-complex morphology one expects in all adult EEGs prior to age forty years.

Approximately at age three years, K-complexes are well-individuated, with full predictable morphology and vertex dominance, while spindles occur in regular, brief bursts lasting about one second, occurring one or two times every ten seconds; spindle bursts usually are seen in the EEG following each K-complex episode.

Progressively between three and six years, increasing numbers of children show deviations from the previous stable and expectable patterned K-complex and spindle relationship outlined above and also expected in the mature EEG. In the individual child, these deviations first occur as minimal departures from previously well-developed patterns. Initially only a few of the many K-complex spindle combinations in each EEG will be deviant. With increasing age, usually over 3.5-4.5 years, there is a steady increase in the number of deviant discharges during sleep, and the individual K-spindle patterns become more markedly deviant. In general, the deviant "sleep patterns" consist of a variety of combinations of single K-complex-spindle variations.

It is convenient first to describe separately the spindle variations and K-complex variations before describing the combination-variants which are termed "distorted paterns."

SPINDLE VARIATIONS
Sharp Spindles

After age three years, there is an increasing occurrence of spindles which are sharply contoured. The mean age of onset for sharp spindles is four years; sharp spindles in any individual may exist for three or four years, and they are seen in 50 to 60 percent of all children between the ages of three and seven years. In general, the individual sharp spindle waves show the sharp component at either the positive or negative peak with the opposite peak being more smoothly rounded, although this is not necessarily the case. These spindles almost always have good bilateral voltage symmetry and stable frequency control with the expected anterior vertex focus. Sharp spindles are seen almost exclusively during early and mid Stage II sleep and generally give way to smoother spindles during deep Stage II and III sleep. Sharp spindles at this time are generally seen following K-complexes; they rarely override or intermingle with K-complexes.

Irregular Frequency

In the three-year to nine-year age group there is an upsurge of spindle activity showing increased variability of frequency (increased bandwidth) within a single spindle burst. This almost always occurs simultaneously with and is part of noteworthy variability in voltage regulation and loss of inter-hemispheric synchrony. Such spindle bursts, therefore, appear to be very irregular in control of amplitude and periodicity within one hemisphere and irregular in terms of the expected voltage and frequency synchrony between the two hemispheres.

High Amplitude Sharp Spindles

Sharp, high voltage spindles $(100\mu v\text{-}200\mu v)$ are seen in slightly older children and show a mean age of onset of five years as compared with four years for sharp spindles. Sharp high voltage spindles, as with other spindle activity, are usually no more than two seconds duration for any given spindle burst; thus they do not resemble "extreme spindles" (Gibbs). When sharp high voltage spindles are seen, it is quite common for an individual spindle wave to be distinctly higher amplitude than surrouding waves and thus resemble a solitary spike or sharp wave discharge. Such occurrences may be numerous in one record and may occur several times during a ten-second epoch. Quite often, this type of spindling is recorded at independent temporal electrodes some distance from the vertex. This appears to be a function of the absolute voltage of the spindles at the vertex. Although this may also be a function of head size, evaluation of our EEG data in terms of cranial circumference, and length and width measurements on our subjects does not confirm this suspicion.

Spikes in Spindles

Between the ages of six and ten years, increasing numbers of children (20% of our subjects) show spike discharges within spindle bursts. These spikes are usually part of a burst of high voltage sharp spindles; rarely they are seen within otherwise "normal," "smooth" spindle episodes. In general, these spikes are transient and randomly shift between the hemispheres, only rarely occurring bilaterally and synchronously. They occur most often during early and middle Stage II sleep and disappear during deeper stages of sleep. On occasion, within one spindle burst, spindling will commence with fairly smooth spindle waves, each wave becoming successively sharper, so that toward the end of the spindle burst, the waves are sharp and high voltage with one or two spike discharges appearing within the terminal portion of the spindle burst. Careful localizing techniques using reference methods, transverse linked bipolar series, anteroposterior linked bipolar series, and combinations of these methods reveal that spike discharges associated with spindles are a product of the high parasaggital region, have the same scalp locus as spindles, and in all ways appear to be part of the spindle-physiology.

SPINDLE-K-COMPLEX INTERRELATIONSHIPS

Within a single EEG the interrelationships of timing and scalp distribution of K-complexes and sleep spindles have a definable developmental course. At approximately age three years and then again after adolescence, spindle bursts usually are primarily localized to the anterior vertex region and tend to follow directly upon a K-complex episode. K-complexes are usually dominant in the posterior vertex (or parasaggital) region. This development is less evident under age 1.5 years than between two and three years. Between ages three and nine years, most often between five and seven years, increasing numbers of spindle and K-complex combinations occur at the same or almost the same point in time so that with montages which supply poor topographical differentiation around the vertex, spindles and K-complexes appear to override and intermingle with one another. Exploration of scalp distribution suggests that at this time spindle episodes are more dominant near the true vertex rather than anterior vertex, while K-complexes also tend to be more dominant near the true vertex rather than posterior vertex. It is apparent, therefore, that not only do K-complexes and spindles tend to occur simultaneously in time at this age, but also manifest themselves in the same scalp regions; this was not the case previously. In the descriptive sense, this temporal and topographic overlap of K-complexes and spindles produces sleep pattern episodes which may appear to take the form of overlapping and intermingled K-complexes and sleep spindles. After age nine years this temporal and topographic overlap of spindles and K-complexes gradually abates. The EEG returns to the more differentiated K-complex-spindle relationship which was also evident at age three years before these temporary distortions took place.

Sharp Waves and Spikes in the K-Complexes

Between ages four and seven years it is common for K-complexes to contain intermingled, superimposed sharp, and/or spike discharges. These discharges are not part of a normal K-complex configuration; they represent an intrusion of waveforms which are an addition to the normally expected biphasic and triphasic K-complex morphology. The spikes may be small, or large and prominent. The vertex spike discharges associated with K-complexes, usually are not persistently lateralizing, but show random shifting between the hemispheres and are rarely seen at independent lateral electrodes. The spikes may appear during any portion of the K-complex. Most of these transient vertex discharges are true spikes, but many are properly defined as sharp waves. K-complexes containing spike discharges are not in themselves morphologically unique, but assume any of the forms found during normal K-complex ontogenesis at the age in question. The timecourse for the development of these disturbances is such that when they first take place, usually between four and five years, only a few of the K-complexes in an EEG contain spikes or sharp waves. However, one year later there may be many such spike-containing K-complexes. The duration of this disturbance is variable, ranging from one to four years.

DISTORTED SLEEP PATTERNS

Thus, it is evident that a number of variants of spindle and K-complex morphology can be individually differentiated. *"Distorted sleep patterns"* is our designation for patterned combinations of two or more of these components, such as repetitive K-complexes combined with random spikes and sharp spindles. Some distorted sleep patterns are restricted to the vertex regions and clearly represent minor, recognizable deviations from ideal expectable vertex sleep activity. Other distorted patterns involve so many deviant elements simultaneously (including abrupt spread to lateral regions) as to strongly resemble "epileptiform" discharges. Our purpose here is to describe these distorted patterns in some detail and to discuss the differentiation from abnormal patterns as well as to discuss some matters of technique to help in this differentiation.

Minimal distortions deviate only slightly from expectable vertex patterns, and contain sharp repetitive irregular K-complexes combined with sharp intermediate and high voltage spindles. The spindles may co-mingle with the repetitive K-complexes and/or may override terminal portions of the K-complexes and extend past the end of the K-complex. More marked distortions in approximate order of increasing "severity" (with no imputation of "abnormality") are as follows:

(1) Sharp, repetitive K-complexes and sharp spindles with the addition of occasional, random spikes within the K-complexes.

(2) Activity similar to above with the added factor of spread of the discharge to lateral regions. This spread involves only the distorted K-complex activity and does not in this instance include the intermingled spikes and spindles which remain limited to high central regions.

(3) Activity similar to (1) and (2) above with the addition of variable frequency, high voltage, spikey spindling rather than the more regular, intermediate voltage, sharp spindles of previous categories. These patterns often appear as extreme and possibly "epileptiform" because of the plethora of spike-like spindles which, although limited to the vertex, interfere seriously with most other aspects of the K-complex and spindle morphology. If lateral "spread" of the K-complex activity also occurs, these patterns begin to resemble EEG pathology by adult standards.

(4) Patterns similar to (3) with the addition of increased numbers of random spikes not only as part of the K-complex discharge, but also as isolated discharges within the episodes of spindling.

(5) Patterns similar to the above, but also spreading to distant (fronto-temporal and temporo-occipital) scalp regions and including occa-

sional lateralizing spikes in frontotemporal and temporotemporal derivations.

(6) Sometimes the above distorted patterns (especially [4] and [5]) spread so abruptly as to appear virtually simultaneously in all scalp regions, rather than occurring first at the vertex and a little later in temporal regions. Differentiation of such distorted, abruptly spreading, spike-containing discharges from patterns with "epileptic connotation" becomes difficult and sometimes impossible on EEG grounds alone.

Once the more "severe" distortions develop in the EEG, all the "lesser" distortions are usually found in the same record. Distorted patterns occur most often during early Stage II sleep and progressively less often during deep Stage II and Stage III and IV sleep.

How may these "abnormal appearing" EEG patterns, so common in normal children, be differentiated from patterns with true pathological implications? It should be remembered at this point, that our clinical database is such that we know that we are dealing with a clinically "normal," asymptomatic population. Our subjects were asymptomatic throughout this longitudinal study (birth to age 10-15 years in each case). All subjects were seen several times a year for history, physical examinations, etc. EEGs were done once or twice a year on each child. Subjects were enrolled in the study by virtue of parents volunteering prior to the second trimester of pregnancy.

Morphology

This is a critical differentiating factor. Some of these patterns, although possibly similar to atypical spike and slow bursts, are readily differentiated because of their morphological similarity to normal vertex sleep patterns. Thus, the slow waves are highly irregular in form and voltage in all regions within a burst and from burst to burst. Spikes included in the slow waves are equally variable and unpredictable for this spike and slow relationship.

Temporal

In general, distorted discharges can be seen to occur first at the vertex and secondarily elsewhere. Abrupt and "synchronous paroxysmal" onset and termination of generalized polysharp and slow bursts without vertex primacy in time or voltage was rare and is, therefore, a minor suspicious finding. Discharges of this sort are common in our normal group; they generally can be demonstrated to share enough features in common with lesser distorted patterns to be unequivocally placed in the normal category.

Topographic

This refers to involvement of distant scalp regions in the variable polysharp and slow bursts. Assuming virtually simultaneous and synchronous onset and termination of such a burst as in "Temporal," above, the bursts most resemble "true normal distortions" when the vertex recording is clearly higher voltage and morphologically different (i.e. more and better developed sharp waves) from the distant recording discharge.

Conditions Prevailing for Abnormal Bursts

Bursts continue to tend further away from clear normality when the following series of conditions prevail additively in order of their ranking:

(1) Involvement of anterior temporal electrodes.
(2) Involvement of frontal-polar electrodes.
(3) Involvement of occipital electrodes.

Thus, a burst involving only vertex and midtemporal regions will be more acceptable than a similar burst with simultaneous involvement of frontal-pole, temporal, occipital, and vertex electrodes. Following this, other criteria, such as age, morphology, etc. would contribute to final judgement.

Loss of vertex voltage dominance, vertex morphology-dominance, and vertex temporal dominance results in patterns more closely resembling "traditional" epileptiform discharge. Their probability for normality is thus reduced.

Duration

Generally, "normal distorted sleep patterns" are of brief duration, usually no longer than two seconds. As noted earlier, the most minimal distortions are vertex dominant in time and morphology. As the duration of a discharge increases, its probability for being within the normal range of variation decreases. Thus, discharges regardless of vertex dominance or morphology, if persisting for more than five or six seconds, pass the point of being readily acceptable. Usually, distorted discharges of over five seconds unbroken duration also have further deviant characteristics so that judgement about them is made easier because of the presence of abruptness, atypical spike and slow wave morphology, etc.

It should be emphasized that these "severe," virtually "epileptiform," long duration distortions are seen in a few of our normal cases and that occurrence of such discharges is not alone sufficient evidence to judge an EEG to be abnormal.

Ontogenic Factors

Distorted patterns of any sort, whether minimal or severe, are extremely rare under age two years. The younger the child who shows such distortions, the more likely he is to represent significant central nervous system pathology. Weight is added to this judgement by virtue of the fact that one child in our normal series who showed such distortions under age two years ultimately developed epilepsy (at age 4.5 years). Furthermore, it is our experience that children with phenylketonuria and prematurely born infants tend to have distorted sleep patterns under the age of two years. The most common EEG disturbance associated with phenylketonuria and with premature birth is the early onset of distorted sleep patterns and their long persistence. Distorted patterns have their own natural developmental course tending to be first seen at around the age of three years and then occurring more commonly through approximately the age of seven years, after which their incidence decreases. The incidence of distorted patterns drops precipitously with the first onset of puberty (often associated with a spurt in alpha development) and is rarely seen after adolescence is under way. The oldest normal children in whom distorted sleep patterns were seen were two children, one of them age thirteen and the other age fourteen; all others stopped showing distorted patterns by the age of eleven years.

Sleep Stage

In general, distorted patterns are most often seen in early Stage II and mid Stage II sleep. They are occasionally seen in Stage III or Stage IV sleep, but this is so rare as to be considered in itself deviant and suspicious. Still further from normal is the occurrence of deviant vertex discharges or distorted patterns during Stage I sleep. This is a difficult judgement to make inasmuch as the occurrence of any K-complex combination during Stage I may force the judgement that this is now early Stage II sleep. However, it is usually possible to make a reliable sleep-stage judgement. When these severe distortions occur in what is otherwise unbroken Stage I sleep, this is considered a maximum sleep stage deviation seen extremely rarely in our normal group.

Lack of Precedence or Predictability

The general background of an EEG lends some predictability and/or expectation to the EEG evaluation. One is never surprised to see one or more types of distortions in an EEG when most of the sleep patterns are distorted. However, by an "unprecedented" distorted discharge, we mean the occurrence of distorted sleep discharges (usually of one of the more severely deviant varieties) in a record where all sleep patterns are otherwise smooth, regular, and very normal and mature. Severe distortion within the context of an otherwise very unremarkable EEG has never been seen in our normal group and therefore would strongly suggest underlying pathology. Patterns of this sort are commonly seen in children with significant clinical complaints and was one of the outstanding features of the one child in our series to develop epilepsy.

More "Classical" Epileptiform Discharges

As sleep discharges show a closer and closer approach to the more typical "epileptiform" patterns, particularly spike and slow bursts with minimal morphological variability, the judgement regarding normality decreases sharply. Ultimately, regular, synchronous, relatively invariant spike and slow discharges, whether vertex dominant or not, would be judged abnormal. This would be further strengthened if the discharges are in the 3/sec range. Thus morphology becomes the ultimate critical criterion in evaluating this trend away from normality.

We believe that it is important for clinicians and investigators to recognize the normal occurrence of a high incidence of deviant sleep EEGs in children between the ages of three and nine years. We have shown that many of these deviations ("epileptiform" by adult standards) are within the normal range of variation for children. We have furthermore indicated how these distorted patterns can usually be differentiated from abnormal patterns.

Appropriate EEG technique is very helpful in establishing such differentiations. Briefly, a combination of standard bipolar and reference linkages are quite helpful. If reference montages (particularly ear or vertex references) are used exclusively during sleep, distorted vertex patterns are given a more abrupt, generally paroxysmal appearance and tend to resemble more closely spike and slow wave bursts. Also, a parasaggital, linked bipolar-series tends to emphasize vertex activity, again tending to lend the EEG a paroxysmal appearance when distorted discharges are present. It is helpful during Stage II sleep in children to use some type of montage which does not "contaminate" distant scalp regions with vertex activity and permits activity at lateral, posterior and frontal polar regions to be clearly differentiated from activity originating at the vertex. Several "standard" montages commonly used in EEG laboratories are useful for these differentiations. At the very least, some variant of the "Queens Square" or "Temporal Ring" montage associated with independent high central recording is useful. One such montage (for an 8-channel recording) is indicated here. There is no problem in arranging analogous and better montages for a 16-channel instrument.

Channel No.—	1	2	3	4	5	6	7	8
Electrodes—	F_{p2}-F_8;	T_6-O_2;	F_{p1}-F_7;	T_5-O_1;	F_4-C_4;	F_3-C_3;	F_4-F_3;	P_4-P_3

These findings emphasize the extreme caution which must be used in interpreting apparently abnormal children's EEGs. This is particularly important because deviant but normal EEGs occur with maximal frequency during an age period when children "normally" have an increase of a variety of complaints unrelated to EEG findings. These include learning disturbances, abdominal pain, dizzy episodes, severe headaches, behavior disorders, and fainting spells. Discovery of EEG disturbances of these types (distorted sleep patterns) in association with a clinical suspicion of "minimal brain disturbance" does not suffice for a diagnosis of central nervous system disturbance. Additionally, 6 and 14/sec positive spikes also occur during this age period, generally coincident with the occurrence of the previously described deviant patterns. Again, similar caution is advised. Six and 14/sec positive spikes as well as the deviant sleep patterns show no association with clinical symptoms. It may be that the most extreme distortions and/or the presence of numerous, high amplitude 6 and 14/sec positive spikes connotes a different physiological and clinical situation. Further careful work with clinically normal and deviant children is required to clarify this issue. We do suspect that further investigation will reveal a group of children whose deviant EEGs show quantitative or qualitative features that do bear a meaningful relationship to borderline organic CNS dysfunction. To date, however, despite these strong suspicions, the burden of proof must be on the claim that deviant EEG findings in the three to nine year age group represent abnormality. In other words, such EEGs must be considered to be within the broad range of normal variation unless clearly and firmly proven otherwise by rigorous clinical, historical, and physiological criteria. It should furthermore be emphasized that the alleviations of symptoms with potent psychotropic or anticonvulsant medication, such as phenothiazines or diphenylhydantoin, is *not a diagnostic test*. These medications can have a significant impact on many serious symptoms and signs of behavioral, cognitive, or physiological dysfunctions in the absence of specific CNS involvement. We do not suggest *against* the exhibition of useful medication, but rather, make a plea for the intelligent, rational use of potent medications without making this part of a diagnostic test in an area of incomplete and inadequate knowledge. Lastly, we again caution clinicians against attributing a diagnosis of epilepsy or nonspecific organic brain dysfunction to children who present with "peculiar" and "possibly epileptiform" EEGs in conjunction with a clinical picture "suggestive" of CNS dysfunction. In this age group it is more likely that one is dealing with a series of normal developmental variants which will disappear (as will possible associated symptoms) after age twelve or thirteen years.

REFERENCES

1. Berger, H.: On the electroencephalogram of man. In Berger, H.: *The Electroencephalogram of Man*. Translated and edited by Gloor, P.: *Electroenceph Clin Neurophysiol, Suppl. 28*, 1969.
2. Dreyfus-Brisac, C.: The bioelectric development of the central nervous system during early life. In Falkner, F. (Ed.) : *Human Development*. Philadelphia, Saunders, 1966.

3. Emde, R. N. and Metcalf, D. R.: An electroencephalographic study of behavioral rapid eye movement states in the human newborn. *J Nerv Ment Dis, 150*:376-386, 1970.

4. Emde, R. N., Harmon, R. J., Metcalf, D. R., Koenig, K. L., and Wagonfeld, S.: Stress and neonatal sleep. *Psychophysiology* (in press).

5. Gibbs, E. L., and Gibbs, F. A.: Extreme spindles: Correlation of electroencephalographic sleep pattern with mental retardation. *Science, 138*:1106-1107, 1962.

6. Lenard, H. G.: The development of sleep spindles in the EEG during the first two years of life. *Neuropadiatrie, 1*:204-276, 1970.

7. Metcalf, D. R.: EEG sleep spindle ontogenesis. *Neuropadiatrie, 1*:428-433, 1970.

8. Metcalf, D. R. and Emde, R. N.: Ontogenesis of sleep in early human infancy. *Psychophysiology, 6*:264, 1969.

9. Metcalf, D. R., Mondale, J., and Butler, F. K.: Ontogenesis of spontaneous K-complexes. *Psychophysiology* (in press).

10. Monod, N., Dreyfus-Brisac, C., Morel-Kahn, F., Pajot, N., and Plassart, E.: Les premières étapes de l'organization du sommeil chez le prématuré et le nouveau-né. *Rev Neurol, 110*:304-305.

11. Parmelee, A. H., Jr., Schulte, F. J., Akiyama, Y., Wenner, W. H., Schultz, M. A., and Stern, E.: Maturation of EEG activity during sleep in premature infants. *Electroenceph Clin Neurophysiol, 24*:319-329, 1968.

Chapter 9

Quantitative Pharmaco-Electroencephalography Using Frequency Analyzer and Digital Computer Methods in Early Drug Evaluations*

T. M. ITIL, F. GÜVEN‡, R. CORA†, W. HSU, N. POLVAN,
A. ÜÇOK†, A. SANSEIGNE, AND G. A. ULETT

Eighteen years after the introduction of chlorpromazine, the first major tranquilizer, marking the beginning of the era of classical psychopharmacology, there is still no useful scientific approach for assessing new psychotropic drugs. Knowledge of the chemical structure, animal pharmacology, and physiology may be of benefit in predicting its effect, but the final evaluation of a compound remains largely in the hands of the clinicians. Even in recent years, many important psychotropic drugs have been discovered by accident in clinical practice.

Since the recording of bioelectrical potentials by means of the electroencephalogram is the only method by which we can obtain continuous information about cerebral function and since behavioral changes are related to changes in brain function, it would appear that the application of electroencephalographic techniques in the study of psychotropic drugs offers the greatest potential. After studying hundreds of compounds using conventional visual evaluation of EEG records, we demonstrated that any drug which affects behavior also produces changes in the scalp-recorded EEG. The quality and quantity of these changes are dependent upon the type of drug, the dosage, the route and rate of administration, and the subject's predrug EEG pattern. Since intraindividual and interindividual variability of the resting EEG pattern interferes significantly with the drug effect, we investigated different drugs in the same group of subjects using standard dosages, routes, and rates of administration. Based on this study of up to twenty-eight phenothiazines, we defined several EEG reaction types which characterize phenothiazines with similar chemical structures and pharmacological and clinical effects (Itil, 1961).

Strong "anticholinergic" phenothiazines produce a decrease of alpha waves, increase of fast as well as some slow waves, decrease of amplitude,

*Supported, in part, by the Psychiatric Research Foundation of Missouri and E. R. Squibb and Sons.
†Involved only in SQ 11, 290 investigation.
‡Involved only in chlorazepam investigation.

and increase of desynchronization in EEGs with alpha dominance. Since these kinds of changes were most characteristic of promethazine, we called this type of drug-induced EEG syndrome the "promethazine reaction type" (Fig. 9-1.) Drugs producing these types of EEG alterations have some sedative effect and may be effective in treating agitation and depressive mood, but they are not effective in controlling psychotic symptomatology, particularly in schizophrenic patients.

RESTING EEG

	Stage I	Stage II	Stage III (sleeplike state)
Promethazine type	with Promethazine (0.7 mg/kg)		
Chlorpromazine type	with Chlorpromazine (0.7 mg/kg)		
Piperazine type	with Butaperazine (0.7 mg/kg)		

St. M. 39 years old
Diagnosis: neurotic reaction

T. Itil   med. exp. 5, 347 (1961)

MIP/241

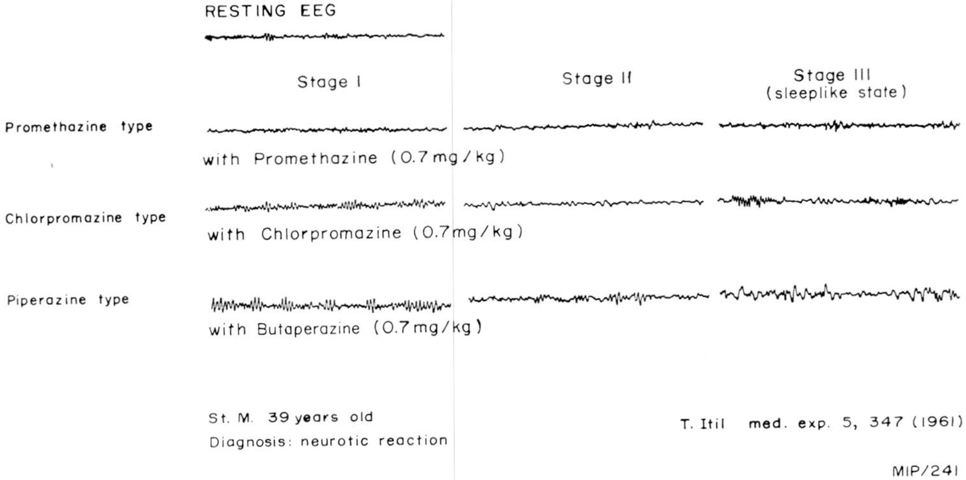

Figure 9-1. Types of EEG reactions with phenothiazine derivatives. Promethazine (given over 10 min, i.v.) induces first a decrease of alpha activity (Stage I), later an increase of low-voltage slow waves (Stage II), and finally sleeplike EEG patterns with slow waves and fast spindle activity (Stage III). Despite slow activity, fast beta waves are present. After chlorpromazine there is first an increase in alpha activity, then marked slowing, and finally slow waves and spindle activity are seen, also increased synchronization and rhythmic activity. After butaperazine, there is a marked increase of rhythmical, slow alpha activity followed by high-voltage slow waves. Marked rhythmic activity and high-voltage slow waves appear with less spindle patterns during sleeplike states.

Phenothiazines with aliphatic and piperidyl side chains induced slow waves with an increase of amplitude, an increase of synchronization and rhythmical tendency, and an increase of sleep-like patterns in the EEG. Since chlorpromazine systematically produced these changes, we called this EEG syndrome the "chlorpromazine reaction type." Clinically, phenothiazines which produce this reaction type have a sedative effect and are effective in treating agitation, anxiety, and also psychotic symptoms of both depressive and schizophrenic patients. In high dosages they produce a "parkinson-like" syndrome in man.

EEGs following the administration of phenothiazines with a piperazine side chain showed a marked increase in the percentage of alpha activity with synchronization and a rhythmical tendency, and an increase of amplitude. In high dosages they may produce slow waves, but in low dosages they induce superimposed fast activity. These drugs have a predominant effect in the treatment of a "typical" florid schizophrenic symptomatology involving thought disorders, perceptual distortions, and delusions. They induce extrapyramidal side effects, predominantly of a hyperkinetic-hypertonic type, such as akathesia, restlessness, and dyskinesia.

We observed that some of the anticholinergic phenothiazines, as well as nonphenothiazine compounds, produce another EEG syndrome: an increase of slow as well as fast activity, a decrease of rhythmical pattern, and a decrease of amplitude, all associated with an increase or decrease of alpha waves. Since most of the compounds eliciting these EEG changes are effective in the treatment of the typical depressive mood, we designated this EEG syndrome the "thymoleptic reaction type." In recent years we have added three more reaction types to the EEG classification of psychotropic drugs (Itil, 1968) :

(1) All compounds which produce hallucinations without altering consciousness decrease the percentage of alpha activity, produce desynchronization, decrease amplitudes, accelerate background activity, and frequently increase fast waves. We called this EEG syndrome the "hallucinogenic reaction type."

(2) Drugs which produce a confusional-delirious syndrome decrease the percentage of alpha activity, decrease the rhythmical pattern, increase amplitudes, and increase very slow and very fast activity with labile amplitude and frequency. Since the basic representatives of this EEG syndrome are anticholinergic hallucinogens, we called this EEG syndrome the "anticholinergic reaction type." The EEG profile of this group of drugs is similar to the "promethazine reaction type" and "thymoleptic reaction type" EEG changes.

(3) After establishing that all of the available minor tranquilizing compounds decrease alpha waves and produce fast spindle activity (highly rhythmical waves with stable frequency and amplitude), predominantly in the anterior area, we called this the "minor tranquilizer reaction type."

The EEG classification of drugs, which was developed by "classical" visual evaluation of records, did not receive general acceptance. Considering the fact that the scalp-recorded EEG represents only a small part of the total bioelectrical activity of the brain and that psychotropic drugs or their metabolites are present in very minimal amounts in the brain, it is difficult to believe that drugs produce any systematic changes in brain function which could be detected in the scalp-recorded EEG, much less which could be called "specific" for a particular drug or group of drugs. The necessity of developing objective methods for the study of drug-induced EEG changes was obvious.

In recent years we have systematically applied quantitative analysis and statistical methods in our resting and all-night sleep EEG investigations. We have been able to differentiate the changes induced by the main representatives of the three EEG reaction types (chlorpromazine, thymoleptic, and minor tranquilizers) from both saline and from one another using analog frequency analyzer and digital computer period analysis (Figs. 9-2, 9-3, 9-4, 9-5) (Itil *et al.*, 1968a, 1969a). The resting and sleep EEG profiles of various compounds, including trifluperidol (Itil and Fink, 1969), haloperidol (Itil *et al.*, 1970), thiothixene (Itil *et al.*, 1969b), fluphenazine (Heinemann and Itil, 1970; Itil *et al.*, 1969b), molindone (Itil *et al.*, in press a), cinanserin (Itil *et al.*, 1971), pinoxepine and perphenazine (Holden

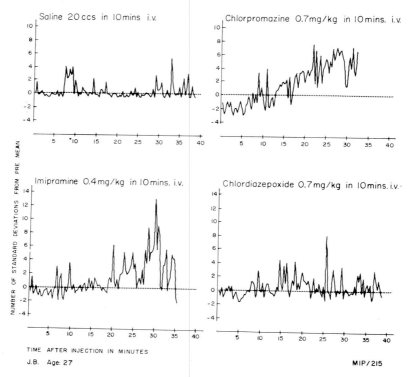

Figure 9-2. EEG drug-response curves based on period analysis baseline cross-frequency band 0-3 cps. Increase of 0-3 cps activity after chlorpromazine and imipramine. (Itil, T. M. *et al.: The Psychopharmacology of the Normal Human.* Springfield, Thomas, 1969, pp. 219-237.)

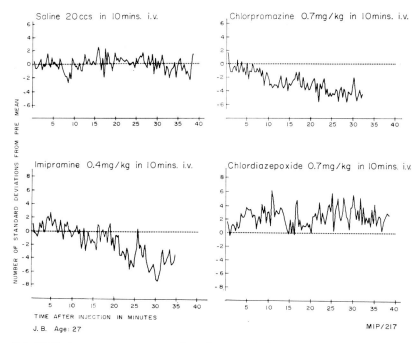

Figure 9-3. EEG drug-response curves based on period analysis baseline cross-frequency band 16-26 cps. Decreases in 16-26 cps activity after chlorpromazine and imipramine, but increases after chlordiazepoxide. (Itil, T. M. *et al.: Psychopharmacology of the Normal Human.* Springfield, Thomas, 1969, pp. 219-237.)

et al., 1969), metronidazole (Itil *et al.,* 1968b), cycloserine (Simeon *et al.,* 1970), cyclazocine (Fink *et al.,* 1969), fluphenazine enanthate and decanoate, (Itil *et al.,* in press b), and combined drugs, such as Dilantin and thioridazine (Itil *et al.,* 1967a), thioridazine and chlordiazepoxide (Itil *et al.,* 1967b), and chlorpromazine and Quide (Holden *et al.,* 1970), have been studied using quantitative EEG analysis. Recently we developed a method for determining qualitatively and quantitatively the central effects of drugs based on EEG drug profiles, which established effective dosage ranges after oral administration of single doses, based on drug response curves using analog frequency analyzer and digital computer EEG analysis and statistical procedures. We called this method "quantitative pharmacoelectroencephalography."

Although in the past we had been able to correctly predict the clinical efficacy of a new compound based on the EEG alone (Bente and Itil, 1960; Flügel *et al.,* 1961; Itil, 1965; Fink *et al.,* 1970), these predictions failed to satisfy sufficiently the requirements of a scientific approach. The replication of these investigations was impossible, because of the absence of objective

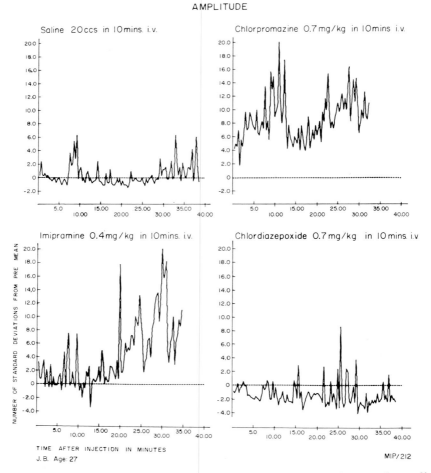

Figure 9-4. EEG drug-response curves based on period analysis. Increased amplitudes after chlorpromazine and imipramine (period analysis). Slight decrease of amplitudes after chlordiazepoxide. (Itil, T. M. *et al.: The Psychopharmacology of the Normal Human.* Springfield, Thomas, 1969, pp. 219-237.)

methods for evaluating the EEG and determining the clinical efficacy of the compound. Only recently, following development of objective methods with which to evaluate clinical and EEG findings, have we been able to carry out prospective studies to predict the clinical value of drugs based on the scalp-recorded human EEG alone.

To date we have completed two major studies:

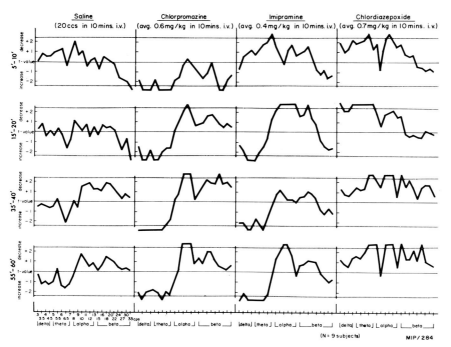

Figure 9-5. Pattern of differences between predrug and postdrug EEG power spectra. (Differences are in terms of t-values; dotted lines imply significance at .05 level or better.) In contrast to the predrug means in an average of nine investigations, there was no significant difference after saline injection in any of the frequency bands (except 33 cps) in any of the four time periods.

After administration of chlorpromazine, significant increases in theta and delta frequencies (compared to predrug means) appeared in all four time periods; at the same time, there was a significant decrease of alpha activity in three of the four time periods (15-20 min, 35-40 min, and 55-60 min).

After administration of imipramine, a significant increase of slow waves occurred during the second, third, and fourth time periods. There was also a significant increase in alpha activity during the second and fourth time periods (compared to predrug means).

After chlordiazepoxide, a decrease in theta and delta activity appears in all four time periods. There is also a decrease of alpha activity in time periods 3 and 4. (Itil, T. M. *et al.: Agressologie,* no. 2, pp. 267-280, 1968.

INVESTIGATIONS WITH SQ-11,290
Introduction

SQ-11,290 is a derivative of the dihydrodibenzoxazepine heterocycle and was chosen for this study because it belongs to a novel tricyclic group (Fig. 9-6). From animal pharmacology data, SQ-11,290 was predicted to be effective in anxiety syndromes, schizophrenic pathology, manic disorders, and agitated-depressive states. The single effective oral dosage range was estimated to be 5-1000 mg.

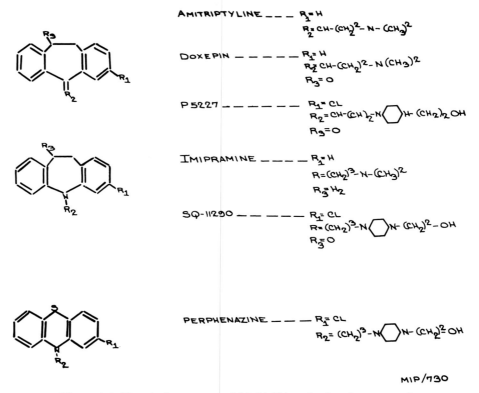

Figure 9-6. Chemical structure of SQ-11,290 and related compounds.

EEG Investigations

Single dose investigations with SQ-11,290 were carried out using quantitative electroencephalography.

Material and Method

Twelve male volunteers between the ages of twenty-one and thirty years were included in this study. Each volunteer was investigated on two different treatment days—one active medication day and one placebo day—approximately one week apart. Two patients received placebo on both treatment days, and the other ten were divided into five groups of two patients, each receiving 5 mg, 25 mg, 50 mg, 100 mg, or 200 mg of SQ-11,290 and placebo on the two respective days. The study was double-blind. EEG recordings were taken before and at the first, third, and sixth hours after drug administration. Several clinical assessments and rating scales were completed in the same time periods. In each EEG session a twenty-minute recording was taken for ten minutes during the resting period and for ten minutes while the patient's reaction time was tested. The reaction time measurements were included to maintain the vigilance of the patient at a certain level.

Results

In the dosage range of 5-200 mg (mean 76 mg) SQ-11,290, slow activity increased significantly (ANOV), and fast activity and alpha waves decreased, particularly three hours after administration (right occipital to right ear during resting EEG) (Fig. 9-7). The EEG profile of SQ-11,290, based on frequency analyzer data (Fig. 9-8) of change scores from predrug to postdrug, also showed an increase of slow waves and decrease of fast activity. These changes are significantly different from those produced by placebo.

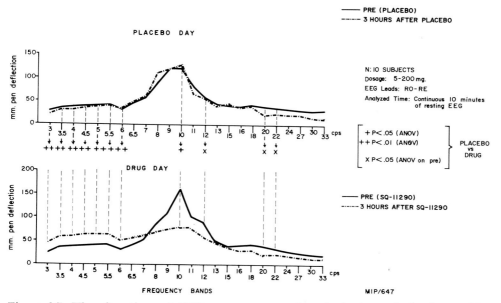

Figure 9-7. The alterations of EEG power spectra after single dose of placebo or SQ-11,290. Differences are in terms of t-values; dotted lines imply significance at .05 level.) In the abscissa frequency bands in the ordinate millimeter pen deflection. Before and three hours after placebo no marked differences were found in the analog power spectra. Three hours after SQ-11,290 however, in comparison to predrug an increase of power in the slow frequencies, decrease in alpha bands, and decrease in fast frequency bands. There were significant differences between placebo and SQ-11,290—induced changes.

Further analysis of the data demonstrated that the changes in the mean values of the computer EEG measurements became evident at a dosage level of 50 mg (during resting [Fig. 9-9] and reaction time EEGs). However, single doses of 100 or 200 mg produced little further change than the 50 mg dosage. Placebo-induced changes were very limited. (The detailed results will be reported elsewhere.)

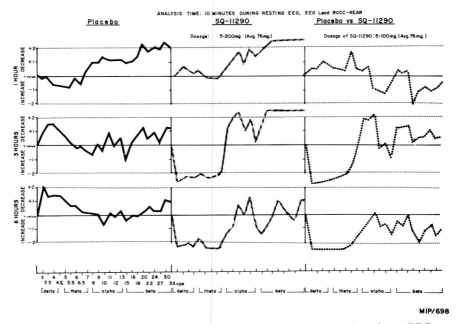

ANALYSIS TIME: 10 MINUTES DURING RESTING EEG, EEG Lead: ROCC-REAR

MIP/698

Figure 9-8. Pattern of differences between predrug and postdrug based on EEG power spectra. In the abscissa the frequency bands. In the ordinate changes from predrug (or placebo) at one, three, and six hours. After placebo only a few frequency bands showed significant changes (decrease of power in fast frequency bands during one hour, as well as decrease of 3 cps band during six hours after placebo administration). In contrast, after SQ-11,290 (average 7/6 mg) in all three time periods significant changes were observed. During the first and third hour a significant decrease in power in several fast frequency bands, and during the third and sixth hour an increase of power in several slow frequency bands were seen. An increase of power in slow frequencies was significantly different between placebo and SQ-11,290-induced changes.

Summary

The two types of quantitative analysis demonstrated that (a) SQ-11,290 produces significant changes in the EEG (increase of slow activity, decrease of alpha and fast waves) recorded from the right occipital lead, and these changes are significantly different from those produced by placebo; and that (b) the changes are similar to those seen with drugs which induce the "chlorpromazine reaction type" EEG syndrome (see Fig. 9-5). Consequently, we predicted that SQ 11,290 would have a clinical effect similar to chlorpromazine. The effective dosage based on the quantitative EEG starts at 50 mg single dose.

Clinical Investigations During Chronic Oral SQ-11,290 Treatment

Three separate studies were conducted to determine whether SQ-11,290 is a clinically effective drug. The first investigation studied the effect of SQ-

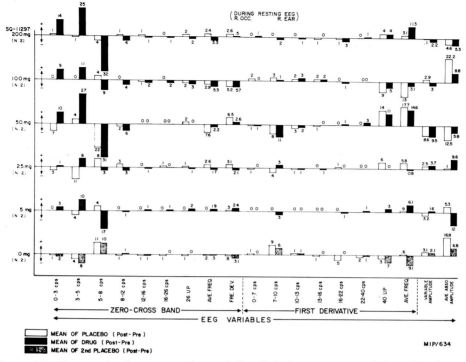

Figure 9-9. Changes in the mean values of the digital computer period analyzed EEG measurements of the different dosages of SQ-11,290 in comparison to placebo. In the abscissa EEG variables. After placebo (0 mg), 5 mg and 25 mg SQ-11,290 did not produce marked changes in any of the 19 EEG variables. After 50, 100, and 200 mg SQ-11,290 an increase of 0-3 cps and 3-5 cps activity and a decrease of 5-8 cps waves were seen.

11,290 on depressive patients with marked anxiety (12 subjects, 21-50 years of age); the second, the effect of SQ-11,290 on acute schizophrenic patients with anxiety (11 patients, age range 19-55); and the third, its effect on chronic schizophrenic patients with florid symptomatology (10 patients, age range 17-33 years). The length of treatment ranged from twenty-three to thirty-one days.

These studies were conducted by investigators who did not know the chemical structure, animal pharmacology, or possible EEG effects of SQ-11,290. They were told only that SQ-11,290 is presumably an antipsychotic drug and that they could start with 25 mg twice daily and go up to 1,000 mg daily. At the end of the study period, ten of the twelve depressive patients showed moderate to marked improvement; seven of the ten acute schizophrenics exhibited moderate to marked improvement, while only three of ten chronic schizophrenics showed moderate to marked improvement

(Table 9-I). The optimally effective doctor's choice average daily dosages for the respective groups were 106 mg for the depressive group of patients, 500 mg for acute schizophrenics, and 750 mg for the chronic schizophrenics.

TABLE 9-I

SUMMARY OF THE CLINICAL TRIALS
WITH SQ-11290

GROUPS	Sex M.	Sex F.	Age Range	Age Mean	Length of Illness Range	Length of Illness Mean	Length of last Hospitalization Range	Length of last Hospitalization Mean	Out-patient	SQ 11,290 TREATMENT Length of Treatment (Range)	SQ 11,290 TREATMENT Daily Dosage (Range)	SQ 11,290 TREATMENT Total Dosage (Range)	Outcome 0	Outcome +	Outcome ++	Outcome +++	Discharge D	Discharge SD	Discharge N	Dropped
GROUP I Endogenous and Reactive Depressives with Marked Anxiety N: 12	12		21 – 55 years	25.8 yrs.	4 – 416 weeks	131 weeks	4 – 35 days	21 days	2	31 – 34 days ***	25 – 600 mg. mean: 106.38 ***	2900 – 5600 mg. mean: 3559.09 ***	1	0	4	6	8*	0	1	1
GROUP II Acute Schizophrenics with Anxiety N: 11	10	1	19 – 55 years	24.7 yrs.	45 – 417 weeks	203 weeks	4 – 120 days	28 days	1	30 – 34 days	100 – 700 mg. mean: 500.27	12,300 – 19,100 mg. mean: 16,463.63	2	2	5	2	6*	3	1	0
GROUP III Chronic Schizophrenics with Florid Symptomatology N: 10	10		17 – 33 years	26 yrs.	5 – 624 weeks	203 weeks	4 – 2180 days	457 days	0	23 – 24 days ***	200 – 1000 mg. mean: 750.46 ***	16,000 – 17,400 mg. mean: 17,088.88 ***	1	5	2	2	1	1	6	1

```
   *   2 Outpatients started to work
  **   1 Outpatient started to work
 ***   These figures do not include the patients
       who were dropped from the study.
```

KEY:
0	= no improvement	D	= medically discharged
+	= slight improvement	SD	= socially discharged
++	= moderate improvement	N	= not dischargeable
+++	= marked improvement		

MIP/728

SQ-11,290 was significantly effective for many of the depressive symptoms (Table 9-II) but effective for only a few symptoms of the acute schizophrenics (Table 9-III) on the Brief Psychiatric Rating Scale (BPRS). Although some improvement was noticeable, none of the symptoms of the chronic schizophrenics (BPRS) improved during SQ-11,290 treatment at a level of statistical significance (Fig. 9-10).

Conclusion

The clinical trials with SQ-11,290 confirmed our prediction based on quantitative pharmacoelectroencephalography. It was demonstrated that SQ-11,290 is indeed a psychotropic drug which has a predominant effect on either depressive patients with anxiety or acute schizophrenics. The most effective dosage range for depressive patients was shown to be 50 mg twice daily. As predicted by quantitative electroencephalography, SQ-11,290 was also found to be clinically similar to chlorpromazine with a broad spectrum effect in psychiatric disorders. It also showed side effects similar to chlorpromazine, such as extrapyramidal symptoms (dystonic reactions), a sedative effect, hypotonic reactions, and increase of SGOT in the laboratory investigations. The electroencephalographical findings during chronic oral administration showed a very similar pattern to that seen after single

TABLE 9-II

CHANGES IN PSYCHIATRIC SYMPTOMS
(BPRS)
AT DIFFERENT DOSAGE LEVELS OF SQ-11,290 TREATMENT

GROUP II: (N:11) (Acute Schizophrenic Patients)

PERIODS COMPARISON / VARIABLES	PLACEBO					I				II			III	IV	
	1	2	3	4	5	2	3	4	5	3	4	5	4	5	5
1. Somatic Concern															
2. Anxiety															
3. Emotional Withdrawal			=	=	=		=	=	=						
4. Conceptual Disorganization															
5. Guilt Feelings															
6. Tension															
7. Mannerisms and Posturing															
8. Grandiosity															
9. Depressive Mood															
10. Hostility															
11. Suspiciousness															
12. Hallucinatory Behavior			=	=	=		=	=	=						
13. Motor Retardation															
14. Uncooperativeness															
15. Unusual Thought Content			=	=	=		=	=	=						
16. Blunted Affect				=					=						
17. Excitement															
18. Disorientation															

-: Decrease at the .05 level of significance (ANOV)
=: Decrease at the .01 level of significance

Period 0: Placebo
Period 1: 2-10 days (100-400 mg. AVE. 228.18 mg.)
Period 2: 10-14 days (400-600 mg. AVE. 563.63 mg.)
Period 3: 5-9 days (300-700 mg. AVE. 554.54 mg.)
Period 4: 4-6 days (300-700 mg. AVE. 545.45 mg.)
Period 5: 5-7 days (300-600 mg. AVE. 536.36 mg.)
            (Rating completed 1 - 2 days post drug.)

MIP/743

dosages, such as increase of slow activity, decrease of fast waves, and decrease of alpha activity, all at a level of statistical significance (ANOV). As does chlorpromazine, SQ-11,290 produced synchronization, rhythmical activity, and a significant increase of sharp waves and dysrhythmic groups in the EEG. (The detailed results will be reported elsewhere.)

INVESTIGATIONS WITH CHLORAZEPAM AND DIAZEPAM
Introduction

Based on our previous investigations, all presently available minor tranquilizers seem to produce typical alterations in the EEG, including an increase of rhythmical fast activity (in the frequency ranges of 16-40 cps),

TABLE 9-III

CHANGES IN PSYCHIATRIC SYMPTOMS
(BPRS)
AT DIFFERENT DOSAGE LEVELS OF SQ-11,290 TREATMENT

GROUP I: (N:12) (Depressive Patients with Anxiety Symptoms)

PERIODS COMPARISON / VARIABLES	PLACEBO					I				II			III		IV
	1	2	3	4	5	2	3	4	5	3	4	5	4	5	5
1. Somatic Concern				■	■	■	■	■							
2. Anxiety		■	■	■	■	■	■	■	■	■	■				
3. Emotional Withdrawal			■	■	■	■	■	■							
4. Conceptual Disorganization															
5. Guilt Feelings				-				-							
6. Tension		■	■	■		■	■	■							
7. Mannerisms and Posturing															
8. Grandiosity															
9. Depressive Mood		■	■	■	■	■	■	■	■	■	■				
10. Hostility															
11. Suspiciousness															
12. Hallucinatory Behavior															
13. Motor Retardation				■	■		■	■	■						
14. Uncooperativeness															
15. Unusual Thought Content															
16. Blunted Affect															
17. Excitement								-							
18. Disorientation															

-: Decrease at the .05 level of significance (ANOV)
■: Decrease at the .01 level of significance

Period 0:   Placebo
Period 1:   4 days (25-400 mg. AVE 116.66 mgs.)
Period 2:   8-14 days (100 mg. daily, AVE 100 mg.)
Period 3:   7-10 days (100-150 mg., AVE 104.54 mg.)
Period 4:   6-7 days (100 -150 mg., AVE 104.54 mg.)
Period 5:   4-7 days (100 mg., AVE 100 mg.)
          (Rating completed 1 - 2 days post drug.)

MIP/736

decrease of very slow delta waves and very fast activity (over 40 cps), decrease of alpha activity, increase of average absolute amplitude, and decrease of amplitude variability (Itil, 1968; Itil *et al.*, 1968). In the past two years we have tested the predictive value of quantitative pharmacoelectroencephalography for minor tranquilizers. We conducted various prospective studies with new drugs, which had never been tested before in man. One of these compounds was chlorazepam, which actually is not a new compound, but a chemical entity resulting from the reaction combination of diazepam and chloralhydrate in equimolecular proportions. The chloralhydrate element represents 36.8% of the molecular weight of this compound. Chlorazepam behaves qualitatively much like its diazepam moiety. On a milligram-to-milligram basis in animal studies chlorazepam was found to be more potent than diazepam.

GROUP 3 (N:10)

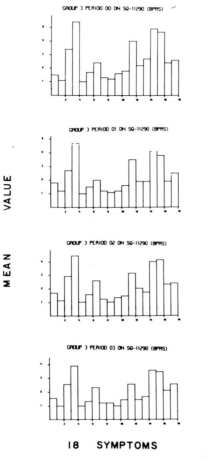

18 SYMPTOMS

MIP/760

Figure 9-10. Psychopathological changes during SQ-11,290 treatment (BPRS Rating). In the abscissa eighteen symptoms of BPRS rating. In the ordinate the mean values. Before SQ-11,290 treatment (00 Period) marked symptoms were seen. During the course of treatment, particularly at the end of the treatment (Period 03), symptoms were decreased. The improvement in none of the symptoms reached the level of statistical significance.

Single Dose EEG Investigations

Single dose investigations were carried out using quantitative electro-encephalography to answer the following questions:

(1) Does chlorazepam have any central effect?

(2) Does this effect have any similarity to diazepam?

(3) Are there any differences in the electroencephalographical effectiveness of equivalent doses of diazepam and chlorazepam?

(4) What is the effective dosage range of diazepam and chlorazepam?

Material and Method

Thirty-two female and male subjects in the age ranges of eighteen to fifty-four years with minor anxiety syndromes were included in this study. Before patients were included in this study, they had an adaptation EEG and, based on this EEG, subjects with abnormal EEGs were excluded from the study. Patients were randomly assigned to single oral doses of placebo, 1 mg, 2 mg, 5 mg, 10 mg, and 20 mg diazepam or chlorazepam. Each patient received these two compounds or placebo at weekly intervals. Clinical evaluations (rating scales, neurological examinations, and tests of the autonomic nervous system, such as blood pressure and pulse rate) and electroencephalographical recordings were carried out before, and one hour, three hours, and six hours after placebo or drug. The EEG recording ran from ten to twenty minutes (5-10 min during resting EEG, and 5-10 min during reaction time measurements). The right occipital to right ear lead, as well as the anterior vertex to right occipital lead, were recorded on tape and analyzed with a digital computer system (IBM 1710) using period analysis. The right occipital to right ear lead was also analyzed using an amplitude integrator (Drohocki method).

Results

Both diazepam and chlorazepam, given in single does of 1-20 mg (mean 6.4 mg), produced typical EEG changes in twenty-four subjects with an increase of fast activity, decrease of alpha and theta waves, and increase of average frequency and frequency variability (Fig. 9-11). The first hour recording after diazepam showed no significant changes in the right occipital to right ear lead during resting time. However, during the third and sixth hours after diazepam the EEG changes (increase of fast activity and decrease of slow waves [only in first derivative measurements]) were at a level of statistical significance (t-test). Chlorazepam (dosage range 1-20 mg, mean 6.4 mg) showed EEG profiles almost identical to diazepam in the same group of subjects. However, in contrast to diazepam, chlorazepam also produced significant changes the first hour after the drug. The differences between the EEG profiles of chlorazepam and diazepam appeared only in the 3-5 and 5-8 cps activity. which increased after chlorazepam but not at a level of statistical significance. In contrast to chlorazepam and diazepam, the placebo produced no significant changes in any of the nineteen computer EEG variables during any of the three time periods. Analysis of the data during reaction time measurements, including the right occipital to anterior vertex recordings,

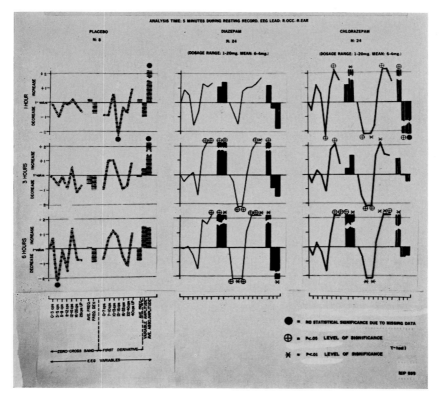

Figure 9-11. Pattern of differences between predrug and postdrug based on digital computer period analysis. (Differences are in terms of t-values; dotted lines imply significance at .05 level.) In the abscissa EEG variables of the period analysis. In the ordinate differences from predrug (or placebo) recordings and EEGs at different time periods. After placebo, in none of the time periods, none of the EEG variables showed significant changes. After diazepam (average 6.4 mg) during the third and sixth hour recording, a significant increase of fast frequencies and a decrease of slow frequencies (the latter only in first derivative measurements) were seen. After diazepam, in all, first, third, and sixth hour recordings, significant changes were observed, which included increase of fast and decrease of slow activity (the latter only in first derivative measurements) were observed. In contrast to diazepam, chlorazepam (in the same dosage range of 6.4 mg mean) produces significant changes also during the first hour recordings (note the very similar profiles of diazepam and chlorazepam-induced changes, particularly during the third and sixth hour recordings) .

demonstrated practically the same results. Simple regression analysis revealed no significant differences between diazepam and chlorazepam at any time; however, discriminant function analysis showed differences between the two drugs in various frequency bands at various time periods. These suggest that chlorazepam has a greater effect on the EEG in the initial time period than diazepam, including slight differences in quality (increase of

slow waves). However, during the third and sixth hours, changes induced
by chlorazepam seem to be almost identical to diazepam induced changes,
but much fewer in quantity. The evaluation of the EEG data following
different dosages demonstrated that during the first hour after drugs, 1 and
2 mg dosages produced very few changes, however more than did placebo.
In 5 and 20 mg dosages, chlorazepam and diazepam produced similar
changes (although alpha activity increased after diazepam, but decreased
after chlorazepam and average absolute amplitude and amplitude variability
showed reversed changes), while after 10 mg the EEG changes were different than at the other dosages (almost all patients exhibited a sleep pattern
with this dosage and probably these interfered with typical diazepam-in-
duced EEG changes). During the third hour even 1 mg of diazepam and
chlorazepam produced greater changes than placebo (Fig. 9-12). Again,

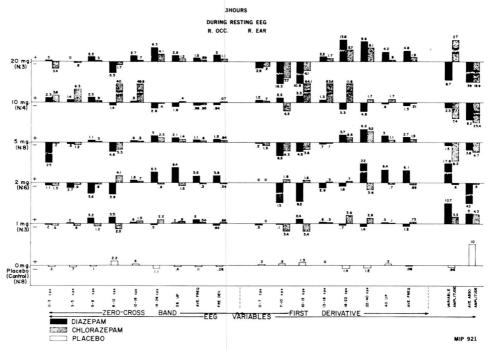

Figure 9-12. Changes in the mean values of the digital computer period analyzed EEG
measurements of the different dosage of diazepam in comparison to chlorazepam. In
the abscissa period analysis EEG variables. In the ordinate changes from predrug (or
placebo) mean values. Three hours after placebo very little EEG changes were observed (except average absolute amplitude). After 1, 2, 5, but particularly 10 and 20
mg, chlorazepam and diazepam produced marked EEG changes in several EEG variables.
Basically, both drugs produce more fast activity, equally slow waves, and decrease average
absolute amplitude. It is interesting that 2 mg diazepam and chlorazepam produce
changes in more EEG variables than with 5 mg of the two drugs.

except after 10 mg, the EEG changes in all dosage groups were similar. However, at the third hour the changes after 2 mg were as great as the changes after 20 mg. Six hours after drug administration, EEG changes could be observed in all dosage ranges, and they were still more marked than placebo (still different changes after 10 mg). Statistical analysis of the data, using analysis of variance, demonstrated that the higher the dosage range the greater the number of EEG variables which changed at a level of statistical significance. (The detailed results of the study will be reported elsewhere.)

Summary

Based on the quantitatively analyzed EEG, it was demonstrated that chlorazepam indeed has a significant central effect. The types of chlorazepam-induced changes are almost identical to those produced by diazepam. Chlorazepam differs from diazepam only during the first hour recording. In this time period chlorazepam produces more EEG changes. Later, diazepam induces more frequency significant EEG alterations. The effective doses of chlorazepam seem to be 1 mg (3rd hour) and 5 mg (1st hour) which is very similar to diazepam.

Clinical Investigations During Chronic Oral Treatment of Diazepam and Chlorazepam

To test our EEG predictions, a double-blind clinical study was carried out with diazepam and chlorazepam in a group of outpatients suffering from anxiety. Forty-six male and female patients with an age range of seventeen to fifty-five years were randomly assigned to diazepam (24) or chlorazepam (22). A doctor's choice dosage was given, with a starting dosage of two tablets (each tablet equals 2 mg diazepam or chlorazepam) and a maximum of 18 mg (9 × 2 mg tablets). Patients were evaluated clinically before and during the first, second and fourth week of treatment (global evaluation, psychiatric, and side effects rating scales). During the same time periods, the EEG recordings were done and the records were analyzed visually and with digital computer period analysis.

Results

After diazepam (24 patients completed the study), two patients did not show any improvement; three patients showed slight, six patients showed moderate, and thirteen patients showed marked improvement. After chlorazepam one patient showed no improvement; two patients showed slight, six patients showed moderate, and thirteen patients showed marked improvement. Statistical analysis revealed no differences in the effects of diazepam and chlorazepam. These clinical results, however, were obtained with a smaller total dosage (5198 mg versus 6144 mg), as well as with a smaller daily dosage of chlorazepam (average dose of 8 mg chlorazepam and 9 mg diazepam daily). Because chlorazepam consists of 64 percent diazepam, and the average daily dosage of chlorazepam was 9 percent less than diazepam, it is obvious that approximately 45 percent less diazepam in combination (chlorazepam) was enough for a clinical effect similar to diazepam alone. Statistical analysis of the data based on BPRS and NOSIE rating scales showed that more symptoms improved with chlorazepam than diazepam. (The data will be reported in detail elsewhere.)

Conclusion

This clinical study again confirms predictions based on quantitative pharmacoelectroencephalography. Apparently the potentiation of the effects of diazepam by very small doses of chloralhydrate in chlorazepam during the first hour after single dosages did have a clinical impact on the treatment of anxiety syndromes. To achieve the same or greater therapeutic benefits, patients needed smaller amounts of diazepam when this compound was combined with chloralhydrate in chlorazepam.

The clinical application of pharmacoelectroencephalography was successful with these two drugs. By means of on-going studies with several new compounds we hope, in the future, to demonstrate the significance and limitations of this method in psychopharmacological research and clinical practice.

Summary

Using analog frequency analysis, digital computer period analysis, and statistical methods, the EEG effects of two new compounds were studied. Based on this so-called quantitative pharmacoelectroencephalography, the type, dosage, and onset of the clinical effects of these compounds were predicted. Subsequent, clinical trials confirmed the value of quantitative pharmacoelectroencephalography in the very early evaluation of psychotropic compounds.

REFERENCES

1. Bente, D., and Itil, T. M.: EEG-Veränderungen unter chronischer Medicarion von Piperazinyl-Phenothiazin-Derivaten. *Med exp*, 2:132-137, 1960.
2. Fink, M., Itil, T. M., Zaks, A., and Freedman, A. M.: EEG patterns of cyclazocine, a narcotic antagonist. In Koella, W., and Karczmar, A. (Eds.): *Neurophysiological and Behavioral Aspects of Psychotropic Drugs.* Springfield, Thomas, 1969, pp. 62-71.
3. Fink, M., Simeon, J., Itil, T. M., and Freedman, A. M.: Clinical antidepressant activity of cyclazocine-A narcotic antagonist. *Clin Pharmacol Ther*, *11*:41-48, 1970.

4. Flügel, F., Bente, D., Itil, T. M., and Molitoris, B.: Klinische und elektroencepha-lographische Untersuchungen in der Reihe der acylierten Piperazino-Phenothiazin-Derivate. In: Rothlin, E. (Ed.): *Neuro-Psychopharmacology.* Amsterdam, Elsevier, 1961, vol. 2, pp. 236-243.

5. Heinemann, L. G., and Itil, T. M.: Quantitative EEG changes during high and low dosage fluphenazine hydrochloride treatment. *Int Pharmacopsychist 4*:43-52, 1970.

6. Holden, J. M. C., Itil, T. M., and Keskiner, A.: Comparison of perphenazine and P-5227 in chronic schizophrenics: Clinical and EEG effects. *J Clin Pharmacol, 9*:163-175, 1969.

7. Holden, M., Itil, T. M., Sanford, E., and Ahmed, M.: Clinical and electroencepha-lographical effects of piperacetazine in comparison to chlorpromazine. Presented at 7th Congress of Colleguim Internationale Neuro-Psychopharmacologicum, Prague, Czechoslovakia, August 11-15, 1970.

8. Itil, T. M.: Elektroencephalographischer Befunde zur Klassifikation neuro- und thymoleptischer Medikamente. *Med exp, 5*:347- 363, 1961.

9. Itil, T. M.: Elektroencephalographische Untersuchungen mit einem Triflumethyl-phenothiazin-Derivat. *Arzneimittelforschung, 15*:817-819, 1965.

10. Itil, T. M.: Electroencephalography and pharmacopyschiatry. In Freyhan, F. A., Petrilowitsch, N., and Pichot, P. (Eds.): *Clinical Psychopharmacology, Modern Problems of Pharmacopsychiatry.* Basel/New York, S. Karger, 1968, vol. 1, pp. 163-194.

11. Itil, T. M. and Fink, M.: Electroencephalographic effects of trifluperidol. *Dis Nerv Syst, 30*:524-530, 1969.

12. Itil, T. M., Rizzo, A. E., and Shapiro, D. M.: Study of behavior and EEG correlation during treatment of disturbed children. *Dis Nerv Syst, 28*:731-736, 1967a.

13. Itil, T. M., Holden, J. M. C., Fink, M., Shapiro, D. M., and Keskiner, A.: Treatment of chronic psychiatric patients with combined medications. In Brill, H., Cole, J. O., Deniker, P., Hippius, H., and Bradley, P. B., (Eds.): *Neuro-psycho-pharma-cology,* Amsterdam, Excerpta Medica, 1967b, pp. 1016-1020.

14. Itil, T. M., Shapiro, D., and Fink, M.: Differentiation of psychotropic drugs by quantitative EEG analysis. *Agressologie, 9*:267-280, 1968a.

15. Itil, T. M., Holden, J. M. C., Keskiner, A., and Shapiro, D.: Central effects of metronidazole. *Psychiat Res Rep Amer Psychiat Ass, 24*:148-165, 1968b.

16. Itil, T. M., Shapiro, D. M., Fink, M., Kiremitci, N., and Hickman, C.: Quantitative EEG studies of chlordiazepoxide, chlorpromazine and imipramine in volunteer and schizophrenic subjects. In Evans, W. O., and Kline, N. S. (Eds.): *The Psycho-pharmacology of the Normal Human.* Springfield, Thomas, 1969a, pp. 219-237.

17. Itil, T. M., Gannon, P., Heinemann, L. G., Holden, J. M. C., and Keskiner, A.: The effect of fluphenazine and thiothixene on digital computer sleep prints. In *Scientific Proceedings in Summary Form,* 122nd Annual Meeting, American Psychiatric Association, Washington, 1969b, pp. 274-276..

18. Itil, T. M., Gannon, P., Hsu, W., and Klingenberg, H.: Digital computer analyzed sleep and resting EEG during haloperidol treatment. *Amer J Psychiat, 127*:462-471, 1970.

19. Itil, T. M., Polvan, N., and Holden, J. M. C.: Clinical and electroencephalographi-cal effects of cinanserin, a serotonin inhibitor, in schizophrenic and manic pa-tients. *Dis Nerv Syst, 32*:193-200, 1971.

20. Itil, T. M., Cora, R., Heinemann, L., Keskiner, A., Gannon, P., and Hsu, W.: Digi-tal computer analyzed resting and sleep EEG investigations and clinical changes during molindone treatment, *J Psychiat Res* (in press a) .

21. Itil, T. M., Keskiner, A., Han, H., and Hsu, W.: EEG changes after fluphenazine enanthate and decanoate based on analog power spectra and digital computer period analysis. *Psychopharmacolgia* (in press b).
22. Simeon, J., Fink, M., Itil, T., and Ponce, D.: d-Cycloserine therapy of psychosis by symptom provocation. *Compr Psychiat, 11:*80-88, 1970.

Chapter 10

Limbic Lesion-Induced Changes in Cerebral Excitability*

MARTIN W. ADLER

MANY STUDIES have demonstrated that altered emotional states affect the level of brain excitability, although more than one mechanism is probably involved in the resultant changes. Since the level of excitability of brain tissue is a critical determinant of seizure threshold, it is reasonable to assume that factors affecting emotionality might also affect seizure threshold.

It has long been recognized that the limbic system of the brain is intimately involved in behavior, especially the emotional aspects. Lesions and stimulation of limbic structures result in changes in emotionality as, for example, the hyperreactivity to stimuli seen following destruction of the septal nuclei.[8,26] On a clinical level, a marked correlation between rage reactions and temporal lobe epilepsy has been reported.[23] In addition to its relationship with behavior, one part of the limbic system, the hippocampus, has a remarkably low threshold for seizure activity (references may be found in the review by Green[15]). The strong anatomical and physiological connections between the various parts of the limbic system thus invited a study of the effects of single and multiple lesions of the limbic system on threshold to convulsions. Although previous reports have indicated that both stimulation and lesions of the hippocampus may give rise to seizure discharges resembling human psychomotor epileptic attacks,[16] few studies have been concerned with the effects of lesions in other limbic areas in relation to seizures. Furthermore, there is an absence of reports involving possible antagonistic or potentiating effects of multiple lesions of the limbic system on seizure susceptibility.

Finally, it is well known that the input to the limbic system is mediated in part through the classic afferent sensory pathways. Earlier studies in this laboratory[1,3] demonstrated that lesions of sensory nuclei, either alone in some cases or combined with other lesions in other cases, could affect seizure threshold. The fact that the olfactory nuclei represent one of the

*This study was supported in part by Grant MH05173 from the National Institute of Mental Health, the General Research Support Grant to Temple University School of Medicine and a grant from Temple University.

167

primary sensory modalities and at the same time are an intimate part of the limbic system presented an intriguing area for investigation in regard to seizure threshold.

METHODS

The subjects employed in this study were adult male albino rats of the Sprague-Dawley (Holtzman) strain weighing 280-330 gm at the time of surgery. Animals were chosen at random for one of seven surgical procedures: (a) sham operation; (b) bilateral lesions of the dorsal hippocampus; (c) bilateral lesions of the amygdala; (d) bilateral lesions of the lateral septal nuclei; (e) bilateral lesions of the olfactory tubercles; (f) bilateral lesions of the dorsal hippocampus, amygdala and lateral septal nuclei; (g) bilateral lesions of the dorsal hippocampus, amygdala, lateral septal nuclei, and olfactory tubercles. Animals were housed in groups of three or four per cage (except during the first three postoperative days when they were housed individually) with food and water allowed *ad libitum* except during the actual test sessions.

Bilateral lesions were produced stereotaxically using unipolar anodal direct current passed through a formvar-coated stainless steel electrode (diameter 0.254 mm) with .5 mm of the tip scraped free of insulation. Stereotaxic coordinates were determined by a modification of the DeGroot[11] atlas. All animals received a single intramuscular injection of sixty thousand units of an aqueous suspension of procaine penicillin G immediately following surgery.

The threshold for convulsions induced by flurothyl (bis-2,2,2-trifluroethyl ether, Indoklon®) was determined at one and fifteen weeks postoperatively. Previous studies in this laboratory[5] showed that three flurothyl-induced seizures could be produced in rats without significant threshold modifications. Rats were placed singly in a one-gallon glass jar closed by a screw cap to which wire mesh containing a three-inch by three-inch surgical sponge was attached. A 10 percent solution of flurothyl in 95 percent ethanol (v/v) was continuously applied to the sponge at a rate of 0.103 ml/min by means of a Harvard infusion pump. The time between the start of the infusion and the onset of a generalized seizure with loss of posture was considered the convulsive threshold.

Histological verification of lesion sites was carried out in all animals. Brains were perfused *in situ*, serially sectioned at 20μ and stained with luxol fast blue and cresyl violet. Designations of the location and extent of the lesions are in accordance with the atlases of DeGroot[11] and Zeman and Innes.[28]

RESULTS

Anatomical

For each lesion site, anatomical criteria for the acceptance or rejection of an animal's results into a particular group were established, and in the few cases where lesions were found not to meet criteria, the results were not included. Hippocampal lesions completely bisected the dorsal hippocampus in a dorsoventral direction about 2.5 mm lateral to the midline. Damage to underlying thalamic structures was absent, and damage to the overlying cortex and corpus callosum, minimal. This is illustrated in Figure 10-1. Lesions of the amygdala were generally in the ventral portions about 3.5 to 4.5 mm lateral to the midline. The primary nuclei involved were the cortical amygdaloid nucleus and parts of the medial nucleus and basolateral nucleus. Damage to the lateral septal nuclei almost always included damage to the medial septal nucleus and a small portion of the hippocampal commissure. Lesions of the olfactory tubercles were in the ventrolateral portions of the tubercle (see Fig. 10-2). Slight damage to the anterior portions of the caudate nucleus were occasionally noted, but no correlation between this damage and the results could be found.

Seizure Thresholds

When animals were tested one week postoperatively, there was an *increase* in threshold in animals with lesions of the hippocampus, the olfactory area or the combination of hippocampus, amygdala, lateral septal, and olfactory. These increases are statistically significant using the method of orthagonal comparisons.[22] This is shown in Table 10-I. When the animals were tested fifteen weeks postoperatively, an entirely different result was obtained. *None* of the lesioned groups had an increased threshold. Rather, a reversal in the lesioned groups had occurred sometime between the first and fifteenth postoperative week, and *all* groups showed a *decreased* threshold to the flurothyl-induced seizures (Table 10-II). Using Dunn's method of multiple comparisons,[12] rats with lesions of the hippocampus or combined hippocampus, amygdala and lateral septal or combined hippocampus, amygdala, lateral septal, and olfactory showed a statistically significant decrease in seizure threshold. The decreases resulting from olfactory or lateral septal lesions were just shy of significance with the test used, although individual comparisons with the sham-operated group would show significance at the .05 level using a standard *t*-test. The decrease in threshold noted with the combined hippocampus, amygdala, and lateral septal lesions can be attributed to the effect of hippocampal damage alone. However, the combined hippocampus, amygdala, lateral septal, and olfactory group showed

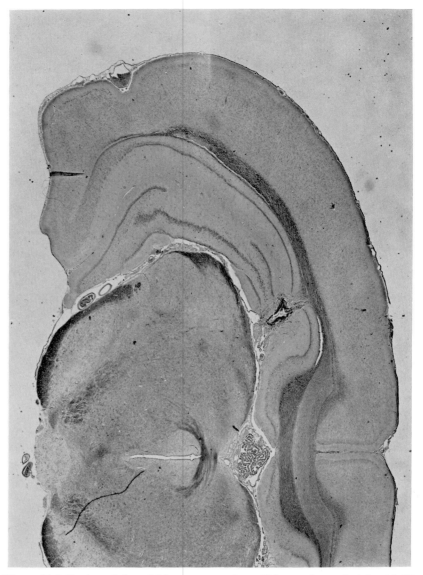

Figure 10-1. Lesion of dorsal hippocampus. Luxol blue and cresyl violet × 15.

a result explainable only on the basis of a potentiating effect of the olfactory damage on the threshold changes produced by the combination of H, A, and L lesions.

Discussion

The present study confirms our hypothesis that important relationships exist between various limbic structures and seizure mechanisms. As has been

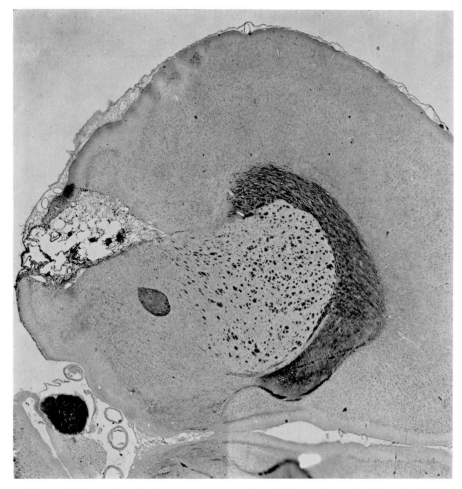

Figure 10-2. Lesion of olfactory tubercle. Luxol blue and cresyl violet × 20.8.

reported by other investigators,[16,24] the hippocampus is an important factor in at least some types of seizure susceptibility. In addition, we noted some rather surprising effects as the result of lesions of other limbic structures and as the result of multiple lesions. We were also able to establish that the changes resulting from the limbic damage developed over a period of time, rather than beginning immediately.

I would like to comment first on this latter finding. For many years, the concept of denervation supersensitivity as expounded by Cannon and Rosenblueth[9] has been accepted for the peripheral nervous system. However, it is only in the past few years that this concept has been applied to the brain. One of the critical determinants in the application of this law to a

TABLE 10-I

THRESHOLD FOR FLUROTHYL - INDUCED SEIZURES FOLLOWING LIMBIC LESIONS
(Time in Sec ± S.D.) One Week Postoperative

	Number of Animals	Mean ± S.D.	% Change from Sham-Operated
Sham-operated	20	312±30	. . . . . .†
Hippocampus	6	346±25	+11%*
Amygdala	7	315±33	+ 1%†
Lateral Septal	7	308±39	— 1%†
Olfactory	7	359±24	+15%*
A + L + H	12	325±36	+ 4%
A + L + H + O	7	350±59	+12%*

*H, O, and ALHO do not differ from each other, but differ from each of the groups with the double asterisk at p < .01.[22]

†S, A, and L do not differ from each other but differ from each of the groups with the single asterisk at p < .01.[22]

given situation is the latency before the onset of the increased sensitivity. A period of several days is the minimum time, but several weeks may be required for the maximum effect, especially in the central nervous system. Changes which occur immediately do not constitute an example of denervation supersensitivity, but are often the result of loss of inhibitory influences. The data clearly show that a period of more than one week after surgery is required for the development of the increased susceptibility to seizures. The general picture of a reversal from a decreased responsiveness to an increased sensitivity fits well with Cannon and Rosenblueth's theory. This is reminiscent of our studies with cortical and lateral geniculate lesions.[2,3] The findings may thus be another example of central denervation supersensitivity.

In view of the low threshold for seizure discharge that is characteristic of the hippocampus and in view of the fact that lesions of the hippocampus of cats[16] can result in frank epileptic seizures, the increased seizure susceptibility noted in our rats after bilateral hippocampal damage is not surprising.

TABLE 10-II

THRESHOLD FOR FLUROTHYL - INDUCED SEIZURES FOLLOWING LIMBIC LESIONS
(Time in Sec ± S.D.) Fifteen weeks Postoperative

	Number of Animals	Mean ± S.D.	% Change from Sham-Operated
Sham-Operated	20	324±22	. . . . . .
Hippocampus	6	268±31	—17%*
Amygdala	7	311±25	— 4%
Lateral Septal	7	292±33	—10%
Olfactory	7	300±24	— 7%
A + L + H	12	275±25	—15%*
A + L + H + O	7	241±16	—26%*

*Statistically different from sham-operated at p < .005 with 2-tailed t-test (12) giving overall level of p < .05 for all comparisons.

However, in Green's studies, the epileptic seizures occurred during the first two weeks after surgery and then stopped except in one case. It would be interesting to know if these animals continued to have a lower seizure threshold even in the absence of overt seizure activity. The unexpected was found with other limbic lesions. In all cases, at least a slight drop (albeit not always statistically significant) in threshold was noted fifteen weeks postoperatively, and this drop was just shy of statistical significance in the case of lesions of the olfactory tubercles and the lateral septal nuclei. Since the statistical test employed is rather conservative in nature, a somewhat larger number of subjects per group might have resulted in a statistically significant change. On this basis, one would then logically predict that combined lesions would have an additive effect, and the result would be a drop in threshold greater than that seen with any one lesion alone. It was therefore surprising to find that combined lesions of the hippocampus, amygdala, and lateral septal nuclei did not result in an effect greater than that produced by hippocampal damage alone. A possible explanation is that lesions of the amygdala and lateral septal nuclei somehow cancel out each other's effect. Credence is given to this interpretation by the fact that such lesions are antagonistic on emotionality.[19,20,25] The possibility that hippocampal damage produced the maximum increase in seizure susceptibility that can be measured by our test procedure is obviated by the results seen when olfactory tubercle damage is added to animals with combined lesions of hippocampus, amygdala, and lateral septal nuclei.

Bilateral lesions to all four limbic structures produce a greater effect than that seen with just the combination of hippocampus, amygdala, and lateral septal damage. The increase in susceptibility is, in fact, greater than just an additive effect and the potentiation is statistically significant. A similar finding was noted in our earlier studies with lesions of the lateral and medial geniculate nuclei.[3] It seems possible that since the olfactory area represents a structure involved in both limbic mechanisms of emotion and in sensory input, the potentiating effect that results from this lesion is due to its sensory afferent influence on limbic mechanisms. Although little is known about olfactory pathways beyond the tubercle, the known convergence of multiple sensory inputs on single neurons[21] presents an intriguing situation for future studies.

With regard to some of the intimate mechanisms involved in the altered seizure susceptibility resulting from damage to limbic structures, the effects of such lesions on food, water, and sodium intake that have been demonstrated by others[10,13,14,17,27] invite experiments on ionic balance and the chemical composition of the brain in regard to limbic seizures.

Because of the peculiar susceptibility of the hippocampus and the rhinencephalon to damage during the prenatal period and during delivery, comparative studies of the effects of limbic damage on seizure thresholds in immature versus mature brains should be carried out. Differences would be expected on the basis of anatomical studies showing different patterns of neuronal degeneration following brain damage in animals of different ages[7] as well as studies in animals and humans demonstrating differences in behavior following limbic lesions at different ages.[6,18,23]

Finally, alterations in durg response are known to occur following destruction of various areas of the brain including the limbic system.[4] Indeed, preliminary studies in this laboratory indicate that there is an increased sensitivity to the anticonvulsant actions of ethosuximide in rats with lesions in certain limbic structures. This is most striking in groups with lesions of the olfactory or lateral septal nuclei or with combination lesions involving these structures.

SUMMARY

In order to gain further insight into the relationships between the limbic system and cerebral excitability, the threshold for flurothyl-induced seizures was determined in rats with lesions in various parts of the limbic system. Bilateral damage to the dorsal hippocampus resulted in a markedly lower threshold for convulsions. Bilateral lesions of the amygdala, lateral septal nuclei, or olfactory tubercles resulted in some lowering of threshold, but these changes were not statistically significant. Combined lesions of the amygdala, hippocampus, and lateral septal nuclei yielded results comparable to the changes noted with hippocampal damage alone. Adding olfactory lesions to the above resulted in a potentiation of the threshold-lowering effect. The decrease in seizure thresholds following the lesions took more than one week to develop.

It can be concluded that marked changes in cerebral excitability, as determined by alterations in seizure susceptibility, occur following certain single and multiple lesions of the limbic system.

ACKNOWLEDGMENTS

The author wishes to thank Mrs. Phyllis Cooper and Mrs. Ruth Tresky for their assistance throughout the course of the studies reported and Mrs. Shirley Braverman of the Department of Biometrics for her invaluable assistance with the statistical evaluation of the results.

REFERENCES

1. Adler, M. W.: Increased sensitivity to pentylenetetrazol and flurothyl following cortical ablations in rats. *J Pharmacol Exp Ther, 148:*131, 1965.
2. Adler, M. W.: Time course of altered sensitivity to flurothyl following cortical ablations in rats. *J Pharmacol Exp Ther, 153:*396, 1966.

3. Adler, M. W.: Lowered thresholds to flurothyl seizures after lateral geniculate lesions in rats. *Int J Neuropharmacol, 8:*393, 1969.

4. Adler, M. W.: Drug response following brain damage. In Smith, W. L. (Ed.) : *Drugs and Cerebral Function.* Springfield, Thomas, 1971.

5. Adler, M. W., Sagel, S., Kitagawa, S., Segawa, T., and Maynert, E. W.: The effects of repeated flurothyl-induced seizures on convulsive thresholds and brain monoamines in rats. *Arch Int Pharmacodyn, 170:*12, 1967.

6. Aird, R. B.: Clinical syndromes of the limbic system. *Int J Neurol, 6:*340, 1968.

7. Bleier, R.: Retrograde transsynaptic cellular degeneration in mammillary and ventral tegmental nuclei following limbic decortication in rabbits of various ages. *Brain Res, 15:*365, 1969.

8. Brady, J. V. and Nauta, W. J.: Subcortical mechanisms in emotional behavior: affective changes following septal forebrain lesions in the albino rat. *J Comp Physiol Psychol, 46:*339, 1953.

9. Cannon, W. B. and Rosenblueth, A.: *The Supersensitivity of Denervated Structures.* New York, MacMillan, 1949.

10. Covian, M. R.: Studies on the neurovegetative and behavioral functions of the brain septal area. In Adey, W. R., and Tokizani, T. (Eds.) : *Progress in Brain Research, Vol. 27: Structure and Function of the Limbic System.* Amsterdam, Elsevier, 1967.

11. DeGroot, J.: The rat forebrain in stereotaxic coordinates. *J Trans R Neth Acad Sci, 52:*1, 1959.

12. Dunn, O. J.: Multiple comparisons among means. *J Amer Stat Ass, 56:*52, 1961.

13. Gentil, C. D., Antunes-Rodrigues, J., Negro-Vilar, A., and Covian, M. R.: Role of amygdaloid complex in sodium chloride and water intake in the rat. *Physiol Behav, 3:*981, 1968.

14. Giammanco, S., LaGrutta, V., Tessitore, V., and DiBernardo, C.: Effects of ablation of the olfactory bulbs in very young rats. *Electroenceph Clin Neurophysiol, 27:*102, 1969.

15. Green, J. D.: The hippocampus. *Physiol Rev, 44:*561, 1964.

16. Green, J. D., Clemente, C. D., and DeGroot, J.: Experimentally induced epilepsy in the cat with injury of cornu ammonis. *Arch Neurol Psychiat, 78:*259, 1957.

17. Grossman, S. P. and Grossman, L.: Food and water intake following lesions or electrical stimulation of the amygdala. *Amer J Physiol, 205:*761, 1963.

18. Isaacson, R. L.: When brains are damaged. *Psychol Today,* p. 38, Jan., 1970.

19. King, F. A., and Meyer, P. M.: Effects of amygdaloid lesions upon septal hyperemotionality in the rat. *Science, 128:*655, 1958.

20. Kleiner, F. B., Meyer, P. M., and Meyer, D. R.: Effects of simultaneous septal and amygdaloid lesions upon emotionality and retention of a black and white discrimination. *Brain Res., 5:*459, 1967.

21. Murata, K., Cramer, H., and Bach-y-Rita, P.: Neuronal convergence of noxious, acoustic and visual stimuli in the visual cortex of the cat. *J Neurophysiol, 28:*1223, 1965.

22. Nair, K. R.: The studentized form of the extreme mean square test in the analysis of variance. *Biometrika, 35:*16, 1948.

23. Ounsted, C.: Aggression and epilepsy: rage in childen with temporal lobe epilepsy. *J Psychosom Res, 13:*237, 1969.

24. Passouant, P. and Cadilhac, J.: The hippocampus in epilepsy. *World Neurol., 1:*500, 1960.

25. Schwartzbaum, J. S., and Gay, P. E.: Interacting behavioral effects of septal and amygdaloid lesions in the rat. *J Comp Physiol Psychol, 61*:59, 1966.
26. Stark, P., and Henderson, J. K.: Increased reactivity in rats caused by septal lesions. *Int J Neuropharmacol, 5*:379, 1966.
27. Vilar, A. N.; Gentil, C. G., and Covian, M. R.: Alterations in sodium chloride and water intake after septal lesions in the rat. *Physiol Behav, 2*:167, 1967.
28. Zeman, W., and Innes, J. R. M.: *Craigie's Neuroanatomy of the Rat.* New York, Academic Press, 1963.

PART IV

CHILDHOOD PSYCHOPHARMACOLOGY

Chapter 11

Stimulant Drugs and Cortical Evoked Responses in Learning and Behavior Disorders in Children

C. KEITH CONNERS

INTRODUCTION

STIMULANT drugs, such as methylphenidate and dextroamphetamine, produce a variety of perceptual, cognitive, and motor changes in children. Many of these changes have been described in the previous symposium of this series (Conners, 1970; Werry, 1970) and will not be reviewed here. However, a recently completed study will serve to illustrate the empirical findings and problems emerging from the body of data now available.

The recent study involved the comparison of methylphenidate, dextroamphetamine, and placebo. The subjects were seventy-one children with a mean age of 9.5 years, with a range of six years. The children were referred for treatment either because of severe behavior problems at home or school, or because they were failing academically. No children with known organic brain syndromes, retardation, or medical illness were included in the sample. The children were randomly assigned to one of the three treatments. A battery of neurological, psychological, and physiological tests was administered prior to drug treatment and one month after the beginning of treatment. Figure 11-1 shows the results for the psychological tests.

In general, there were few significant differences between the two active drugs, though methylphenidate was significantly better on two subtests of the WISC and generally did slightly better for several other tests. There was a definite superiority of methylphenidate in terms of side effects, however. Figure 11-2 shows the weekly report of any degree of side effect mentioned by the parents, and the superiority of methylphenidate is even more clearly evident in more detailed analyses of severe side effects. Both drugs produce many highly significant improvements over placebo.

Some of the effects of the drugs are quite dramatic. Figure 11-3, for example, shows the kinds of qualitative changes which some children showed on the drawing of a man. Some children showed IQ gains of thirty or more points, and reading changes of two or more years in grade level.

However, the data raise some important issues regarding the generality of such findings: (a) While some subjects change dramatically for a given test, others may show no change or even decrements in performance for that test; and a patient may change in one test, but not in others. (b) Some of

179

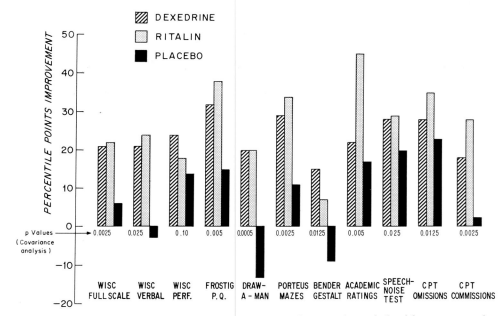

Figure 11-1. Changes in psychological tests over a three-week period with treatment by dextroamphetamine, methylphenidate, or placebo. Changes are in terms of percentile points of the normal curve for the entire sample.

the most significant improvements, as for the graphomotor tests of figure drawing and copying Bender Gestalt designs, had failed to show significant drug effects in previous drug studies. (c) Some of the tests which did not show significant changes in this study, such as the test of auditory synthesis and rote learning, and previously shown sensitivity to these drugs. (d) Several other investigators have now conducted similar studies in which sometimes one and sometimes another objective test measure fails to replicate.

It is always possible to try to explain such variability from one study to another in terms of differences in dosage, length of treatment, techniques of measurement, etc. But it has seemed to us that this type of finding is substantive and more than experimental error. The findings raise the question of the way the various changes in test measures are related to one another, whether these changes are predictable from characteristics of the subjects, and whether there might be important underlying physiological variables to account for individual differences between dramatic responders and nonresponders. *Perhaps differences between and within studies are due to different kinds of changes in different kinds of patients.*

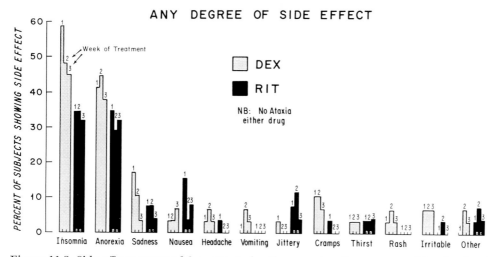

Figure 11-2. Side effects reported by parents for three weeks of treatment with stimulants or placebo. Table shows any degree of side effect, whether mild or severe.

RELATIONSHIP AMONG THE CHANGES PRODUCED BY DRUGS

In three of our studies we have used either methylphenidate or dextro-amphetamine over a three-week to four-week treatment period and with a

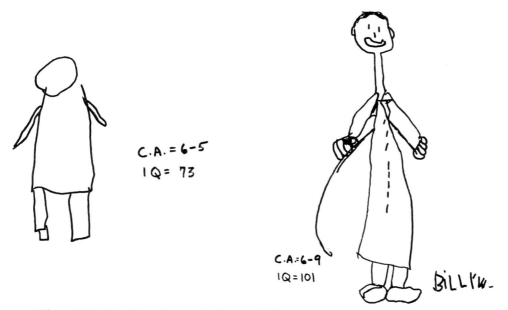

Figure 11-3. Drawing of a man before and after treatment with methylphenidate.

number of psychological tests in common. In each study the children were randomly assigned to drug or placebo under double blind conditions. By pooling the data from these three studies, we have a total sample size of 178, with 107 drug-treated patients, and 71 placebo treated patients, each having predrug and postdrug test scores on thirty-two separate variables.

The first feature of the gain scores—that is, the prescores minus the postscores—that comes to one's attention is the low degree of relationship among the change scores for separate measures. These correlations are seldom larger than .2 or .3. A factor analysis of these change scores gives a smaller number of variables to work with and clarifies the nature of the changes which are occurring together. A principal components solution, with varimax rotation to simple structure produces six factors. The first factor is very clearly the set of changes associated with the teacher questionnaire. This is a thirty-nine-item symptom list filled out by the teacher, which is divided into academic behavior, classroom behavior, and attitude towards authority. The second factor appears to reflect attentional processes. It is loaded most highly by errors made during paired-associate learning, errors of omission on the continuous performance test, and to a lesser extent by errors of commission. The third set of gains appears to be a perceptual-motor factor, with highest loadings from the changes in the Bender Gestalt, drawing of a man, Porteus Mazes, and errors of commission.

The fourth gain factor is essentially a reading improvement factor, which has, besides the reading changes, changes associated with improvement in the qualitative score of the Porteus Mazes, suggesting perhaps a type of reading enhancement associated with more careful attention to detail, better control over impulsiveness, and eye-motor coordination.

The fifth factor is associated with gains in spelling and arithmetic, while the sixth factor has only one substantial loading, auditory synthesis (sound blending) . Thus, it would appear that for this sample, although most of the variables show statistically significant drug-placebo differences, *a number of separate kinds of drugs changes are occurring;* there is no general, global effect of the drugs. Rather, it seems that the drugs may produce a change in one set of test scores quite independently of other test scores. Although the reliability of *change* scores is always substantially lower than the reliability of the original measures, all of the tests are reliable enough that it seems unlikely that one can account for the independence of these changes on the basis of unreliability. One must, perhaps, entertain the hypothesis that the drugs can produce certain changes depending either on the prior physiological state of the organism or some behavioral characteristics of individual subjects. The next question then becomes whether one can predict these drug changes from something known about the individual patients.

PREDICTION OF CHANGES INDUCED BY DRUGS

There are many characteristics that one could use to predict drug changes. At present we have investigated the utility of the various psychological tests, parent and teacher ratings of symptomatology, and age as predictors of the change factors previously described. Each subject is assigned six change factor scores (these are standardized scores weighted by the factor loading contribution of each of the variables).

We then computed six stepwise multiple regression equations with the six gain factor scores as the dependent or criterion variables, and the tests and ratings as predictors. The stepwise regression procedure starts by taking the variable most highly predictive of the criterion, with all other scores partialled out, and successively adds the next most contributory predictors until the gain in prediction is no longer significant.

The overall result of these analyses was most surprising: All of the regressions were highly significant. For the six problems the multiple Rs were .73, .82, .64, .58, .70, and .57, respectively. The results are summarized in Table 11-I.

Let us consider the most successful prediction, that for gain-factor number 2. It will be recalled that this factor appears to measure those changes which are suggestive of improvements in attentional state, being most highly loaded by failures to detect signals during a continuous vigilance task, and errors made during the lengthy paired-associate learning task. The first two variables entered into the equation are the pretest scores on paired-associate errors and the continuous performance tests. In other words, changes in this factor are most predicted by initially poor performance on the pretest scores most strongly contributing to the gain factor itself. This is in general true of the other prediction equations. A subject with poor performance in a given area is most likely to improve in that area. This certainly makes sense, both from the point of view of pathology that is in need of improvement, but also from the statistical point of view since one would expect regression to the mean to produce such effects.

However, after these two variables have been entered into the equation, there are still several significant additions to the predictability. The first of these is the pretest score on arithmetic. It is generally believed that arithmetic performance is also highly dependent on attention and concentration. Next in importance is the parent's rating of hyperactivity. The next variable is most surprising and perhaps clinically important: The drug condition of Dexedrine® or Ritalin® enters in as a significant predictor. In other words, more attentional change occurs as a result of methylphenidate than dextroamphetamine. This gain factor is the only one in which the drug condition seemed to be of much consequence. Another feature worth noting

Drugs, Development, and Cerebral Function

TABLE 11-I

REGRESSION ANALYSIS: REGRESSING SIX IMPROVEMENT FACTORS
ON TWENTY PRETREATMENT VARIABLES

(Pooled Dexedrine and Ritalin Subgroups)

Factor I (Teacher Questionnaire): multiple $r = .73$, $r^2 = .54$

		weight	gainers are
Predicted by:	SQ Academic	.25	bad
	SQ Classroom	.31	bad
	Frostig PQ	.17	good
	SQ Authority	.26	bad
	WISC Perf. IQ	.22	good
	Bender	.21	bad
	CPT Omit	—.14	good
	Porteus IQ	—.11	bad

Factor II (Attention?): multiple $r = .82$, $r^2 = .67$

Predicted by:	PA Errors	.59	bad
	CPT Omit	.57	bad
	WRAT Arithmetic	.20	good
	WISC Perf. IQ	.12	good
	PQ Hyperactive	.17	bad
	Drug	.11	on Ritalin
	CPT Commit	—.11	good

Factor III (Perceptual): multiple $r = .63$, $r^2 = .40$

Predicted by:	Bender	.24	bad
	CPT Commit	—.50	good
	Porteus IQ	—.36	bad
	PA Errors	—.25	good
	Qualitative	—.18	good
	CPT Omit	.21	bad
	SQ Academic	.08	bad

Factor IV (Reading +): multiple $r = .58$, $r^2 = .34$

Predicted by:	Age	.48	older
	PQ Neurotic	—.30	good
	Qualitative	.25	bad
	CPT Commit	.31	bad
	CPT Omit	—.19	good
	WISC Verbal IQ	.12	good
	SQ Classroom	—.19	good
	Frostig PQ	.11	good
	SQ Academic	.20	bad
	SQ Authority	—.15	good
	WRAT Reading	—.11	bad

Factor V (?): multiple $r = .70$, $r^2 = .48$

Predicted by:	CPT Commit	.44	bad
	WRAT Spelling	—.88	bad
	WRAT Arithmetic	.59	good
	CPT Omit	—.43	good
	Porteus IQ	—.27	bad
	PQ Neurotic	—.20	good
	Age	—.39	younger
	WRAT Reading	.41	good
	WISC Verbal IQ	—.11	bad

TABLE 11-I *(Continued)*

	Bender	—.19	good
	WISC Perf. IQ	—.13	bad
Factor VI (?) : multiple r = .57, r^2 = .32			
Predicted by:	SQ Authority	.47	bad
	SQ Academic	—.38	good
	D-A-P IQ	.23	good
	WISC Perf. IQ	—.22	bad
	WISC Verb. IQ	.20	good
	Bender	.24	bad
	WRAT Arithmetic	.16	good
	Porteus IQ	.08	good

All regressions have an overall F significant of at least the .0005 level.

for changes in this area, is that they are not at all predictable from academic status or teacher's appraisal of classroom behavior.

Let us consider gain-factor number one: the factor involving changes in academic and classroom behavior. As mentioned, the first predictors are the pretest scores on the teacher questionnaire itself. But other variables which significantly contribute to this prediction are the perceptual quotient of the Frostig Test of Developmental Visual Perception, the WISC Performance IQ, and the Bender Gestalt Test. The prediction coefficients indicate that patients who have good performance IQs, good perceptual quotients, but *poor* Bender Gestalt performance are most likely to be rated by teachers as improving in response to the drugs. This would seem to indicate that some other characteristic than perceptual ability and perceptual organization associated with Bender performance is contributing to the prediction. Perhaps it is the poor planning ability of the Bender performance that is involved. This is supported by the fact that also entering into the prediction—though to a somewhat smaller degree—is the pretest Porteus Maze score, which has an important element of planning ability. In other words, children who are perceptually intact but are impulsively responding on the Bender, can be expected to show changes in academic and classroom behavior. Note, however, that actual improvement in *achievement* tests does not occur in this factor.

If we turn to gain-factor number four, which appears to measure mainly changes in reading or word recognition, we see that this is most successfully predicted by age, the parent's rating of neurotic traits, Porteus Q scores, and errors of commission on the CPT. In other words, the older, more impulsive neurotic child can be expected to benefit in reading from the drugs. Note also that errors of omission has a negative prediction coefficient, indicating that these patients are not inattentive.

We are, of course, dealing with predictions based on the entire sample of subjects which is undoubtedly a heterogeneous collection of types of children; and such predictions will be biased by any large aggregates of children who happen to predominate. We know, for example, that the patients have a bias towards being hyperactive, so that one would like to know whether the changes we have been predicting are due to certain types of children. This is the next problem to which we turn.

TYPOLOGICAL CLASSIFICATION OF PATIENTS AND DRUG RESPONSE

Our procedure for classifying patients into types is based on well-established quantitative procedures of taxonomic classification in the biological sciences (Sokal and Sneath, 1963). The procedure involves separating subjects into groups on the basis of the distance between them as determined by their location in the space defined by a number of independent dimensions. Consider, for example, a case in which we have four individuals, t_1, t_2, t_3, and t_4, who each have scores on two sets of independent characteristics, x and y. The distance between those individuals can be expressed geometrically and algebraically as in Figure 11-4: the Euclidean distance between any

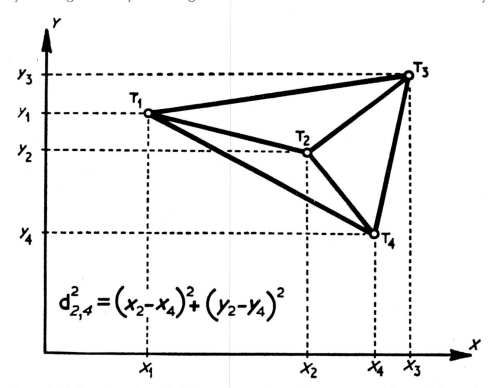

$$d_{2,4}^2 = (x_2 - x_4)^2 + (y_2 - y_4)^2$$

Figure 11-4. Procedure for calculating linear distance between two of four subjects who are characterized by scores on two dimensions, x and y.

two of those individuals is given by the sum of the squared distances between the coordinate points defining their position. Similarly, if one has three independent attributes or traits to describe the individuals, the distances between the individuals in three-dimensional space can be specified by the linear distance formula involving the three coordinate values. This procedure may be generalized to n-dimensional space.

Now if one considers that two individuals in this space who are closest together form a natural group because their test profiles are most similar, the total number of groups, N, is now reduced to N-1. If we now take the average distance between this small two-member group and the rest of the individuals, and successively add to the group other members in order of their nearness (similarity), whenever there is a large gap in the successive average distances, we may infer that some natural group has been identified. If the individuals are randomly distributed in the n-dimensional space or are essentially equidistant from one another, the successive reductions of average within-distance values will form a smooth, unbroken function. If, however, there are natural groups in the hyperspace, the plot of average within-group distances will have breaks in it, indicating that adding a new member to the group has produced a large reduction in the distance between the remaining group members.

In order to describe our subjects by independent dimensions, their pre-test scores on ratings and psychological tests were factor analyzed and rotated to simple structure. The resulting factor scores serve as the coordinates for estimating distances between subjects. This is then, essentially a kind of profile analysis, which groups subjects on the basis of their test profiles.

The results of performing the iterative measures of distance reduction by grouping the successively most adjacent individuals, is shown in Figure 11-5. We see that at the point of the arrow, there begin to appear large gaps, indicating the occurrence of natural groups. From this analysis seven groups of individuals are identified. Figure 11-6 shows the mean factor score profiles for the seven groups. Note, for example, group six: The children in this group are slightly younger than the other groups, are low in achievement tests, very poor in classroom and academic behavior, and poor in concentration and attention. This group may be contrasted with group four who are also quite poor in achievement tests, but are older and actually rated as performing well in the classroom. They appear to have no particular attentional deficit, but are somewhat low in cognitive tests, especially performance IQ.

If we now turn to the effects of drugs in these seven groups of children, we see that there are highly significant differences between the groups in the kind and amount of change produced by the drugs. These drug effects are shown in Figure 11-7. We find that groups two and six are showing signif-

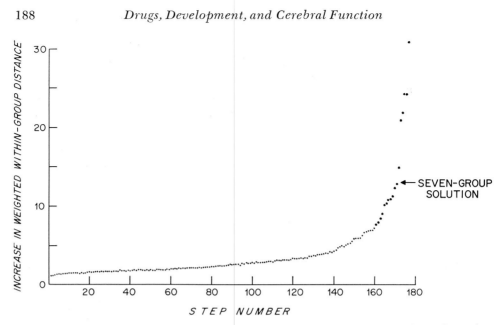

Figure 11-5. Plot showing average reduction in distance among group members. Grouping procedure finds distance between the two nearest subjects, and considers them as a subject to the group, etc. Plot shows the size of reductions at each step.
group. The distance between this two-member group is then calculated for the nearest

icant improvement in classroom ratings by teachers, and group two is also showing a marked improvement in attention.

Table 11-II shows the test changes which are significantly different for drugs and placebo in the seven groups. The most important feature of these findings is that some tests show highly significant changes attributable to drugs in one group, but no changes in other groups. Thus, the net effect of lumping all subjects together is to obscure drug effects that are occurring for some of the subjects, and not occurring for other subjects.

Group *one* shows significant changes for spelling, Porteus IQ, academic ratings, classroom behavior, and paired-associate learning. Group *two* shows significant improvement in ratings of academic behavior and errors of commission on the continuous performance test (CPT). Group *three* shows marked improvement in Porteus IQ, and in paired-associate learning. Group *four* shows change only in the Bender Gestalt Test. Group *five* shows no significant drug effects, although auditory synthesis approaches significance (p <. 06). Group *six* shows the most dramatic improvement in ratings by the teacher of classroom behavior, academic status, and attitude towards authority, as well as changes in paired-associate learning. Group *seven* shows highly significant gains in draw-a-man IQ and errors of commission. Unfortunately, we did not have enough postdrug ratings from parents to de-

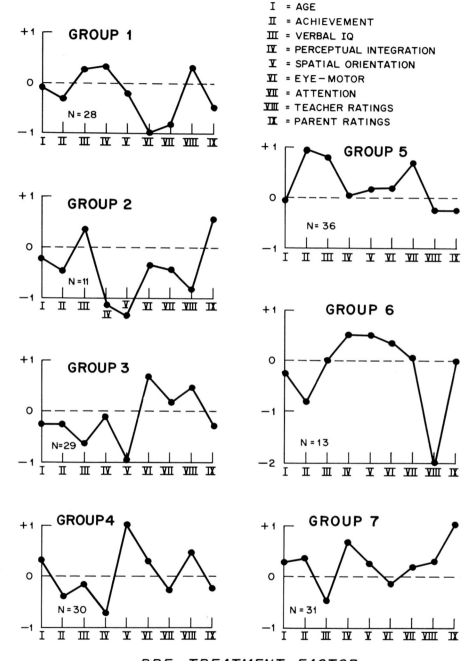

I = AGE
II = ACHIEVEMENT
III = VERBAL IQ
IV = PERCEPTUAL INTEGRATION
V = SPATIAL ORIENTATION
VI = EYE-MOTOR
VII = ATTENTION
VIII = TEACHER RATINGS
IX = PARENT RATINGS

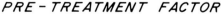

Figure 11-6. Factor profiles (pretreatment status) of seven groups identified by cluster analysis.

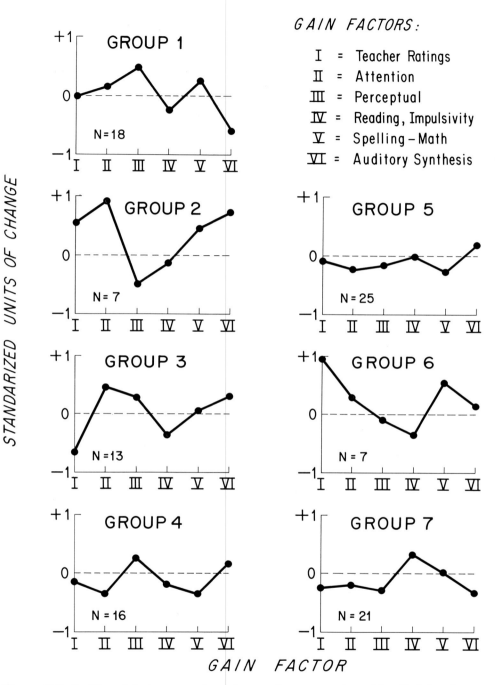

Figure 11-7. Profiles of factor score drug changes for seven groups identified by cluster analysis of behavior tests.

TABLE 11-II

WITHIN-GROUP DIFFERENCES IN RESPONSE TO TREATMENT CONDITION
(Significant Differences in Drug and Placebo Group Gains)

Measure	t-value	one-tailed- p
Group I (drug n = 18; placebo n = 10)		
Spelling	3.161	.002
Porteus IQ	3.851	.001
SQ Academic	3.155	.002
SQ Classroom	3.323	.0015
Paired Assoc.	2.372	.013
Group II (n = 7, 10)		
SQ Academic	2.429	.021
SQ Classroom	1.801	.0545
CPT Commit	2.998	.009
Paired Assoc.	1.888	.046
Bender	1.490	.049
Group III (n = 13, 6)		
Porteus IQ	3.107	.0025
CPT Omit	1.695	.057
Paired Assoc.	2.561	.008
Group IV (n = 15, 13)		
Bender	2.290	.015
Group V (n = 25, 11)		
Auditory Synth.	1.939	.031
CPT Commit	1.840	.037
Group VI (n = 6, 6)		
SQ Academic	6.231	.000
SQ Classroom	3.816	.0015
SQ Authority	3.884	.0015
Paired Assoc.	2.342	.021
Group VII (n = 21, 10)		
Spelling	1.741	.046
Draw-A-Man	2.967	.003
CPT Commit	2.153	.020

termine which of these groups showed the most improvement in behavior at home.

It is of considerable practical importance that group five, which constitutes 20 percent of the sample, showed no improvement attributable to the drugs. The test profile of this group shows them to be above average for the sample in achievement, intelligence, perceptual functioning, and attentional performance. They are low only in parents' ratings of behavior and academic performance in the classroom (though not in actual achievement scores). Thus, they appear to constitute a group who may be referred because of parental overconcerns and possibly some neurotic inhibitions which prevent them from showing up as well in class as they are capable of.

In summary, it appears that the grouping procedure is highly successful in identifying types of children who differentially respond to pharmacologic intervention. We will wish to characterize further these groups in terms of their medical and social histories, and determine whether variables other than the behavioral measures which we have employed can discriminate between these groups. One of the areas which we have begun to explore is direct measures of brain function, as measured by bioelectric recordings of cortical evoked response, a problem to which we now turn.

VISUAL EVOKED RESPONSES

There is a growing body of evidence to suggest that the late waves of the cortical evoked response are intimately associated with cognitive processes of attention and arousal, as well as emotional states. It is generally felt that these late evoked response components may be closely related to the significance of a stimulus for a subject, and possibly even to his intellectual capabilities. Of especial relevance in this regard, for the study of children, is the finding that evoked responses from the left hemisphere are more affected by semantic and symbolic stimuli, while evoked responses from the right hemisphere tend to be more affected by geometric and spatial information processing, in normally left-hemisphere dominant subjects.

We have been interested in three questions: (a) the relationship between the evoked response parameters of latency and amplitude, and behavioral features of children; (b) the effects of stimulant drugs on these electrophysiological variables; and (c) the relationship of evoked response changes to changes in behavioral performances. Moreover, it was felt that a crucial test of the validity of our grouping procedures would be the possible discovery of unique evoked response characteristics in the groups, since the evoked response was not used in any way in the determination of the group structure.

Before describing the effects of drugs and before considering the variations between groups, let us consider some suggestive information from studies of children with reading disorders. Figure 11-8 shows four visual evoked response tracings from an eleven-year-old boy with a severe reading disorder. The recordings are from 01, 02, P3, and P4, referenced to Cz, with a ground at Fz. Note the remarkable attenuation of the left parietal amplitudes. This child also had some acalculia, finger agnosia, and difficulties with sequential spatial memory, though he was of above-average intelligence. The next figure shows tracings from several of his family members, all of whom except the mother are extremely poor readers.

The tracings shown in the next figure (Fig. 11-10) are from another child with a severe reading disorder who has four siblings who also are all

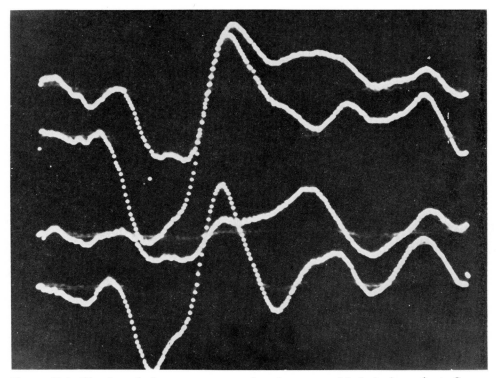

Figure 11-8. Visual evoked response waves for eleven-year-old dyslexic patient. Curves from top to bottom are left occipital, right occipital, left parietal, and right parietal. Locations are 01, 02, P3, and P4 in the international 10-20 system of referencing. Recordings are bipolar to Cz with ground at Fz. Negativity upwards. Time base 512 msec. Averages based on sixty-four trial (1.6 sec intertrial intervals).

poor readers. His father was a mirror writer as a child, and though a college graduate, still considers himself a poor reader and very bad speller.

Following these leads, we subsequently conducted three studies on children with reading disorders. Two of the samples were from special reading instruction programs, and one sample of twenty-six children was from our clinic. The latter were matched on Full Scale IQ, age, and sex, and had either a low verbal, high performance IQ, or a high verbal, low performance IQ.

Consistently for all three studies, the following findings emerged: The significant relationships with reading and spelling performance were found only with the visual evoked response, left parietal area amplitudes. However, in the Verbal-Performance study there were also significant differences in latencies of evoked visual response (p < .001). Children with low Performance IQ had significantly slower right-sided latencies. These studies

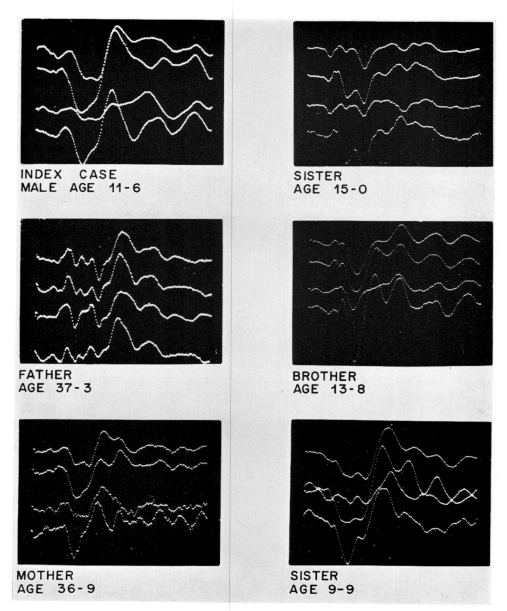

INDEX CASE
MALE AGE 11-6

SISTER
AGE 15-0

FATHER
AGE 37-3

BROTHER
AGE 13-8

MOTHER
AGE 36-9

SISTER
AGE 9-9

Figure 11-9. Visual evoked responses for index case and his immediate family with reading disorders, showing flattening of left parietal curve for siblings. Note the anomaly in father's left parietal curve. Father and all siblings are all poor readers. Mother is a normal reader. (Curves top to bottom are left occipital, right occipital, left parietal, and right parietal.)

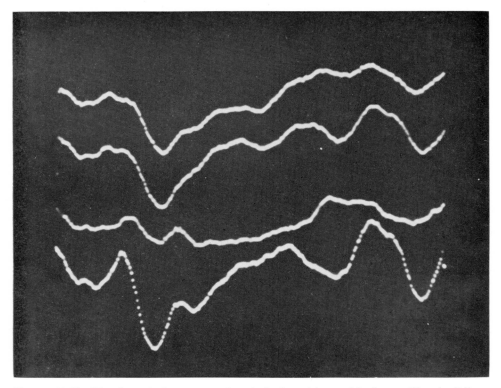

Figure 11-10. Visual evoked response for dyslexic subject with four afflicted siblings, showing left parietal flattening.

have been reported in detail elsewhere (Conners, 1971). Suffice it to say that we were somewhat surprised at the magnitude of the correlations between reading and spelling and evoked response measures. We then asked the question of the effect of the stimulant drugs on these evoked response measures.

Measures were obtained before and at the end of the Dexedrine-Ritalin-placebo study described earlier. The results were analyzed by multivariate analysis of variance for the three groups. There were almost no changes of any kind attributable to the drugs in the amplitudes of either auditory or visual evoked responses. However, highly significant effects on latencies were found. Figure 11-11 shows the latency reductions plotted for the two drugs against placebo. It is especially notable that the two drugs produce changes primarily in the visual evoked response.

The next Figure shows the nature of these changes as regards the two hemispheres. The figure shows that the major source of actual change is the slowing of the placebo group, while the drug groups are showing some

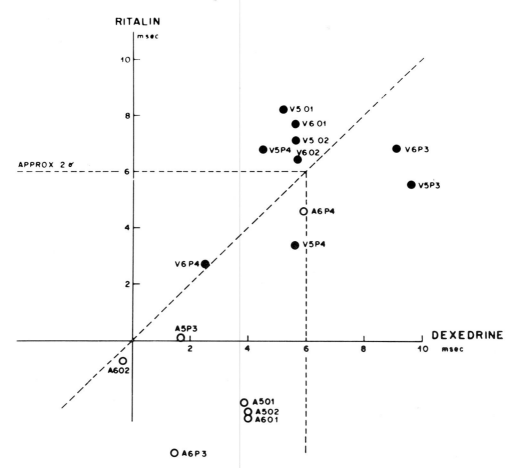

Figure 11-11. Latency reductions of evoked response measures resulting from drugs, relative to placebo. Placebo is plotted at the origin. V = visual; A = auditory. Digits 5 and 6 refer to waves 5 and 6 in Gastaut's system (approximate latencies of 180 msec and 240 msec, respectively). (Signs are reversed to give latency reduction.)

changes in the hemisphere dominance—changes perpendicular to the diagonal indicate a change in the ratio of hemispheric activity.

Next, we were interested to determine whether the subtypes of children we had identified on the basis of their test profiles, would differ in evoked response variables. The results of this analysis were most rewarding, for not only were there highly significant differences between groups in their initial evoked responses, but the kind of differences were specific enough to be informative. In brief, all of the differences were accounted for by Wave VI of the visual evoked response, with the exception of two differences for auditory latencies of wave VI. Despite the relatively small N in the groups

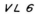

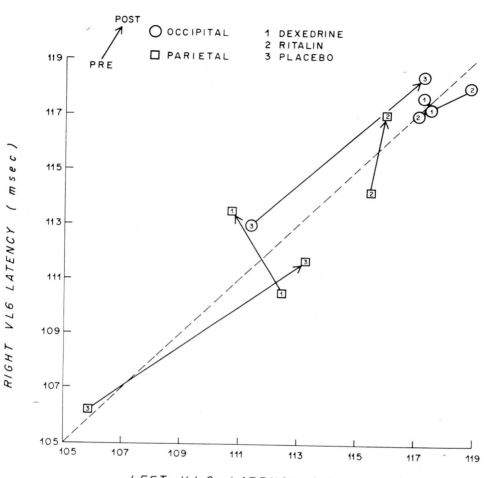

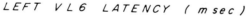

Figure 11-12. Changes in latency for left and right hemispheres. Changes parallel to the diagonal indicate no change in relative speed of response in the two hemispheres; changes perpendicular to the diagonal indicate changes in relative left-right activity.

when subdivided, some of the differences are very impressive, suggesting that the groups are indeed homogeneous for some neurophysiological characteristics. Both amplitudes and latencies show differences among groups, and the groups are also significantly different in the *changes* which occur as a result of drug treatment. For example, there *are* significant drug effects on the left parietal amplitudes of Wave VI, as well as on several of the latency measures. Just as with the psychological measures, the grouping procedure has had the effect of revealing drug effects that were obscured in the overall sample.

One of the analyses that was particularly revealing has to do with the question raised earlier of the role of the left and right hemispheres. In order to examine the relative role of the two hemispheres we expressed both latency and amplitude data from the two sides in terms of left/right ratio. The higher the score then, the larger the amplitude or longer the latency on the left side. Analysis of variance showed that the seven groups differed ($p < .001$) very markedly on the ratio of the amplitudes for Wave V in the parietal area: Especially of note is the contrast between group 4, which has a small Wave V amplitude, and group 1 which has a large Wave V amplitude on the right side. Now it will be recalled that group 4 is especially low on Performance IQ and extremely high on the Frostig Test of Visual Perception; while group 1 is average in Performance IQ but low in a number of the spatial-motor tests, such as Frostig figure drawing, Bender Gestalt Test, etc. The groups also differ significantly ($p < .05$) for the parietal amplitudes of Wave VI. These results suggest that the several clinical subgroups may be differing, among other things, in the degree and direction of cerebral dominance.

Finally, we have examined the relationship among all of the psychological test variables and evoked response variables. The pattern of relationships from this large matrix is too complex to describe in detail here. However, it does seem clear from the results that there are a great many more relationships than can be accounted for by chance. And most importantly, the strongest relationships appear to occur with reading, spelling and arithmetic measures. There appear to be a number of highly significant relationships between *changes* in evoked response and changes in the psychological test scores. For example, there are a number of significant relationships between changes in the right parietal latencies, and improvement in arithmetic after stimulant drug treatment. These data will be presented more fully at another time.

In summary, then, we have the following facts:

(1) The stimulant drugs significantly alter test performances for a variety of variables;

(2) These changes are highly predictable from combinations of the test scores themselves, with different patterns of change being predicted from different pretest measures;

(3) The children can be characterized by the similarity of their test profiles, and subdivided into homogeneous groups;

(4) These groups are found to differ, not only in the changes in test scores due to drugs; but also in several parameters of evoked response, especially the late component identified as Wave VI;

(5) Changes in evoked response due to drugs are mainly in the direction of shortened latencies when all groups are considered;

(6) The groups differ on several parameters of the evoked response in terms of left and right hemispheric activity especially amplitudes; and

(7) Several evoked response changes are found to occur in some of the groups that did not appear before the grouping procedures were undertaken.

ACKNOWLEDGMENTS

This study was supported by Grant No. MH 14432 from the Psychopharmacology Section of the National Institute of Mental Health and by Research Scientist Development Award No. K2 MH 7839.

The author wishes to acknowledge the invaluable assistance of Mr. Arthur Applebee who prepared many of the programs for data analysis for the study.

The staff of the Child Development Laboratory, including Drs. Michael Murphy, Gerard Rothschild and Joseph Tecce, Miss Myra Woods and Mr. Daniel Stone all contributed significantly to the studies reported in this paper.

REFERENCES

1. Conners, C. K.: The effect of stimulant drugs on human learnings and performance with special reference to children. In Smith, W. L. (Ed.): *Drugs and Cerebral Function.* Springfield, Thomas, in press.
2. Conners, C. K.: Cortical visual evoked response in children with learning disorders. *Psychophysiology,* 7:418-428, 1971.
3. Sokal, R. R., and Sneath, P. H.: *Principles of Numerical Taxonomy.* San Francisco, W. H. Freeman and Co., 1963.
4. Werry, J. S.: Some clinical and laboratory studies of psychotropic drugs in children: An overview. In Smith, W. L. (Ed.): *Drugs and Cerebral Function.* Springfield, Thomas, 1970.

Chapter 12

School Phobia:
Diagnostic Considerations in the Light
of Imipramine Effects*

RACHEL GITTELMAN-KLEIN AND DONALD F. KLEIN

TYPICALLY, the school phobic child has marked distress both during the approach to school and while in school. The anxiety is reduced drastically by avoidance of school. Difficulties comprise various degrees of psychophysiological upset, such as malaise, nausea, stomach pains, and pallor. In addition, besides the school situation, most of the children experience varying degrees of anxiety from mild discomfort to outright panic, while away from their mothers or from home, e.g. at camp, friends' homes, etc. It has been consistently observed that separation anxiety is a central issue among school phobic children.

Separation anxiety takes various forms. For instance, some children are able to go out freely, provided the mother remains at home accessible to their erratic wishes. However, the children do not tolerate the mother's absence if they themselves remain at home. Here, the child's comfortable adaptation depends on always being able to find his mother should he feel anxious and want to be with her.

Exactly the opposite pattern may occur; the child displays separation anxiety from the home rather than the mother per se. As long as he remains at home, the child does not experience anxiety when separated from the mother. However, he feels anxious away from home, more so if alone, but even in his mother's presence.

A yet further pattern is that of the child who defines a circumscribed area within which he feels comfortable, i.e. a home base. This may consist of a one block area, or infrequently, a much larger radius. Outside the extended home base, the child experiences anxiety, sometimes even if accompanied by a parent. The anxiety may engender the fear of being lost, with the fantasy that he will never find his parents.

Other children do not accept any separation and must be in the mother's presence at all times. In one such extreme case, the child accompanied his mother to her part-time job.

*This paper was supported in part by the National Institute of Mental Health, U.S. Public Health Service Grant no. MH 14514-03.

200

In addition to the primary anxiety occasioned by separation, the child also develops marked anticipatory anxiety and refuses to go to school. The anticipatory fear has a gradient of severity, so that some children will refuse to get dressed for school; others will do so easily, but will refuse to go to school; others will walk to school with their parents and then refuse separation. This school refusal is labeled "school phobia;" however, the diagnostic emphasis should be upon the separation anxiety and secondary anticipatory anxiety, rather than upon the school as a specific phobic object, since these children react negatively to all occasions of separation or inaccessibility to their mother.

STUDY BACKGROUND

Our experience in the treatment of phobic children follows practice previously established with adults. In studies at Hillside Hospital, imipramine was regularly effective in the treatment of agoraphobic adults.[10,12] These patients have been given a number of diagnoses, such as phobic-anxiety syndrome, phobic anxiety depersonalization syndrome, or anxiety neurosis, as well as less justified sobriquets, i.e. pseudoneurotic schizophrenia, borderline syndrome, etc. These patients suffer from inexplicable panic attacks, accompanied by hot and cold flashes, rapid breathing, palpitations, weakness, unsteadiness, a feeling of impending death, and occasional depersonalization. They progressively constrict their activities until they are unable to leave the house independently for fear of being suddenly rendered helpless while isolated from help. Phenothiazine treatment not only does not alleviate this anxiety, but frequently exacerbates it. However, imipramine is remarkably effective in blocking the onset of panic attacks. Detailed investigation revealed that within a group of phobic-anxious adults, two developmental courses were observable. About 50 percent of the patients had been fearful, dependent children, with marked separation anxiety and difficulty in adjusting to school, often consisting of a phobic reaction. Such patients' adult onset of phobic anxiety was frequently precipitated by bereavement, separation, or loss of love object. In other patients, early adjustment was unremarkable, and the adult onset usually occurred in the context of altered endocrine homeostasis.[10]

The finding that some imipramine responsive adult phobic anxiety states are historically linked to a childhood history of separation anxiety led to a trial of imipramine in a childhood school-phobic population. We were interested in investigating whether school-phobic children and phobic-anxious adults might share a common psychopathological process. Therefore, a clinical pilot study of imipramine among such children was initiated.

The pilot study enabled an uncontrolled investigation of the therapeutic efficacy of imipramine. Further, it provided guidelines regarding the feasibility of administering imipramine to an outpatient child clinic population, and relevant dosage requirements. The pilot study,[15] as well as the ensuing double-blind study, were conducted at a large municipal child psychiatric clinic, whose referrals come largely from school personnel.

In the course of the pilot study, twenty-four (86%) of twenty-eight children who completed a six-week drug trial return to school. Dosage varied from 75 to 200 mg per day. The pilot study justified, indeed required, a double-blind, placebo-controlled investigation of the clinical efficacy of imipramine in school-phobic children. So far, only one controlled study of antidepressant chemotherapy, among phobic children, has appeared.[5] Frommer has reported global improvement of thirty-two depressed children, fifteen of whom were phobic, in a double-blind cross-over study of phenelzine-chlordiazepoxide combination and phenobarbital for a two-week period each. The combination of the antidepressant and minor tranquilizer was superior to the sedative. Treatment response for each drug treatment is not presented for the phobic subgroup.

Procedure

The study presented below is ongoing and expected to continue for another year. At this point, we are presenting findings on thirty-five patients who have completed a six-week treatment period of either placebo or imipramine.

Clinical Criteria

Children ages six to fourteen inclusive, classified as follows, were accepted for study: (a) The child is afraid to attend school and completely refused to go to school, has been absent for two weeks, and displays manifest separation anxiety. (b) The child is similar to type (a), but less severe. He may be able to go to school intermittently, or go under great duress and experience severe discomfort while in school. He displays manifest separation anxiety. (c) The third type consists of children who have refused to go to school for at least two weeks; they are afraid of school and clearly phobic. However, they display no separation anxiety.

The inclusion of the third group of children without separation anxiety stemmed from the fact that, while screening, an occasional child showed clear-cut phobic reactions to school, characterized by severe anxiety leading to avoidance behavior, but no reports of separation anxiety could be elicited from the mother or the child. We included these children to determine whether imipramine was effective only when separation anxiety was present, or whether its clinical action was independent of this factor. Parenthetically, since we added this third clinical category, we have had practically no suitable children. Therefore, our hopes of analysing imipramine effect along the separation-anxiety dimension will probably not materialize.

Treatment Program

Children accepted for study were randomly assigned to matching imipramine or placebo pills. The drug assignment was stratified by age and sex so the drug and placebo groups should not differ with regard to these two variables. At baseline, the child was rated on a number of measures; these were repeated after six weeks of treatment. In addition, school attendance and global improvement were rated after three and six weeks of treatment. A complete blood count, urine analysis, and liver profile were obtained prior to giving medication and after a six-week interval.

The treatment program consisted of giving the child medication with dose ranges from 25 to 200 mg per day. Dosage was fixed for the first two weeks: 25 mg for the first three days, 50 mg for the next four days; 75 mg per day during the second week. Thereafter dosage was adjusted weekly. The medication was given in two daily doses, one in the morning, and the other in the evening. At the end of six weeks, dosage ranged from 100 to 200 mg per day (mean = 152 mg /day).

The patient and family were seen weekly. At the beginning of treatment they were told to expect an abatement of fear. The case worker instructed the family to maintain a firm attitude promoting school attendance. The treatment program was also explained to the school personnel with whom the social worker maintained continuous contact so that no discrepancies occurred between our instructions and the school's expectations. In most cases, a family member was advised to accompany the child to school and maintain the child's presence there until there was reduction of the child's anticipatory anxiety that severe discomfort might recur while he was in school, and the child could attend school alone. The treatment recommendations varied depending upon the severity of the anticipatory anxiety, and of the mother's ability to set and enforce limits.

To give an example, upon screening, one child was refusing to get dressed in the morning; if the mother dressed him, he ran out of the house. The mother was felt to be anxious, distraught, and confused in the face of her child's behavior. Therefore, for the first week, the child and mother were instructed that the child was to get ready for school, but no attempt be made to take him to school. The second week he was to get ready and go to school, again without entering the building; this process (essentially one of desensitization) continued gradually, until the child eventually went to school on his own. The steps selected reflect a hierarchy of approach to school, each step causing some anxiety, but to a degree tolerable both to child and mother. Therefore, the overall results of our study represent the effect of a combination of treatments: persuasive and desensitization techniques coupled with either an active drug or a placebo.

Sample

A total of thirty-five children completed the six-week study, nineteen on placebo, sixteen on imipramine. There were nineteen girls and sixteen boys with a mean age of 10.8, range six to fourteen years. The group is not racially typical of the clinic population; only one (3%) was Negro, whereas 50 percent of the referrals at the clinic consist of Negro children. The reasons for this discrepancy are not clear.

All except one were at least within the normal range of intellectual functioning, as estimated by school performance. One girl was attending a class for mentally retarded children.

The distribution of school phobia types was as follows: Type 1, N=23 (11 on placebo and 12 on imipramine); Type 2, N=6 (5 on placebo, 1 on imipramine); Type 3, N=5 (3 on placebo, 2 on imipramine). One child was rated as Type 1 and 3 simultaneously.

Measures

SCHOOL ATTENDANCE. Return to school was the major criterion of change. It was rated by the mother, on a scale from 1 to 7 (Table 12-I), from complete refusal to regular asymptomatic attendance. After six weeks of treatments, only one child received a score reflecting intermittent school attendance; the others either attended regularly or not at all; an outcome distribution that calls for appropriate statistical analysis.

Therefore, for analysis, the scores were dichotomized between "not back to school" and "back to school."

GLOBAL IMPROVEMENT. The children's overall improvement was evaluated by the psychiatrist, mother, and child, after three and six weeks of treatment. This rating reflects a global impression of the degree of change which has taken place. It is recorded on a seven point scale from "Very Much Worse" to "Completely Well." When a therapist makes the judgment, considerations, such as level of anxiety, mood state, interpersonal functioning, and target symptom changes, all enter into consideration.

Mothers asked to evaluate their children's improvement are more likely to take into consideration the child's tractability and manageability in the home both in the process of sending him to school and in situations not related to school. When a mother felt her child was better, she almost invariably reported that he was no longer "nervous," that he was calmer and more relaxed.

When the child rates his own improvement, he is communicating his subjective sense of well-being, and it is difficult to say what accounts for his

TABLE 12-I

SCHOOL ATTENDANCE

	Attends classes regularly—goes by himself and feels comfortable	7
How well has child been doing for the past week	Attends classes regularly—goes by himself with some minor complaints	6
	Attends classes regularly—must be brought to school or else won't go	5
	Occasional absence because afraid to go to school	4
	Frequent refusal to go to school—about 2 days a week	3
Circle correct rating at right	Almost complete refusal to go to school— 3 to 4 days a week	2
	Complete School Refusal	1
	A. Goes to classes if mother stays in principal's office	
	B. Goes to classes if mother stays outside classroom (nearby)	
	C. Goes to classes if mother stays in classroom	
	D. Will not go to classes no matter what arrangements are made	

judgment. When asked why they were better, children, depending on their age, would generally reply that they no longer had "bad feelings," were not scared, were able to go to school, or just felt good.

The manner in which a child's self-rating was obtained varied with the child's level of comprehension. Among older children, the form is shown and read to them to insure that they know its entire contents, and they are asked to fill it out. Younger children are also shown the form; in addition they are interviewed so that the therapist may fill out the form for them. There is no leading of the witness. Statements such as, "I think you're much better, don't you think so?" are never used, nor are the converse. Rather, questioning goes approximately as follows: "Can you remember how you felt when you first came to the clinic?" "Do you feel the same, better, or worse?" If the children says better, further questioning determines how much better.

PSYCHIATRIC RATINGS OF SYMPTOMATOLOGY. In addition to global ratings of school attendance and improvement, children were rated on three instruments by the psychiatrist: a modified version of the Lorr IMPS, where items are scored from 1 to 9, Rutter's Children's Behavior Questionnaire (CBQ)[16] in which items are on a four-point scale, and our own Psychiatric Interview Rating Form (PIRF) which has been devised to record the specific characteristics of this population, but which was not intended as a measure of change, and therefore items are marked present or absent only.

Ten scores were selected for this analysis because of the expectation that they might be affected by imipramine treatment:

Items 1-3 are from the IMPS; 4-7, from the CBQ; 8-10, from the PIRF.

IMPS.

Item   1. Exhibits in his general demeanor or in his verbalization an attitude of self-depreciation, inadequacy, or inferiority.

Cues: talks about faults, failures, or his uselessness to others; belittles what he does.

Item   2. Manifests verbally or in demeanor a dejection or depression in mood and a despondent or despairing attitude.

Cues: says he does not want to talk, complains of loss of interest, enjoyment, lack of energy; discouraged about being helped; expresses lack of hope; may wish he were dead; expects the worst; everything seems flat and stale.

Item   3. One or more specific irrational morbid fears (phobias) of objects persons, or situations. (Avoid confusing phobias with anxieties.)

CBQ.

Item   4. Often worried, worries about many things.

Item   5. Often appears miserable, unhappy, tearful, or distressed.

Item   6. Five items of the Children's Behavior Questionnaire reflect the child's physical complaints.
   a. Complains of headaches.
   b. Complains of abdominal pains.
   c. Complains of nausea or vomiting.
   d. Complains of dizzy spells.
   e. Complains of vague not feeling well or cold symptoms or other aches and pains.

Item   7. Temper tantrums when threatened with separation from family.

PIRF.

Item   8. Child ventures freely without mother.
Child ventures out alone to close-by, familiar areas only.
Child requires mother to accompany him in order for him to leave the house.

Item   9. Does child report physical discomfort when he goes to school?

Item 10. Does child report fear when he goes to school?

Mothers' Ratings of Children's Behavior. Mothers filled out the Children's Behavior Questionnaire[16] at the beginning of treatment and six weeks later. The items are scaled from 1 to 4. Unfortunately, at the beginning of the study the research secretary failed to give the form to some mothers. As a result, the number of subjects for whom a baseline and posttreatment is available is reduced, leading to small N's in each group (12 *Ss* in each group).

Ten items, all felt to reflect aspects of functioning usually associated with phobic disorders, were selected for analysis of drug effects. They are:

Item 1. Often worried, worries about many things.

Item 2. Often appears miserable, unhappy, tearful, or distressed.

Item 3. Tends to be fearful or afraid of new things or new situations.

Item 4. Has had tears on arrival at school or had refused to come into the building for two weeks.

Item 5. Has extreme fear when attempts to go or goes to school.

Item 6. Has extreme fear at separation from family members at all times, including nighttime.

Item 7. Demands to be accompanied by family members in threatening circumstances.

Item 8. Complains at school of missing family and wants to go home.

Item 9. Five items tapping physical complaints were combined to yield a global rating of physical complaints.
   a. Complains of headaches.
   b. Complains of abdominal pains.
   c. Complains of nausea or vomiting.
   d. Complains of dizzy spells.
   e. Complains of vague not feeling well or cold symptoms or other aches and pains.

Item 10. Temper tantrums when threatened with separation from family.

RESULTS

School Attendance

As may be observed in Table 12-II, imipramine was significantly superior to placebo in effectuating a return to school. It is interesting to note that a period of placebo treatment leads to school return in almost 50 percent of the cases. Therefore, using school attendance as a criterion of drug effect, any psychoactive medication would have to be extremely effective to exceed placebo, using samples of fifteen to twenty patients.

TABLE 12-II

SCHOOL ATTENDANCE AFTER SIX WEEKS TREATMENT

(Mothers' Report)

(N = 35)

	Back to School	*Not Back to School*
Placebo	9 (47%)	10 (53%)
Imipramine	13 (81%)	3 (19%)

P < .05, Fisher-Exact, one tailed

The school attendance data were further examined to see whether, among the school returns, those treated with imipramine returned to school sooner than those treated with placebo. Of the nine placebo patients who were in school after six weeks, seven (77%) were back in school after the three-week treatment period. Therefore, it would appear that if parental pressure and a placebo are going to be effective, they will be so relatively quickly. A different pattern emerges among the twelve imipramine treated children who were in school after a six-week treatment period. Among them only six (50%) were in school after three weeks of treatment. It appears, therefore, that a three-week treatment period of imipramine is not distinguishable from placebo, as far as school attendance is concerned, and that a six-week period of active drug treatment is necessary for the child's school attendance to be affected by the drug.

In the school phobia literature much has been said regarding the different psychological meaning of the disturbance in prepuberty versus puberty years. It is generally stated that school phobia is more pathological if it occurs in the later years. On the basis of this assumption it could be anticipated that older children should be refractory to treatment. To test this possibility, we examined the relationship between age and the rate of school return. There was no significant difference in the proportion of children eleven years and less, and those above the age of eleven who returned to school after six weeks of placebo treatment ($X^2 = 0.04$, Yates correction). However, using a *t test* a trend is found in the expected direction (t = 1.68, $.05 < P < .10$, one tailed). A relationship might be observed between school return and age given larger samples. It may be that the relationship between school return and age is further limited in this study by the fact that we did not include children of fifteen years and above. However, it must be noted, that if age is somewhat related to school attendance, it is completely unrelated to global improvement on imipramine treatment.

Global Improvement

For purposes of analysis, scores of "Slightly Worse," "No Change," and "Slightly Improved" were combined as were the "Much Improved" and "Completely Well" ratings. No child was rated "Definitely" or "Very Much Worse."

As may be noted in Tables 12-III, 12-IV, and 12-V, the psychiatrists, mothers, and children all reported significantly greater improvement among

TABLE 12-III

PSYCHIATRISTS' RATINGS OF GLOBAL IMPROVEMENT
AFTER SIX WEEKS OF TREATMENT*

	No Change and Slightly Better	Much Improved
Placebo	13 (68%) †	6 (32%)
Imipramine	4 (27%)	11 (73%)

P < .025, Fisher-Exact Test, one tailed.
*N of thirty-four reflects missing ratings of 1 S on imipramine.
†One child rated "slightly worse" included.

TABLE 12-IV
MOTHERS' RATINGS OF GLOBAL IMPROVEMENT
AFTER SIX WEEKS OF TREATMENT*

	No Change and Slightly Better	Much Improved
Placebo	11 (58%)	8 (42%)
Imipramine	2 (13%)	13 (87%)

P < .01 Fisher-Exact, one tailed.
*N of thirty-four reflects missing ratings of 1 S on imipramine.

TABLE 12-V
CHILDREN'S SELF-RATINGS OF IMPROVEMENT*

	No Change and Slightly Better	Much Improved
Placebo	15 (79%)	4 (21%)
Tofranil	0 (0%)	15 (100%)

P < .005, Fisher-Exact, one tailed.
*N of thirty-four reflects missing ratings of 1 S on imipramine.

the imipramine group. The degree of perceived improvement, however, varies among raters, the children on imipramine all reporting they had been much improved.

Among the placebo-treated children, a few felt they had remained the same, most felt slightly better, few felt much better.

To see to what extent return to school is associated with the children's reports of feeling better, the school attendance and the self-rating of improvement were jointly examined (Table 12-VI), revealing interesting patterns of improvement. Though children receiving imipramine all reported feeling better, this improvement was not always associated with school return.

TABLE 12-VI
RELATIONSHIP BETWEEN SCHOOL RETURN AND SELF-RATINGS
OF IMPROVEMENT
(N = 34)

	Back to School and Feeling Better	Back to School but not Feeling Better	Not Back to School but Feeling Better	Not Back to School and not Feeling Better
Placebo (N = 19)	4	5	0	10
Imipramine (N = 15) *	12	0	3	0

*Self-ratings of 1 S missing.

The picture presented by the placebo-treated children is markedly different. Relatively few reported feeling better (4, 21%), but a larger proportion (9, 47%) went back to school. Therefore, feeling better is not a necessary condition for school return since five (26%) of the children went back to school in spite of the fact that they reported no overall improvement.

The small number of subjects within each type does not allow for statistical analyses of the relationship between this variable and improvement.

Self-Ratings of Improvement after Three and Six Weeks of Treatment

Having established that after a six week-period imipramine is significantly superior to placebo, the question arises as to whether imipramine has similar therapeutic efficacy after a three-week period. The three-week self-ratings of children who rated themselves as "Much Improved" after six weeks of treatment were examined regardless of which treatment they had received. Of the four patients on placebo who felt much better at the six week point, two already felt much better at three weeks; one felt slightly better. Among the eleven patients on imipramine who felt much better after six weeks of treatment, only three reported feeling much better after three weeks of drug intake. Therefore, drug and placebo are indistinguishable after three weeks, and a six-week treatment period seems necessary to elicit the drug's true effect. The difference between three and six weeks may be similar to that in depression where frequently improvement requires several weeks from the beginning of drug intake. On the other hand, the difference might be dosage-related rather than time-related since patients were taking less medication at three weeks (mean daily dose = 107 mg; range: 75-125 mg/d) compared to six weeks (mean daily dose = 152 mg; range: 100-200 mg/d). This difference in dosage is unavoidable since careful medical practice prevents the prescription of sudden high doses of imipramine, since some patients may be sensitive to the drug and have behavioral side-effects, such as motor restlessness, jitteriness, flight of ideas, etc. on too rapid drug initiation. As described in the study procedure, to prevent the occurrence of too rapid over-prescription, the dosage prescribed cannot exceed 75 mg/day over the first two-week period. It is only during the third week of treatment that the psychiatrist is free to prescribe as much as he wants, up to a maximum limit of 200 mg per day. However, he is unlikely to increase the dose suddenly within a one-week period. Interestingly, the cautionary guidelines are derived from data on imipramine treatment of adults. None of the children in the study displayed drug sensitivity, and our procedures may be over-conservative for this population.

In conclusion, given the usual precautions necessary in dosage increments, an imipramine effect in self-perceived overall improvement cannot be detected after three weeks of treatment, but is clearly present after six weeks.

Psychiatric Ratings of Symptomatology

The pretreatment and posttreatment differences of the psychiatrist-rated scale items were analyzed by means of Mann-Whitney U tests. Of the eight items thus analyzed, three significantly favored imipramine:

Item 2, from the Lorr, IMPS, reflecting observable depression ($p < 01$, one tailed).

Item 3, from the Lorr, IMPS, reflecting the severity of phobic behavior ($p < .01$, one tailed).

Item 8, from the PIRF ($p < .025$, one tailed), reflecting the child's venturesomeness from the mother.

Group comparisons of posttreatment ratings of two psychiatric ratings from the PIRF (Items 9 and 10) rated "present" or "absent" were done by chi square analyses. For this analysis, only scores of children rated at baseline to have physical distress, and fear before going to school were included; the expectation being that significantly less complaints of physical distress and fear would be present after treatment in the imipramine group.

At baseline, twenty-nine of the thirty-four children rated (post data missing on one S) reported experiencing physical distress when going, or trying to go, to school; five denied it; of these, three were in the imipramine, two in placebo groups. All children reported being afraid when going to or trying to go to school. The unanimous report of fear is to be expected since children must be afraid of school to be accepted in the study.

Tables 12-VII and 12-VIII summarize the results. As may be noted, both physical complaints and fear before going to school are significantly reduced by imipramine ($p < .005$ and $< .02$, respectively, Fisher-Exact Test, one tailed).

TABLE 12-VII

POSTTREATMENT PSYCHIATRIC RATINGS OF PHYSICAL COMPLAINTS
AMONG CHILDREN WITH PHYSICAL COMPLAINTS AT BASELINE
(N = 29)

	Present	Absent
Placebo (N = 16)	11	5
Imipramine (N = 13)	2	11

P < .005, Fisher-Exact, one tailed.

Mothers' Ratings of Children's Behavior

The pretreatment and posttreatment differences of the ten items from the mothers' ratings were analyzed by means of Mann-Whitney U tests.

TABLE 12-VIII

POSTTREATMENT PSYCHIATRIC RATINGS OF REPORTED FEAR
WHEN GOING TO SCHOOL

(N = 32)

	Present	*Absent*
Placebo (N = 17)	12	5
Imipramine (N = 15)	4	11

P < .02, Fisher-Exact, one tailed.

Only one item differed significantly between two groups indicating a lessening of depression among the imipramine-treated children, compared to those on placebo (p = .05, one tailed).

The other items reflecting various aspects of phobic behavior were not drug-sensitive. Many of the items are too specific, leading to a low prevalence of children rated as pathological within each category. Due to the low frequency of most ratings, all the items tapping separation anxiety and fearful reactions were summed (mothers' Children's Behavior Questionnaire, Items 1, 3, 4, 5, 6, 7, 8, 10). The predifference and postdifference of the summed scores between the two treatments is significant at the .05 level (U test, one tailed). Therefore, imipramine does appear to affect the child's phobic anxiety; however, it is difficult to demonstrate this effect since placebo treatment coupled with other therapeutic interventions is also relatively effective. Thus, of the twelve children on placebo, six (50%) had lower scores after treatment; however, of the 12 children on imipramine, eleven (92%) had lower scores (p < .04, Fisher-Exact, one tailed).

Side Effects

Side effects were recorded on a standard form at every visit. Of the sixteen patients on double-blind imipramine treatment, three (19%) had no side effects during the six-week treatment period. Among the nineteen placebo patients, ten (53%) reported no side effects.

The difference between the number of patients with side effects differs significantly between the placebo and drug-treated groups (p < .025, Fisher-Exact Test, one tailed). Further, when placebo-treated children report side effects, they report fewer than children treated with imipramine.

As noted in Table 12-IX, a total of thirty-three side effects were elicited; eight of these (nos. 1-8) were found in the placebo group only. Some of them may reflect complaints associated with the patient's presenting problems that may be interpreted as side effects. It might therefore be useful to obtain a list of complaints at baseline, recorded on a side effects form, to see whether the so-called treatment emergent symptoms are being accurately evaluated.

TABLE 12-IX
SIDE EFFECTS REPORTED ANYTIME DURING
SIX-WEEK DOUBLE-BLIND TREATMENT
(N = 35)

		Placebo (N = 19)		Tofranil® (N = 16)	
		N	%	N	%
1.	Excitement	1	5	0	0
2.	Irritability	1	5	0	0
3.	Abdominal Cramps	1	5	0	0
4.	Epigastric Pains	1	5	0	0
5.	Heartburn	1	5	0	0
6.	Headache	1	5	0	0
7.	Blurred Vision	1	5	0	0
8.	Hiccups	1	5	0	0
9.	Nightmares	1	5	2	6
10.	Anorexia	3	16	2	12
11.	Indigestion	1	5	2	12
12.	Insomnia	6	31	1	6
13.	Dry Mouth*	1	5	8	50*
14.	Bad Taste	2	11	1	6
15.	Constipation	1	5	5	31
16,	Increased Appetite	1	5	2	12
17.	Drowsiness	6	31	10	62
18.	Dizziness	2	11	4	25
19.	Nausea	2	11	3	19
20.	Nasal Congestion	0	0	1	6
21.	Muscle Pains	0	0	1	6
22.	Urinary Frequency	0	0	1	6
23.	Apathetic	0	0	1	6
24.	Hypotension	0	0	1	6
25.	Vomiting	0	0	1	6
26.	Mild Tremor	0	0	3	19
27.	Tired	0	0	1	6
28.	Weight Loss	0	0	1	6
29.	Gastrointestinal Pains	0	0	1	6
30.	Fever	0	0	1	6
31.	Flushed Face	0	0	1	6
32.	Sweating	0	0	2	12
33.	Listlessness	0	0	1	6

*Treatment difference, p < .003, Fisher—Exact, one tailed.

From Table 12-IX it appears that complaints of dry mouth, constipation, dizziness, and tremor (Nos. 13, 15, 18 and 26) are more prevalent among the imipramine subjects. Sixty-two percent of the imipramine children reported feeling drowsy, but so did 31% of the placebo-treated children. The side effect of dry mouth is the only one which is found significantly more often in the drug group (p < .005, Fisher-Exact Test, one tailed). The difference between placebo and imipramine for the other three side effects just misses significance. A side effect found in one subject only deserves mention. Orthostatic hypotension was significant in a girl treated with 125 mg/day of imipramine; it subsided when the dose was reduced to 100 mg. After a few days the drug dosage was raised to 150 mg without any further hypotension. This is the only double-blind imipramine case which required dosage adjustment because of interfering side effects; other side effects disappeared without any dose alterations.

On the whole, our experience indicates remarkably little difficulty resulting from side effects in using relatively large doses of imipramine in an outpatient group of children.

Blood Tests

Blood tests and urinalyses were performed prior to drug administration and after six weeks of treatment.

Blood analyses include CBC and liver profiles. In addition, we have been taking positional blood pressures and EKG's. The exact values of the above procedures have not been analyzed; however, a perusal of the data reveals no abnormality using generally applied clinical guidelines.

COMMENT

This study establishes that imipramine is superior to placebo in the treatment of school phobic children between the ages of six to fourteen years. Using school return as a measure of drug effects, the superiority of the drug just achieves statistical significance $(p < .05)$. However, this does not indicate a minor drug effect, but rather the fact that with a major placebo effect, only large drug effects can be detected in samples between fifteen to twenty subjects. Imipramine induced school return in 81 percent of the children; placebo, in 47 percent. If a 34 percent difference in efficacy truly exists between the two treatments, seven out of ten study replications would detect it even using our small sample sizes.

By Cohen's[2] standards, a large treatment effect has an "h" index of .80, whereas a medium effect is characterized by an "h" of .50. The "h" index in this study is .73 indicating a sizeable drug effect.

Using global ratings of improvement, especially the children's self-ratings, the superiority of imipramine is marked. In view of our findings, the drug's action cannot be viewed as one which automatically leads to renewed school attendance. Rather, it has to be seen as modifying the child's self-perception probably because of an alteration of mood state and experience of panic attacks. This change may enable the child to return to the classroom; however, the maintenance of strong anticipatory anxiety may block this action. The case of one child who was much improved on imipramine but refused to go to school is given illustratively: Mark had separation anxiety, morbid concern about his mother, numerous compulsive habits, and had had difficulty attending school throughout his school career. Absences had been frequent, but the child had never refused to go to school over any length of time. In September, 1969, Mark entered junior high school. He was beaten up twice on his way to school, for no apparent reasons, by unknown groups of older children. Mark developed an obsessive preoccupation with the possibility of violence and completely refused to go to school. When he entered the study he was rated as Type 1 (separation anxiety), as well as Type 3 (school phobia independent of separation anxiety).

During the course of study treatment, Mark received imipramine and became completely free of separation anxiety, felt much less anxious in general, but retained a morbid obsessional fear of the possibility of being beaten up in school and was unable to return to school. He was eventually hospitalized in an effort to mobilize him.

Therefore, return to school is a complex behavior related to factors independent of drug effect. Some of these factors probably consist of anticipatory anxiety, the school's attitude toward the child, the parents' management of the child, the nature of the psychotherapeutic contact, etc.

In addition to the controlled report by Frommer,[6] a recent clinical report of antidepressants among phobic depressive children by the same author, corroborates the usefulness of this drug type.[6] Frommer favors MAO inhibitors versus tricyclics. However, the dosages reported for the two drugs are not equivalent. Regular adult doses of MAOI (Phenelzine, 45 mg/day) were used, but imipramine dosage was far below that which we found effective. Thus, the effects of 60 mg/day for children of at least ten years of age are reported, with lower doses among younger children; our lowest dose was 100 mg/day. In our experience, doses below 100 mg/day are indistinguishable from placebo, given an extensive nonpharmacological therapeutic program. In view of the greater risk involved in the use of MAO inhibitors, a tricyclic antidepressant is felt to be the drug of choice. Since we observed a 100 percent rate of improvement with imipramine, the MAO inhibitors could only be useful in the rare exception who might not respond adequately to imipramine treatment. A recent British article[9] reports uncontrolled results of MAO inhibitors among a large group of adult phobic patients. The rate of improvement fall far below that found by Klein in a placebo-controlled double-blind study of imipramine in the same population.[10] The discrepancy in therapeutic effectiveness between imipramine and the MAO inhibitors is further support for recommending the former. Frommer's viewpoint regarding dosage reflects the persisting notion that age should be a guide to dose levels in child psychopharmacology. There is no evidence to support such an assumption. Though we have found no child who responded to doses of less than 75 mg/day, children vary widely in their response to imipramine beyond this level. In one instance, during drug follow-up, dosage had to be increased from 200 mg to 300 mg/day in a twelve-year-old child who had been stabilized, but was relapsing. The effect of the added dosage was dramatic; medication was later reduced to 200 mg again, but had to be raised to 250 mg. In this case 250 mg appeared to be the minimum stabilizing dose. Age has not been one of our useful criteria for determining dosage level. As a matter of fact, no criterion seems to be clearly relevant.

In the same article referred to above[6] recent onset and early morning awakening are positive prognostic signs; in our work, length of illness is not related to treatment response, and only one child had early awakening. It must be noted that only three of sixteen children did not return to school on imipramine. Further, all these children reported being much improved. In dealing with so few treatment failures, it is unlikely that reliable criteria of variation in treatment response will be found. More relevant is a study of treatment response to placebo since greater variation in outcome was observed in this group.

The return to school of placebo-treated children who feel better is easily understood. However, it is difficult to identify the causes of school return among children who do not feel improved. Here again, a number of variables are probably involved. Our assessment of parent attitudes made by the social worker at the beginning of treatment are not helpful, since, except for one exception, all parents were rated as wanting the child back in school. This is hardly surprising since the treatment program is voluntary, and no external threats exist such as court actions, as is often the case in truancy or other antisocial behavior.

As mentioned, in the age range studied, age was not a statistically significant factor, though it might be so if children fifteen years and above were included. The fact that older children tend to remain out of school, but that they improve just as much as younger children is further indication that school return partly depends upon nondrug factors. In the case of the older children, the parent cannot be used as forcefully in getting the child to school. As a result, successful treatment depends to a larger degree upon the patient's cooperation, rather than the parents. Therefore, the tendency for older children to fail in a treatment program does not necessarily indicate greater psychopathology. Length of illness was not contributory either in predicting return to school. We plan to examine other familial and patient characteristics, such as child's motivation and parents' marital accord, to search for clues as to what factors may play a role in school return among placebo-treated patients.

Eisenberg[4] reports a greater rate of success in return to school than was found in this study, using essentially the same therapeutic procedures without pharmacological treatment (72% versus 47%). However, a large group of the children were preschoolers; comparing this study's nineteen placebo patients who received weekly individual psychotherapy, parental counseling, and school casework, to Eisenberg's fifteen children above the age of six years, it appears that we were less successful than Eisenberg in getting the elementary school age children back in school. The success rates of both studies are equivalent for the older age group.

The results obtained in the placebo group of this study are consonant with those reported by Hersov[7] in fifty youngsters between the ages of seven and sixteen. Forty-eight percent returned to school within six months of treatment comparable to ours and Eisenberg's; another 20 percent resumed school attendance between seven and twelve months of therapy. No age-outcome relationship was found. In the absence of restrictions because of research designs, school phobic children are treated for much longer periods of time. Obviously, rates of success derived from six weeks versus months or years of treatment are not comparable.

Frommer refers to children such as the ones described in this study as phobic depressives, since they show "typical" depressive symptoms of weepiness, tension, explosiveness, and instability. However, she goes on to point out that to the lay observers and to themselves, the children do not appear depressed.[5,6] Why Frommer considers the above symptoms more characteristic of depression than of other psychiatric syndromes such as tension states, hysterical episodes, emotional instablity, etc., is not clear.

We have found that, as a group, the children are not depressed, using the definition of depression which emphasizes inability to experience pleasure and a sense of incompetence.[11] Many of the children do weep easily; they may be explosive and irritable, but only in the context of threatened or actual separation. When no demands for independent functioning are exerted, they can enjoy themselves and may be active, capable, and gregarious. Many children restrict their peer interaction and seem "withdrawn." However, for the most part, retreat from peer groups is manifest during the school year only. During summer months the children are active and show no aversion to being with their peers. Our impression is that the children are concerned about having to justify their school absences, and therefore avoid being with their friends to avoid any possible embarrassment. Thus, the social withdrawal of phobic children, when it occurs, appears to be largely an attitudinal change due to the anxiety-producing qualities of the peer situation, rather than the secondary manifestations of a depressed mood state.

Of the thirty-four children rated by the psychiatrist, twelve were rated as quite depressed (IMPS, Item 2, Manifests verbally or in demeanor or dejection or depression in mood and a despondent or despairing attitude, scores 6-9). Yet, a crucial distinction between this sample of phobic children and depressed adults is that none of the children had lost the capacity to anticipate pleasure or lost all sense of competence. Remarkably, almost all children had the conviction that somehow, at some point in the future, the next day or next week, they would miraculously be able to attend school without any difficulty. The conviction that everything will turn out well (often referred to as magical thinking in children) is singularly lacking among depressed adults; for that matter, its presence would preclude a psychiatric diagnosis of depression.

Therefore, though depression appears in a good proportion of phobic children (about 30% in our sample), the characteristic pessimism and anhedonia of the adult depressive is not a predominant clinical factor. Therefore, it seems erroneous to us to equate these children's disorder with that of the adult depressions.

Our treatment of school phobia was prompted by the knowledge that imipramine was useful to adult agoraphobes, whose retrospective histories revealed a high prevalence of childhood phobic disorders. The clinical picture of the phobic children resembles that of the adult agoraphobes, but also differs from it in important ways. Like the adults with a history of childhood separation anxiety, almost all the children's onset (28 of 35) could be related to bereavement, illness, or some object losses. However, unexplained, out of the blue, sudden panic attacks do not seem to occur in children as they do in adults. Thus, the child may become panicky if separation is attempted; however, panic never occurs outside the context of separation. Among adult agoraphobes, panics are markedly reduced by the presence of a companion or by being at home, but are not eliminated.

The constant possibility of a panic episode regardless of the external circumstances is clearly not true for the children. We have seen only one child, aged fourteen, who seems identical to adult agoraphobes. Further, the panic experienced by the phobic children seems physiologically different from that reported by adult agoraphobes. The children do not report getting dizzy, faint, or depersonalized; there are no palpitations with a feeling of impending death. On the other hand the children frequently experience stomachaches, which are not reported by adults. It may be that children and adults are undergoing the same initial stages of their disorders, but that the children's physiological makeup has not matured to a point which allows for the adult process to take place, leading to a different phenomenological experience.

In any case, just as school phobias cannot be conceived of as miniature depressions, they cannot be viewed as miniature phobic anxiety states. Their symptomatology and treatment responses are related to the adult depressive states and obviously to adult phobic states, but they do not appear to be identical phenomenologically or psychophysiologically. From cross-section evaluation it is impossible to obtain conclusive evidence regarding the significance of a disorder. Only long-term studies of phobic children can elucidate to what degree this childhood disorder is a precursor to adult depressive disorders or adult anxiety syndromes.

The fact that only one child was Negro, given that 50 percent of the clinical population is Negro is puzzling. Marks reports that adult agoraphobes come from stable families.[13] Others have also commented on the fact that phobic children come from homes where the mothers are close-knit. This has certainly been our observation as well. It might be argued that the socio-familial environment among lower class Negroes who form the bulk of the clinic patient population does not provide the type of setting which favors the development of pathological attachment to the parent or the home. This possiblity might deserve examination if it had been clearly demonstrated that, compared to other groups, families of phobic children are more child-oriented, foster to a greater degree the child's dependence on the family, and that the mothers or fathers of phobic children experience greater anxiety at separation from their offsprings.

One study[7] compared various parental and familial characteristics of three patient groups: two groups of school refusers who had been out of school for at least two months (one group showed a preference for staying home, the other consisted of truants), and a control group of random clinic cases without school refusal and gross brain damage. The first group is equated with school phobia. The results support the hypothesis that the families of phobic children are most stable in that the children in this group experienced less extended separation from their parents. Further, the mothers of the phobic children were rated as being less rejecting and more overprotective. However, the groups were not equivalent for social class, the phobic group being significantly superior; further the phobic children had higher I.Q's and had fewer siblings compared to the truant group. In addition, the ratings were not made without the knowledge of the child's group membership possibly leading to bias, especially with regard to ratings of parental attitudes. It has been noted that child-rearing practices differ in various social classes. Therefore, it is conceivable that much of the variance observed among the groups could be because of this factor. In a further controlled study, Hersov describes three patterns of parental management: (a) overindulgent mother and an inadequate passive father, (b) a severe controlling mother and a passive father and (c) a firm controlling father and an overindulgent mother.[8]

In the absence of adequate controlled comparisons, impressions, though they may eventually prove of scientific value, remain only interesting anec-

dotal evidence. Thus, as mentioned, our observations of the family are consonant with those of others regarding the fact that a large proportion of the
families functioned as a total unit. The parents rarely went out without
their children, and only if necessary. If the mother worked, most often she
did so during school hours only and had stopped working when the child
started having difficulties. On the whole, the feeling was that the children
were included in all the family's social activities, and that much of the parents' satisfaction was derived from being with their children.

However, one of us spent three years working with outpatient psychotic
children of similar ages, and exactly the same impression had been noted at
the time. The groups are not strictly comparable since it can be argued
that in the psychotic group, families need to be extremely attached to their
offspring to tolerate the severely disruptive influence of the psychotic member. In any case, the experience of working intensively with such differing
pathological groups has led to a skeptical attitude toward conclusions regarding parental characteristics based upon uncontrolled, biased observations. The limited number of controlled studies dealing with this issue in
children with a variety of characteristics certainly underlines the need for
avoiding premature closure concerning what type of parent is associated
with what type of child.

Another possible hypothesis regarding the low prevalence of Negroes in
our sample is that schools may not respond to a Negro child's school refusal in
the same manner as to that of a white child. A nonwhite child who is not in
school may be stereotyped as a truant by the school personnel and may never
come to the attention of psychiatric clinics. We know of no epidemiological
surveys conducted through bureaus of attendance investigating this
problem.

Several theories of the mechanisms underlying separation anxiety and
phobic behavior have been postulated. Therapeutic interventions are bound
to be determined by the theoretical model adhered to. A large body of
psychoanalytic writing traces the dynamic origin of phobic symptoms and
separation anxiety to such concepts as the sexual significance of the school
resulting from symbolic displacement of libidinal impulses, or the destructive hostile fantasies harbored toward the parents.[14] Such a model calls for
treatment of the child with the goal of resolving intrapsychic conflicts. Another formulation is that the mother transmits to the child her own anxiety
about separation and individuation. Eisenberg[3] who is closely associated
with this view recommends therefore that the child be separated immediately from the mother since the origin of the conflict does not lie in the
child, but in the parent. In addition, he recommends parental counseling to
alter the families' attitudes and anxieties regarding separation.

On the other hand, it has also been suggested that separation anxiety is a biological phenomenon whose evolutionary significance lies in eliciting care and retrieval from the mothering figure.[1,11] It might be argued that wide constitutional variations can occur in the threshold of such a biological mechanism. In this context, severe separation anxiety may be seen as a pathological manifestation of a normal biological developmental process, around which secondary anxieties may be learned. If such were the case, one would expect relatively little alteration of the biological anxiety threshold via verbal or management therapeutic efforts; though the adaptive mechanisms used by the child to cope with the anxiety could be expected to change as a result of various external interventions.

Our design does not allow for clarification of the issues suggested by the psychoanalytic models since no attempt was made to deal with the children's unconscious fantasies. However, our results challenge the model which posits an extrinsic source of anxiety, i.e. it is not the child's anxiety but his family's which is at the root of his refusal to separate from his mother. If parental handling were the crucial variable, no significant difference in improvement between placebo and imipramine should have been noted since parents in both groups received identical counseling. This counseling was effective in getting almost 50 percent of the placebo-treated children back to school; but if one considers the children's feelings of well-being, it did not "work."

Therefore, our results give support to the notion of the presence of a pathological process intrinsic to the child. Whether this process represents a variant of normal biological separation anxiety, or a specific mood disorder coupled with anxiety, is unknown. It could be that the genesis lies in the parental relationship, and that the disorder develops functional autonomy.

In our study, all parents received counseling; therefore we do not know what the value of imipramine would be in treating school phobia without this ancillary treatment. Our impression is that parental cooperation is essential; with imipramine alone, we might have many happy stay-at-home children since anticipatory anxiety might continue to prevent the children from returning to school. Therefore, we see imipramine as instrumental in reducing the primary anxiety, and the parental pressure as forcing the child to venture into danger and by extinction obtain relief from the secondary or anticipatory anxiety.

It has become a platitude to state that both nature and nurture are important in mental illness; this patient group does not escape this truism.

SUMMARY

The results of a double-blind, placebo-controlled study of the effects of imipramine among thirty-five school phobic children between the ages of six and fourteen are reported. The children and families were given a multidiscipline treatment program, concurrently with imipramine or placebo treatment. Imipramine, over a six-week period, was found to be significantly superior to placebo in inducing school return and in global therapeutic efficacy. Doses of medication ranged from 100 to 200 mg/day after six weeks of treatment.

It was found that imipramine effects could not be detected after three weeks of therapy, but were clearly present after six weeks. Of ten items rated by the psychiatrists at baseline and after six weeks of treatment, four which reflect the severity of the child's phobic behavior, the child's venturesomeness from the mother, physical symptoms while going to school, and fear of going to school were significantly improved by imipramine treatment.

Among ten items by mothers, only one reflecting depressive mood showed a significant drug effect. On the whole, side effects were not significant, and only one child required dosage alteration because of orthostatic hypotension.

The diagnostic characteristics of this population are discussed. Further, the relevance of the findings to theories of school phobia is examined.

ACKNOWLEDGMENTS

The study was made possible by the assistance and active involvement of the social worker, Miss Patricia Tierney, and Drs. Albert Buytendorp, Irwin Potkewitz, and Kishore Saraf who treated and evaluated the children. We are thankful to Dr. Charles J. Rabiner, Director of Queens General Hospital Psychiatric Services, and Dr. Sol Nichtern, Director of Children's Services, Hillside Hospital for their helpful cooperation.

Geigy Pharmaceuticals kindly provided us with matching imipramine and placebo medication.

REFERENCES

1. Bowlby, J.: Separation anxiety: A critical review of the literature. *J Child Psychol Psychiat, 1*:251, 1960.
2. Cohen, J.: *Statistical Power Analysis for the Behavioral Science.* New York, Academic Press, 1969.
3. Eisenberg, L.: School phobia: A study in the communication of anxiety. *Amer J Psychiat, 114*:712, 1958.
4. Eisenberg, L.: The pediatric management of school phobia. *J Pediat, 55*:758, 1959.
5. Frommer, E. A.: Treatment of childhood depression with antidepressant drugs. *Brit J Med., 1*:729, 1967.
6. Fromer, E. A.: Depressive illness in childhood. *Brit J Psychiat, Special Publication, No. 2:* 117, 1968.
7. Hersov, L. A.: Refusal to go to school. *Child Psychol Psychiat, 1*:137, 1960.
8. Hersov, L. A.: Persistent non-attendance at school. *Child Psychol Psychiat, 1*:130, 1960.
9. Kelly, D., Guirguis, W., Frommer, E., Mitchell-Heggs, N., and Sargant, W.: Treat-

ment of phobic states with antidepressants: A retrospective study of 246 patients. *Brit J Psychiat, 116:*387, 1970.

10. Klein, D. F.: Delineation of two drug-responsive anxiety syndromes. *Psychopharmacologia, 5:*397, 1964.
11. Klein, D. F., and Davis, J. H.: *Diagnosis and Drug Treatment of Psychiatric Disorders.* Baltimore, Williams and Wilkins, 1969.
12. Klein, D. F., and Fink, M.: Psychiatric reaction patterns to imipramine. *Amer J Psychiat, 119:*432, 1962.
13. Marks, I. M.: *Fears and Phobias.* New York, Academic Press, 1969.
14. Prince, G. S.: School phobia. In Miller, E., (Ed.) : *Foundations of Child Psychiatry.* London, Pergamon Press, 1968, p. 413.
15. Rabiner, C. J., and Klein, D. F.: Imipramine treatment of school phobia. *Compr Psychiat, 10:*387, 1969.
16. Rutter, M.: A children's behavior questionnaire for completion by teachers. *J Child Psychol Psychiat, 8:*1, 1967.

Chapter 13

The Drug Treatment of Childhood Psychosis

DAVID M. ENGELHARDT, POLIZOES POLIZOS, AND REUBEN A. MARGOLIS

IT IS DIFFICULT to estimate the extent to which modern antipsychotic
agents are being used with psychotic children. A sampling of the literature
involving both published articles and abstracts from the National Clearinghouse, encompassing over three thousand children, indicates that only 7
percent of the drug-treated children were labeled as "psychotic." By far,
the largest group of children, 40 percent, were identified as "neurotic" or
"behavior disorders;" 19 percent were labeled as "enuretics;" 15 percent
might best be identified as "organic;" 13 percent, as "retarded," and 5 percent as "hyperkinetic."

It is extremely difficult to interpret the findings presented in the literature. There are very few systematic controlled studies of pharmacotherapy
with schizophrenic children. Populations are highly heterogeneous. In many
studies the sample reported on involves no more than ten to twenty children.
This small sample may include within it as many as five different diagnostic
categories; ages may range from two to twenty; duration of treatment of the
individual patients may vary from two weeks to two years. In some articles
populations are so poorly defined that it is impossible to ascertain whether
the study deals with inpatients or outpatients. Results are generally presented as if the group were homogeneous. Outcome ratings are global in
nature.

Despite these shortcomings in the literature, the reader is impressed with
the consistency with which the published reports reflect a conviction on the
part of authors that pharmacotherapy with children is safe and clinically
effective.

On the issue of safety, there are two relevant review articles by Davis
et al.[1] and McKown et al.[2] dealing with overdosage of psychotropic drugs.
Both articles deal primarily with overdosage in adults, but provide data with
respect to some four hundred children. The toxicity data was derived from
a review of the literature and the Poison Control Branch of the National
Clearinghouse. The data is highly reassuring.

On the whole, fewer children than adults required hospitalization after
overdosage, and fewer children than adults manifested symptoms as a result
of excessive drug ingestion. A major exception to this statement was the
symptom of drowsiness, which was relatively more frequent in children than
adults after ingestion of chlorpromazine, promazine, prochlorperazine, and

hydroxyzine. Promazine ingestion also lead to coma and convulsions more often in children than in adults, and chlorpromazine, more often to convulsions and extrapyramidal symptoms (EPS).

Rather large overdoses of the tranquilizing drugs can be survived by children, especially with proper clinical management. Reported fatalities are extremely rare despite extremely high dosage. Overdosage with antipsychotic agents is clearly less hazardous than with the antidepressants and some of the minor tranquilizers.

Almost all of the antipsychotic agents commonly used with adult schizophrenics were reported as being used with schizophrenic children, including the more recently introduced drugs, such as haloperidol and thiothixene. Dosages, with the exception of fluphenazine, tended to approximate the recommended dosage for adults as given in the package inserts. Reports of clinical effectiveness tend to be positive over this wide range of medications and dosages.

Our interest in pharmacotherapy of children has been concerned exclusively with outpatients, and primarily with psychotic children. Diagnostically these children would be labeled "childhood schizophrenia" or "early infantile autism." Clinically the children we have been working with are among the sickest children seen in psychiatric practice and are indistinguishable from similarly diagnosed children residing in mental institutions.

The children ranged in ages from 4.5 to eleven years, with a mean age of seven. The ratio of boys to girls was four to one. About 50 percent of the children were colored. The parents' social class was between Classes III and V. A significant proportion of children came from broken homes, about 25 percent.

The most consistent problems present in all children were disturbances of speech and communication, mood, attention and concentration, relatedness to peers and to people in general, and motor activity.

Forty percent of the children did not use words; most of these made sounds; only 6 percent approximated being mute. Forty percent were also rated as completely uncommunicative, both verbally and nonverbally. Although 60 percent of the children used words, phrases, and even full sentences, less than 10 percent were rated as having "always relevant and appropriate use of language." Those children with speech presented peculiarities of language, such as echolalia, delayed echolalia, rambling, pronominal reversals, and in general, uncommunicative vocalizations.

Mood disturbances ranged from apathy with severe flattened and constricted affect (present in a few children) to unpredictable, extremely labile, and grossly inappropriate affect display (present in most children).

Disturbances of attention and concentration ranged from mild distractability with short attention span to almost complete lack of attention and ability to concentrate.

All children had disturbances of interpersonal relationships. The childrens' social interactions were characterized by lack of eye contact and aloofness and indifference to the poor of obliviousness.

All children showed disturbances of motor activity; the majority showed hyperkinesis ranging from mild to extremely uncontrollable. Some children showed destructive behavior, assaultiveness, and self-mutilation.

The majority of children showed disturbances of sleeping, eating habits, and severe handicaps in self-management, such as dressing, washing, and toileting.

All children, with only one exception, functioned at a retarded level; three quarters of them were either not testable or severely retarded.

A general physical and neurological examination performed by a pediatric neurologist was part of the initial evaluation. The physical examination revealed no abnormalities except for one child who showed some features of the Teacher Collins syndrome, and another, of achondroplasia. Stigmata of other types were observed; predominant among these were assorted café au lait spots, telangiectasia, abnormalities of fingers and toes, including syndactyly, unusual spacing of large and small toes, abnormalities of the shapes of digits, over-sized and shovel incisors, uneven dentition, late shed of primary teeth, gum overgrowth, and geographic tongue. Asymmetrical and low-seated ears, as well as hypertelorism were seen in at least two subjects.

The neurological examination was often limited because the children were too disturbed for proper cooperation. Of eighty children examined, eight children showed distinct, demonstrable organic lesions, usually in the form of hemiparesis. Overt seizures had been or were present in three cases. Fifteen showed no demonstrable neurologic disease. This group, in general, consisted of the more organized and cooperative children. However, even a few children in this category were considered not adequately examined because of extraordinary hyperactivity. More prolonged independent observations of their behavior during treatment confirmed the negativity of findings. The large majority, fifty-five patients, were rated as showing soft signs suggestive of organic damage but not diagnostic for structural damage of the central nervous system. Two children were totally untestable.

Body movements ranged from minor adventitious movements of the head, trunk, and extremities to gross choreo-athetosis and dystonic posturing. Hyperkinesis, impulsivity, and emotional lability were almost universal. Facial and head asymmetries were noted, and muscular hypotonia was marked in nearly every patient. This was associated with lax joints leading to pronation of the ankles, hyperextension at the knees, and unusual posturing at the wrists and fingers. Examination of the gait revealed consistent abnormalities. These included one or all of the following: pronation of the feet, wide-based shuffling or loping gait, and poor, absent, or distorted automatic associated movements of the arms. Toe walking, with or without manifest shortened heel-cords, was common. Examination of the eyes showed alternating or paralytic strabismus, poor active and sustained eye movements, and nystagmus or nystagmoid jerks. Gross and fine coordination of upper and lower extremities was poor, and hand and finger usage, defective, awkward, and immature, some patients still exhibiting the palmar grasp. Reflex activity was inconsistent; hyperactive reflexes were rare while hypoactive or normal reflexes were common. On repeated testing, varying reflex asymmetries were noted. Speech abnormalities have been previously described.

It is evident that the neurologic findings to date strongly suggest an organic background to the syndrome of the psychotic or autistic child. Based upon observations made thus far, if a greater degree of cooperation could be obtained from these youngsters, more concrete findings would, no doubt, be elicited.

The five single-blind studies with psychotic children that we are reporting on today were guided by several notions. We were interested in producing a positive clinical effect: It was important to help these children and their parents. We wanted to test the effectiveness of inadequately tried or tested agents. We wanted the trials to be long in duration. We wanted to push the dosage. Out of these interests grew a course of action: Children were kept on a treatment as long as it proved effective and if side effects did not outweigh improvement. Where, after a reasonable trial there was no improvement, a change of treatment was instituted. The trials that we are reporting on are still in progress since there is no fixed termination date. We have set ourselves a goal of at least one year per child per drug. Thus, some of the characteristics of the trials, e.g. sample size and duration of treatment, may be or become indirect measures of outcome.

A summary of the duration of treatment and dosage employed in these five single-blind studies is presented in Table 13-I. The different size of the samples is in part related to the doctor's perception of efficacy and side effects: Prochlorperazine was perceived as a "poor" treatment, and the same may be said for trifluoperazine. The high Ns for thioridazine and fluphenazine reflect both positive orientation with respect to efficacy as well as research interest in these two drugs. The low N with chlorpromazine reflects the fact that it followed our completed double-blind study of twenty-four patients on this drug. Despite these varying attitudes, it can be seen that the average duration of trials does not vary greatly. They last between four and five months. Thus, they may be characterized as long trials.

The mean daily dosage per child, the range of these means, and the

TABLE 13-I

SUMMARY OF DURATION AND DOSAGE DATA OF FIVE SINGLE-BLIND STUDIES

	Cpz.	*Thiorid.*	*Triflu.*	*Prochlor.*	*Fluph.*
N (a)	12	24	14	7	28
Duration of Treatment in Weeks					
Mean	17.6	21.8	18.1	18.1	20.0
Range	3-50	2-83	5-38	5-54	4-38
Mg/Day					
Mean	214	288.9	35.2	20.3	12.5
Range of Means	81-496	50-791	7-57	7-50	19-24
Maximum Dose	800	1,000	80	60	40

Cpz.   = chlorpromazine   = Thorazine
Thiorid. = thioridazine   = Mellaril®
Triflu.   = trifluoperazine   = Stelazine®
Prochlor. = prochlorperazine = Compazine®
Fluph.   = fluphenazine   = Prolixin® (Squibb)
                                      Permitil® (White Labs.)

maximum daily dose are also in Table 13-I. As can be seen, they tend to be high; the dose for chlorpromazine is not much different than that employed in our clinic with adult outpatient chronic schizophrenics. By and large all dosages tend to exceed the ones either given or implied for children under twelve in package inserts. Clearly, the data suggests the need for a re-evaluation of our "standards" of appropriate dosage in this population and the establishment of new guidelines based on accumulating data from controlled systematic studies.

Table 13-II presents improvement on ten discrete areas of functioning. Using a cut-off point of 41 percent improvement divided the scales into two thirds showing no effect and one third as having some improvement. The scales on which there was this level of improvement were not evenly distributed among the five treatments. At one extreme was fluphenazine: The cut-off level of improvement was achieved on seven of the ten items. On thioridazine it was achieved on five of the ten items. At the other extreme were prochlorperazine, chlorpromazine, and trifluoperazine, where this level of improvement was only achieved on one or two of the ten items. In every case improvement in sleep pattern was noted. After that the drugs diverged in their efficacy. Three areas of functioning were not touched by any of the treatments using this criteria of improvement: concentration, self-care, and the communicative use of speech.

The difference in the number of trials for each of the five drugs makes it inadvisable to draw any final conclusions from Table 13-II. Nonetheless, the data proved to be somewhat surprising with respect to chlorpromazine

TABLE 13-II

PERCENTAGE IMPROVEMENT ON DIFFERENT ITEMS IN FIVE SINGLE-BLIND STUDIES

Overall N	Chlorpromazine (Thorazine) 12		Thioridazine (Mellaril) 24		Trifluoperazine (Stelazine) 14		Prochlorperazine (Compazine) 7		Fluphenazine (Prolixin-Permitil) 28	
	N with problem	% Impr.	N with problem	% Impr.	N with problem	% Impr.	N with problem	% Impr.	N with problem	% Impr.
Activity Level	12	33	24	45*	14	21	7	42*	28	53*
Frustration Tol.	12	33	24	41*	14	7	6	16	28	57*
Concentration	12	16	24	20	14	21	7	28	28	21
Responsiveness	12	33	24	37	14	14	7	28	28	46*
Eating	6	33	14	64*	10	10	5	40	16	87*
Sleeping	9	77*	22	68*	12	66*	6	66*	22	90*
Self-Help	11	9	23	17	14	7	5	20	26	23
Language Develop.	10	10	20	20	14	7	4	0	21	42*
Communication	12	8	24	25	14	7	7	28	28	39
Mood and Affect	12	41*	24	50*	14	28	7	0	28	60*

*Indicates percentage improvement of 41 or higher.

and fluphenazine: The former proved to be much less effective than anticipated while the latter proved much more effective than anticipated.

We obtained a rating of side effects at each visit. Making such ratings with children is difficult, especially when they are young, disturbed, and nonverbal. Thus, there is little access to subjective data, and the ratings tend to focus on behavior observed by the physician and parent and inferences that they drew. In essence, we were dealing with treatment emergent *signs* rather than *symptoms*.

An indication of the frequency and extensiveness of treatment emergent side effects may be gleaned from the percentage of visits in which there were side effects reported to the total number of visits for children who had any side effects. Here we see that thioridazine, trifluoperazine, and prochlorperazine are relatively high, 41 to 42 percent, and that chlorpromazine and fluphenazine are relatively low, 19 and 28 percent, respectively. If one turns these figures around, one finds somewhat reassuringly that even children showing some side effects were free of side effects for over half of their visits, and that for a drug like chlorpromazine over 80 percent of all their visits were free of side effects. It must be reemphasized that the opportunity for eliciting the full range of side effects, as in adults, was lacking and that, therefore, these "low" figures cannot be taken at face value.

The distribution of side effects for the five single-blind studies is presented in Table 13-III. Chlorpromazine was relatively high in occurrence of adverse behavior effects and EPS. The former occurred primarily in the area of drowsiness and tended to diminish or disappear over time. In only a few

TABLE 13-III

SIDE EFFECTS DATA FOR FIVE SINGLE-BLIND STUDIES

Distribution of Complaints by Symptom Areas: Percentage of Total Complaints in Parenthesis

	Cpz.	Thiorid.	Triflu.	Prochlor.	Fluph.
No. of Trials	12	24	14	7	28
No. of Trials with Positive Treatment Emergent Symptoms	7	17	9	3	19
Total Complaints	14	132	51	13	98
Adv. Behavior Effects	5 (36)	16 (12)	10 (20)	3 (23)	19 (19)
Lethargy - Listless	2 (14)	4 (3)	2 (4)	1 (8)	8 (8)
Increased Appetite	0	46 (35)	8 (16)	1 (8)	14 (14)
Weight Gain	1 (7)	7 (5)	3 (6)	1 (8)	10 (10)
Gastrointestinal Symptoms	0	0	0	3 (23)	0
Anorexia	0	1 (1)	0	2 (15)	4 (4)
Extrapyramidal Symptoms	6 (43)	7 (5)	28 (55) *	1 (8)	33 (34)
Genitourinary Symptoms	0	47 (36)	0	1 (8)	10 (10)
Photosensitivity	0	4 (3)	0	0	0

*This figure is an under-estimate since six of the fourteen children received procyclidine HCl (Kemadrin®) prophylactically and exhibited no extrapymamidal symptoms.

instances was it necessary to control this side effect by dosage reduction. The EPS consisted primarily of rigidity and tremor, drooling or akathesia. The symptoms cleared on administration of procyclidine or on drug reduction. The occurrence of EPS was not age-related, but appeared to be dosage-related.

In the case of thioridazine the bulk of the side effects were in the area of increased appetite and genitourinary symptoms. The G-U complaints were restricted to six children. Side effects ranged from frequency, urgency, and polyuria to enuresis and incontinence. Of the five children who had enuresis, three were reported to be bedwetters on admission. Four children who were reported to be bedwetters on admission did not exhibit this symptom during the thioridazine trial. Thioridazine thus appears to have a very different pattern of side effects than the other medications used with these children. Although the G-U symptoms are probably not as anxiety-provoking as the EPS, they still can be very provocative in a family setting.

The outstanding side effects of trifluoperazine treatment were clearly the occurrence of EPS. In seven of the drug trials EPS ranging from akathesia or drooling to a combination of rigidity, tremor, dystonia, masked facies, and disturbed associative movements were noted. In all seven cases the children were given procyclidine, and this controlled the symptomatology. One child experienced convulsions during the fifth week of treatment on a daily dosage of 50 mg, which he had been receiving for one week, and the trial was discontinued. There was no history of convulsions in this child. However, the child did exhibit an abnormal EEG. In addition, the mother reported that the child had received an unspecified amount of LSD for one week while attending a special kindergarten class for disturbed children approximately two years prior to admission to our clinic. At that time the child did not have convulsions, but had experienced hallucinations which lead to discontinuance of the LSD.

It is difficult to identify a specific profile of side effects for prochlorperazine because of the small sample studied and great variety of effects observed.

The major category of side effects under fluphenazine was EPS. Over one half of these complaints were drooling. In addition, the children exhibited drowsiness, increased appetite, and weight gain, as well as genitourinary symptoms. While the latter did not occur as frequently as under thioridazine, there were two instances of polyuria, four of enuresis, and four of incontinence. With regard to EPS, these occurred in thirteen children, and symptoms were all reversed promptly with 15-20 mg a day of procyclidine. Comparing the children who developed EPS with those who did not, the group with EPS did not start at a higher dosage and was not getting the drug at a faster rate. In fact, we found that the average daily dose for children who developed EPS was lower than for those who did not develop these symptoms. This was especially striking in the younger children under eight years of age where the average dose for children developing EPS was 4.8 mg a day in contrast to an average of 13.2 mg a day for children not developing EPS. Age by itself did not relate to the occurrence of EPS.

Laboratory data was obtained on all children participating in the single-blind studies at a frequency of four to eight weeks and an average of six weeks between laboratory tests. In view of the fact that these were relatively long-term studies, we consider this frequency acceptable although we are currently obtaining laboratory data at each visit. Because the children were extremely ill, only a small number could be exposed to adequate dryout periods prior to the introduction of drug treatment, and therefore proper baseline data is not available for many of the children.

Our findings are highly reassuring. Based on our laboratory norms, the number of abnormal findings of significance is negligible. No abnormal findings were obtained on bilirubin and alkaline phosphatase. Only a single white count exceeded the normal range (3500), out of a total of 322 white counts. There were two abnormal urines out of 180. There were two instances of abnormal hemoglobin, both in the same child, out of 210 readings. There were 17 instances of abnormal hematocrit out of a total of 317 evaluations. None of the abnormal findings referred to represented marked deviations from the normal. With respect to the differential white count there were only a few instances of minor deviations from the normal out of a total of 322 differential counts. There was a tendency for the differential count on monocytes, eosinophiles, and basophiles to exceed the values on our table of norms. These minor abnormalities, assuming that our norms are correct, occurred primarily on fluphenazine and thioridazine.

Reviewing the side effects as well as laboratory data for the five drugs, we are impressed with the absence of serious complications or toxicity during the relatively long, high dosage trials with these potent agents. Almost all difficulties were adequately handled by dose reduction or contramedication. This is not intended to imply that the occurrence of a number of these side effects was not a cause of concern to both physician and parent and undoubtedly a source of discomfort to the child.

Summarizing our work so far, we have come to the following conclusions with respect to pharmacotherapy of psychotic children:

(1) Given cooperative parents, drug research and treatment with severely disturbed psychotic children is feasible at the outpatient level.

(2) Our experience is consonant with that of other investigators that psychotropic drugs are generally safe and effective in these children.

(3) Assuming that our dosage schedules for the various drugs were appropriate and comparable, there seems to be considerable difference in the clinical effectiveness among the drugs in our population.

We were particularly impressed with the effectiveness of fluphenazine and its superiority over the other drugs studied.

(4) The package insert is an inadequate guide for determining dosage for psychotic children under twelve. Dosages tend to be often higher than recommended. In general, our experience has been much the same as that of other investigators; namely, that optimal daily dose for psychotic children seems to be the same as that used with adult schizophrenics.

(5) With regard to side effects, it would appear that the pattern is similar to that observed in adult schizophrenics; however, the impact on the child, and particularly the parents, of certain side effects may be more dramatic and traumatic. We are referring particularly to such side effects as dystonic reactions which are extremely frightening and disturbing to the parents and often lead to visits to emergency rooms of hospitals. Genitourinary symptoms, especially enuresis, are particularly disturbing to parents of children trained after great time, effort, and labor.

(6) With regard to the areas of clinical improvement, none of the drugs tested by us produced improvement in self-management and communication. The most consistent effect among the drugs was improvement in sleeping, mood and affect and activity level. In all cases the amount of residual pathology was significant. Essentially, the action of the antipsychotic agents in this population was to make the children more manageable and easier to live with. Anyone having familiarity with these children will appreciate how meaningfully these symptomatic changes can influence the life of an entire family with such a child in the household.

(7) While our studies have permitted us to observe these children under drug treatment for relatively long periods of time, they have not permitted us to draw any conclusions on the positive or deleterious effects these drugs may be having on the developmental processes of these children. So far there is no information available on the impact of the newer psychotropic agents on developing organisms. Particularly in the case of psychotic children where the course of the illness is chronic, the danger exists of toxicity resulting from long-term administration of drugs.

(8) The results we have reported on are primarily related to drug treatment in the absence of any other meaningful concurrent therapy. The prognosis for more meaningful improvement with drug treatment imbedded in a comprehensive treatment program cannot be judged from our results, but we would consider it likely that improvement would be both quantitatively and qualitatively superior under

the latter conditions. Certainly the drug-induced treatment effects should considerably facilitate involvement of both the parent and the child in more comprehensive treatment programs. Recognizing, however, the limited results obtained so far by other approaches, involving intensive long-term costly treatment programs that have been utilized with some of these children, the effects produced by pharmacotherapy must be viewed as impressive.

REFERENCES

1. Davis, J. M., Bartlett, E., and Termini, B. A. Overdosage of psychotropic drugs: A review. Part I: Major and minor tranquilizers. *Dis Nerv Syst, 29* (No. 3): 157-164, 1968.
2. McKown, C. H., Verhulst, H. L., and Crotty, J. J.: Overdosage effects and danger from tranquilizing drugs. *JAMA,* vol. 185, no. 6, 1963, 87-92.

Chapter 14

Evaluating the Purported Intelligence-Memory Enhancing Pharmacological Agents: Methodological Considerations

FRANK J. MENOLASCINO

INTRODUCTION

MANY DISEASES can be cured, and many diseases which were considered incurable at one time have become curable with new treatment discoveries. Therefore, it is not surprising that laymen as well as many professionals look forward to the discovery of a "cure" of mental retardation. This hope often takes the form of a search for another "wonder drug." People who perceive mental retardation as a disease usually also perceive a potential drug cure. The physician administers a drug to the sick, passive patient who soon improves and eventually "takes up his bed and walks." So far as the condition of mental retardation is concerned, an analogous treatment expectation would be to see an eight-year-old, severely retarded, nonverbal, nonambulatory child suddenly burst forth—talking, walking, and doing the things one would expect the average eight-year-old to do. Not only parents and laymen, but even many professionals and paraprofessional workers, hold such concepts of a potential drug cure of mental retardation and which Yannet in 1957 labeled "the Magic Bullet Theory."

Without explicitly articulating the Magic Bullet Theory, a researcher may adopt an experimental design which clearly implies it. Thus, a number of the glutamic acid studies reviewed by Vogel, Broverman, Draguns, and Klaiber in 1966 had placed retarded subjects on the experimental drug for such short periods of time (e.g. 1 to 2 months) that effects upon global intelligence would have had to be very dramatic in order to reach statistical significance. In 1967, House, Burns, Fensch, and Miller conducted a study of the effects of a single dose of magnesium pemoline on learning. The relevant question here is not so much whether drug effects were actually reported, but why the investigators chose to adopt designs that would assess only quick and dramatic effects, but not the gradual and developmentally equally important ones. The use of adult subjects rather than of children also carries with it the flavor of Magic Bullet expectations. Children generally are believed to be much more plastic than adults, and one can easily perceive a significant increase in their rate of development. In adults, however,

235

a drug effect is difficult to envision except in terms of either performance enhancement or "cure."

The field of mental retardation has witnessed many attempts to improve cognitive functioning by means of drugs, and a number of models of drug action can be discerned. These attempts can be classified as springing from three theoretical models:

(1) *The unblocking model.* Within this model, drugs are employed to treat conditions which interfere with the full use or development of intelligence. Examples are the allaying of anxiety by means of tranquilizers and the control of seizures with anticonvulsants. Especially in psychiatrically-oriented circles, the term "unblocking" may be encountered in this connection.

(2) *The energizing model.* This model implies the use of drugs to stimulate the central nervous system in an effort to improve alertness and/or performance, thereby hopefully maximizing those intelligence-related behaviors that might not be fully utilized even by a well-functioning person. Amphetamines and strychnine have been used in this fashion, and this use has been reviewed by Louttit in 1965 and by Freeman in 1966.

(3) *The direct action model.* The *unblocking model* and the *energizing model* imply an indirect drug effect. However, some drugs are employed in the hope that they will affect cognitive processes directly. Within this model, drugs can be perceived as having a number of possible modes of action. In 1949, Zimmerman, Burgemeister, and Putnam posited a somewhat vaguely conceptualized improvement in higher cognitive processes. A recent and more sophisticated conceptualization envisions improvement in learning and memory processes. Glutamine and glutamic acid (Louttit, 1965; Vogel, Broverman, Draguns, and Klaiber, 1966), vitamins (House, Wilson, and Goodfellow, 1964), sicca-cell treatments (Goldstein, 1956), and combination treatments such as Turkel's 1963 "U Series" of forty-nine drugs have been used within the framework of the direct action model.

While none of the pharmacological agents previously mentioned has been demonstrated to improve the intelligence or the intellectual development of retardates, some of the so-called replacement therapies which aim at the amelioration of specific metabolic syndromes associated with retardation have been effective. For instance, thyroid preparations have been shown to be effective in selected cases of hypothyroidism. Several other metabolic disorders such as phenylketonuria are treated dietetically and apparently with some success (see studies published by Waisman and Gerritsen, 1964, and Kirman, 1965). Though many investigators appear to view replacement therapies as essentially constituting "unblocking," agreement as to the most appropriate model or mode of drug action in these therapies appears to be lacking. On one point only has there been widespread agreement: the success of replacement therapies appears to be correlated negatively with subject's age, i.e. the older the subject, the less successful the therapy.

It is crucially important to be aware of certain other concepts and attitudes which can affect drug study designs in subtle and/or detrimental ways. For example, a curious phenomenon can be discerned in the way people view attempts to improve the intelligence of retarded versus non-retarded individuals. A "pill" to enhance the intelligence of a college student would be expected to improve his learning, memory, and general performance. A moderate and gradually accumulating effect would be considered desirable and quite acceptable. However, with a retardate, a drug would be scorned if it produced anything less than a complete and perhaps even a rapid "cure," unless it produced "normality."

Recently, the hope to enhance intelligence chemically has been re-kindled by reports that RNA, and drugs believed to facilitate the metabolism of RNA in the brain (e.g. magnesium pemoline, registered as Cylert by Abbott Laboratories), result in improved retention and perhaps even increased acquisition in both animals and humans. Other potentially intelligence-enhancing or development-enhancing drugs on which there has been widespread publicity include 5-hydroxytryptophane. Research on these drugs has now moved from animal to human trials, and both the popular press and serious scientists are emitting optimistic forecasts with increasing frequency and widespread publicity. Krech, in 1968, gave optimistic testimony on such drug trials before a congressional committee; also in 1968, Linus Pauling jolted the field by forecasting an era of "orthomolecular psychiatry" wherein drugs play a large role in behavior maintenance and enhancement; and Arthur Koestler, the author of "Darkness at Noon" has joined the ranks of prominent writers anticipating a drug-based utopia.

Inevitably, the question of the possible "cure" of mental retardation by chemical agents arose. It may be timely to recall the past so as not to repeat its errors.

METHODOLOGICAL CONSIDERATIONS

A basic assumption is that we are discussing studies employing a placebo control group and other features of well-designed drug experiments. While there may be a need for uncontrolled exploratory work, the power of the placebo effect has been so convincingly demonstrated that no drug should be accepted as possessing development-enhancing properties unless it has undergone the most rigorously controlled tests.

I am not particularly concerned with those pharmaceutical agents which result in improved performance, such as the central nervous system stimulants or the alleviation of secondary conditions, such as hyperkinesis, seizures, emotional disturbance, etc., that interfere with intellectual efficiency and/or development. The focus in this presentation is primarily on drugs purported to improve directly cognitive functioning or development. When speaking of drug effectiveness studies, it is this type of drug to which I refer.

General Considerations

The first goal of a study designed to assess a drug's ability to accelerate development should be the exploration of whether or not the drug has *any* developmental effect. To demonstrate such an effect is difficult without getting involved in tests of sophisticated and advanced hypotheses, or comparisons of several unproven drugs at the same time.

Since attempts to explore the potential efficacy of drugs are difficult and demanding of time, money, and other resources, experiments should be designed to maximize the discernment of a potential effect. Above all, the study should be designed so as to constitute a fair test of the drug. Many studies in the past have failed in this regard, and whatever the merit of the drug may have been, such studies were simply irrelevant. The history of the field contains instances in which respected and qualified workers enthusiastically embraced belief in the curative action of a drug which was later generally rejected as ineffective, even though neither the original positive nor the later negative studies may have constituted adequate tests of the drug's potential effects. Freeman has pointed out that after twenty-five years of work with glutamic acid and its derivatives, and thirty years with amphetamines, we still do not possess adequate empirical evidence regarding the behavioral effects of these drugs.

Failure to consider certain principles and facts of child development and experimental design account for many erroneous or unpromising research strategies. Much of the rest of this presentation will concern itself with such considerations.

Fallacy of the Magic Bullet Theory

One crucial consideration is that mental retardation is *not* a disease, and that the Magic Bullet model is not appropriate to the drug treatment of mental retardation. Let us recall the example of the severely retarded eight-year-old. Even if it were possible to restore him to normal learning capacity instantaneously, he would, in all likelihood, have to pass through the developmental stages every normal child goes through. There is reason to believe that some behavior skills, such as those in the areas of speech, language, and perceptual development, may rarely, if ever, be mastered unless they are acquired during sensitive, or prior to critical, periods of development. Thus, instead of having a Magic Bullet effect, a development-enhancing drug is more likely to work gradually, additively, directionally, and selectively.

Definition of Drug Effect

Once we have emancipated ourselves from the Magic Bullet model, we can address ourselves more productively to the question as to when a drug (or any treatment) can be considered effective. One orientation encountered in the field of mental retardation is that if a treatment does not cure, or at least result in spectacular effects, it is not worth pursuing. It is important to recall that even a very small change in behavior, or in the rate of development, can have major implications to ultimate functioning and to social and management costs. Being, or not being, toilet trained can mean a difference of two hours work per day to a mother, and this, in turn, can mean the difference between the child remaining in the home or being placed in an institution at great cost to the child, his family, and society as a whole. Since relatively small developmental changes in just one behavior area can have very significant implications to care and management, the efficacy of a drug should not be assessed by its ability to "cure," but on the basis of its having any effect that would not have been achieved, or achieved as efficiently, without administration of the drug.

Nature of the Experimental Variable

A common error in the conceptualization of drug effects, and consequently in the design of relevant experiments, is associated with failure to appreciate the nature of intellectual growth. Some traditional theories of child development have held that behavior unfolds automatically, like a predictable sequence of development in an embryo; one only need sit back and wait for certain behaviors to emerge at specific, almost predetermined ages, and usually little advantage was seen in developmental exercises, drills, activities, etc.

Today a different view prevails. While it is granted that there is a genetic upper limit to development, it is generally believed that a child's current developmental stage is a better predictor of the next milestone to be attained than his chronological age. A child who holds up his head, turns, crawls, stands with support, and walks while being held by one hand is generally ready to learn to walk unsupported, no matter whether he is eight or twenty-eight months old. However, it is also generally believed that a normally endowed child can become retarded if his perceptual, motor, linguistic, and social world is severely restricted. Ordinarily, we would not expect an otherwise normal three-year-old child to walk if he had never been allowed to leave his crib.

Adherence to most contemporary theories and facts of child development would thus lead us to postulate that the effectiveness of a drug in accelerating development cannot be demonstrated, or only very poorly so, unless the child is exposed to favorable environment and to experiences which are stimulating and which are appropriate to his developmental level. This means that drug effect must be tested at the interface of readiness and experience. Indeed, the entire concept that the drug is the experimental variable in drug effect studies should be abandoned. *The interaction between drug and experience should be considered to be the crucial experimental variable.*

Since any factor which jeopardizes the drug-experience interaction may invalidate the study as a fair test of drug potential, we must clearly identify the factors which have their locus in the subject, the drug, or the structure which governs the interaction between the medicated subject and his environment. I will now discuss each of these limiting factors.

Limiting Factors in the Environment

Lack of Appropriate Developmental Stimulation

A common feature of drug studies such as those which involved glutamic acid was the use of perceptually and socially deprived subjects. Thus, residents of institutions appear to have been the main source of subjects to date for many drug effectiveness studies in mental retardation. Retardates living at home in a stimulating environment and engaged in intensive developmental programs would have constituted a more appropriate subject population.

Environmental Effects

If institutional or deprived subjects are used, but are placed in stimulating environments for the purpose of a drug study, a special problem must be kept in mind. We must not only expect an ordinary placebo effect in the control group, but a genuine and substantial acceleration of development due to the nonspecific environmental treatment component. Thus, the experimental subjects must not only improve greatly, but must improve significantly more than the control subjects who may improve significantly themselves.

Limiting Factors in the Subject

Subject Handicaps

There are certain conditions within a person which can constitute limits to the drug-experience interaction. Emotional disturbance, severe seizures, sensory impairment, and orthopedic, esthetic, and health handicaps are of this nature. It follows therefore, that an optimal subject group, at least during early phases of research with a drug, should be free of such limiting conditions.

Optimal Subject Functioning

It is conceivable that some drugs might have an effect only in persons who previously have not functioned near their capacity, while little on no effect might be observed on those persons who are already functioning near their maximal limit. A drug effect that can be conceived rather readily on the theoretical level is one that would counteract or dissipate neural inhibitory processes. Thus, it is possible that some drugs may be more effective in retardates than in normals, and the use of retarded subjects may be a better strategy than the use of normal or even superior subjects such as college students. An analogous phenomenon has been reported by McGough in mice, where maze-dull strains profited more from Metrazol® injections than maze-bright ones. More importantly, the optimal dosage was found to be higher in dull than in bright strains of mice although the drug can have learning-inhibitory effects when administered to maze-bright strains in too high doses.

Subject Age

The subject's age must be considered to be a limiting factor in drug studies. The rate of mental development is generally accepted to be a positive decelerating function which flattens out in the midteens. There is strong reason to believe that most of the growth potential that is not realized during childhood is lost and cannot be recaptured even with intensive stimulation in adulthood. It follows that the younger the child, the more effective a drug-experience interaction should be in promoting development. Conversely, this interaction should decline in effectiveness as the child gets older.

Younger Subjects and Assessment Techniques

The use of younger subjects brings with it the dilemma resulting from limitations in assessment techniques for children of low mental age. Instruments and techniques designed to assess global development are very inadequate for children below a mental age of two years. Even between mental ages of two to five, there are few global tests available, and some of these leave much to be desired. Tests of part or underlying functions of intelligence (e.g. attention, learning, memory, etc.) are even more problematic for this mental age range. This means that even with eight to ten-year-old children, we would have great difficulties if their IQs were below 40-50. The horns of the dilemma are thus constituted of the need for a group young enough to profit considerably from a drug-experience interaction, and the need for children whose mental age is high enough to permit application of appropriate available assessment techniques. Until more and better techniques applicable to subjects of lower mental age are developed, we propose that the optimal solution to the dilemma is to use mildly retarded (IQ 50-80) children between age of five to ten.

Limiting Factors in the Drug

An agent may have toxic or other undesirable side effects, or may be difficult to administer. Further, potentially effective drugs may be effective only if they are available to the nervous system during the learning process, in which case drug administration must be planned with drug characteristics in mind. For instance, a potentially effective drug may be rapidly absorbed and metabolized. An experimental design involving drug administration upon rising at 6 A.M., and upon retiring at 9 P.M., may not constitute a fair test of that drug because the child may not be exposed to highly stimulating activities until midmorning, and to none at all at night. One must thus draw a distinction between the administered and the effective dose, and some drugs may have to be administered in timed release capsules or frequent doses. For this reason, the drug absorption rates should be considered carefully.

The need to give drugs in dosages large enough to be effective creates problems in research, since many drugs given in active dosages have side effects that may reveal the identity of experimental subjects in studies with double or triple blind controls, thereby destroying the utility of these controls. For this reason, some drug studies employ a uniform dosage for all experimental subjects, hoping that drug effectiveness, if any, will manifest itself sufficiently in at least enough subjects so as to yield a statistically significant group difference. Such a design preserves technical purity, but has at least two drawbacks: It may require a large sample before an effect can be accepted as having been adequately demonstrated, and it ignores certain pharmaceutical facts. Thus, the common dosage may be set too low to have a positive and measurable effect on most subjects, or it may be so high as to produce toxic effects which can lead to loss of subjects, or to their identification by the personnel involved. Only a few subjects are likely to receive a dose optimal to them, that is, a dose individualized to their tolerance, sensitivity, metabolic rate, etc.

This dilemma was highlighted in a review of the literature on the effect of glutamic acid on cognitive behavior. The reviewers concluded that current evidence favors a positive effect. However, rather embarrassingly, the positive evidence came mostly from studies which were either uncontrolled or which used individual dosaging techniques which make a double-blind or triple-blind design virtually impossible to maintain. On the other hand, the negative evidence was derived primarily from controlled studies utilizing uniform dosages. A crucial question thus arises: Are the positive results due to the powerful effects of individualized dosaging, or are they due to a placebo effect resulting from loss of subject identity which might have occurred during dosage determination?

Some researchers have attempted to solve the dilemma by separating the clinical management of the subject from the evaluation of drug effect. However, in the light of past experience, one can raise serious doubts about the adequacy of such a technique in maintaining rigorous blind conditions.

Other Experimental Design Considerations

It is desirable that a research design be efficient as well as appropriate. First, let us consider that drug effectiveness studies, by their very nature, must be longitudinal. Experimental and control groups are assessed; a treatment is administered, and then both are reassessed. A statistical design typical for such a study is variously referred to as "repeated measurements of several independent groups" or a "mixed factorial Type I" design. In such a design, the *crucial statistical test* of the drug-experience effect is not of the difference between groups after treatment, but of the statistical interaction between groups and time, i.e. the *differential rate of change*.

Secondly, the efficiency of an experiment is generally related inversely to its duration. Given a potential effect, the design which permits the most rapid demonstration of this effect is, other things being equal, the most efficient one. The adequacy, appropriateness, and efficiency of a drug experiment can be affected by many variables.

Sample Size

In regard to sample size, we need to recall that the larger the experimental and control groups are, the less of a difference between their criterion score means is usually required for statistical significance. Since we have stipulated a gradually additive drug effect over time, larger groups will usually permit a shorter study. One can estimate the approximate minimal duration of an adequate experiment for various assumed improvement rates if one knows the distribution of the "before" scores. Conversely, if one decides to run a study for a given period of time, for example, one year, one can estimate the approximate minimal change needed for statistical significance.

Controls

If there is one thing we should have learned from the history of medicine and of psychology generally, and the history of the management of the retarded specifically, it would be to insist on the most rigorously controlled studies of a new treatment before it is accepted as effective. If one views retardation as a static, hitherto "incurable" condition that will yield only to a Magic Bullet therapy, then controls may appear to be unnecessary because no improvement would be expected unless the Magic Bullet had been found, in which case the expected improvement would be a drastic and self-evident one. For instance, Zimmerman, Burgemeister, and Putnam omitted a placebo control group in their glutamic acid study on the assumption that their retarded subjects were not capable of responding to placebo effects.

The better controlled the control variables are, and the more sources of error variance are eliminated, the more efficient a design becomes. For this reason, matching of subject pairs, though more difficult, appears to be preferable to equation of subject groups. When groups are merely equated (often erroneously referred to as matched), the means of the equated variables are essentially identical, but there may not be a 1:1 correspondence of relevant characteristics between pairs of subjects, and error variance is likely to be higher.

Diagnostic Homogeneity

The above considerations underline the desirability for homogeneity of certain variables. However, some investigators have committed an error in strategy by pursuing homogeneity of variables that should not be homogeneous. For instance, researchers characteristically aspire to constitute subject groups with the same clinical diagnoses (e.g. mongolism). Thus, in their review of glutamic acid studies with retardates, Astin and Ross expressed preference for diagnostic (mostly etiological) homogeneity. Such diagnostic homogeneity is appropriate when there is reason to believe that the drug treatment is of greater benefit in one syndrome than in others. If there is no reason for making such an assumption, diagnostic homogeneity is at best irrelevant and wasteful; at worst it may be destructive to the experiment, for at least two reasons. In some syndromes where biochemical function is disturbed, the drug may be metabolized in atypical fashion and thus may not act as it ordinarily would. Rogers and Pelton have raised the question whether certain types of retardates are capable of metabolizing glutamic acid in the usual manner. In other syndromes, the structure of the brain may be characteristically atypical, and those areas in or upon which the drug ordinarily acts may be impaired. In either instance, there is an increased likelihood that a general effect that might have been observed in a diagnostically heterogeneous group may not take place or may not become measurable. Thus, the experiment would not constitute a fair test for the drug, and might lead to its premature rejection.

Shortcomings of Criterion Measures

A common but questionable feature of drug and other treatment studies has been reliance on assessment of global or very complex behavior. The use of intelligence tests such as the Binet, Wechsler, etc., is of this nature, and may have been a poor strategy. Global intelligence reflects years of learning and experience, and is modified relatively slowly. Lengthy experiments are likely to be necessary to demonstrate changes adequately. A more promising strategy appears to be the assessment of behavior processes which underlie global intelligence, such as arousal, perception (e.g. attention), learning, and retention. For instance, it is conceivable that within a few days or weeks a drug could have measurable effects on vigilance, conditioning speed, or short-term memory, while it might take months and years before such effects are translated into statistically significant improvements on global IQ tests. This point is particularly important if, as suggested by Krech, and as appears reasonable, drugs are more likely to have selective effects on specific conative or cognitive processes.

If underlying processes do not show any change, no change is likely to occur on the global level. On the other hand, once underlying processes have shown improvement, then it is timely to design "second generation" experiments that may involve more global measures.

Personnel Variables

One problem in the design of drug and other treatment studies is rarely mentioned. It is the fact that the before-and-after measurements are often made by technicians or other personnel who do not have a high degree of competence with the assessment technique, or who have not developed a consistent assessment style. For instance, a junior psychologist may be hired to give intelligence tests to subjects before and after administration of the treatment. The examiner may only have had experience in testing a small number of individuals with the particular test involved. Thus, he may improve in competence during the "before" assessments, and may obtain systematically higher or lower scores on the "after" assessments on the basis of his increased skills alone. "Improvement" then may be ascribed erroneously to the treatment, and "loss" to detrimental drug effects or to subject characteristics.

CONCLUSION

In concluding, I would like to return to the distinction made earlier between direct and indirect effects of pharmacological agents. In the light of the foregoing discussion, it is conceivable that this distinction may have limited utility. The difference between such potential agents may lie not so much in their effects as in their mode of action—at least so long as children were used as subjects, and so long as they were exposed to intensive environmental enrichment while on the drugs. I also want to emphasize that I have taken no stand in this presentation in regard to two issues relevant to drug research in retardation: (a) What is the theoretical likelihood that intelligence in retardates can be significantly improved by a pharmacological agent? (b) What emphasis should be given to research of this nature within a global research strategy in mental retardation and/or pharmacology? The stand I *have* taken is that if studies of the intelligence-enhancing effects of pharmacological agents are to be conducted, they should be so designed as to constitute an adequate, fair, and efficient test of such an effect.

ACKNOWLEDGMENT

The author acknowledges the ideological and personal support of his colleague, Dr. Wolf Wolfensberger, in the preparation of this manuscript.

REFERENCES

1. American Medical Association: *Mental Retardation: A Handbook for the Primary Physician.* Chicago, 1965.
2. Anonymous: *Frontiers Hosp Psychiat, 3 (23)*:3, 1966.
3. Association for Research in Nervous and Mental Disease: *Mental Retardation: Proceedings of the Association, December 11 and 12, New York, New York,* Baltimore, Williams and Wilkins, 1962.
4. Astin, A. W., and Ross, S.: Glutamic acid and human intelligence. *Psychol Bull, 57*:429-434, 1962.
5. Birch, H. G., and Belmont, L.: The problem of comparing home rearing versus foster-home rearing in defective children. *Pediatrics, 28*:956-961, 1961.
6. Blackman, L. S.: Toward the concept of a "just noticeable difference" in IQ remediation. *Amer J Ment Defic, 62*:322-325, 1957.
7. Burns, J. T., House, R. F., Fensch, F. C., and Miller, J. G.: Effects of magnesium pemoline and dextroamphetamine on human learning. *Science, 155*:849-851, 1967.
8. Edwards, A. E.: *Experimental Design in Psychological Research.* New York, Rinehart, 1950.
9. Freeman, R. D.: Drug effects on learning in children: A selective review of the past thirty years. *J Spec Educ, 1*:17-44, 1966.
10. Goldstein, H.: Sicca-cell therapy in children. *Arch Pediat, 73*:234-249, 1956.
11. House, M., Wilson, H. D., and Goodfellow, H. D. L.: Treatment of mental deficiency with alpha tocopherol. *Amer J Ment Defic, 69*:328-329, 1964.
12. Kirman, B. H.: Metabolic syndromes. In Hilliard, L. T., and Kirman, B. H.: *Mental Deficiency,* 2nd ed. Boston, Little, Brown, 1965, pp. 486-526.
13. Klerman, G. L.: The social milieu and drug response in psychiatric patients. Paper presented at the annual convention of the American Sociological Society, Miami Beach, Florida, 1966.
14. Koestler, A.: *The Ghost in the Machine.* New York, Macmillan, 1967.
15. Krech, D.: The chemistry of learning. *Saturday Review,* January 20, 1968, pp. 48-50, 68.
16. Lindquist, E. F.: *Design and Analysis of Experiments in Psychology and Education.* Cambridge, Massachusetts, Riverside Press, 1953.
17. Louttit, R. T.: Chemical facilitation of intelligence among the mentally retarded. *Amer J Ment Defic, 69*:495-501, 1965.
18. Mead, M.: *And Keep Your Powder Dry.* New York, Morrow, 1942.

19. Pauling, L.: Orthomolecular psychiatry. *Science, 160:*265-271, 1968.
20. Rogers, L. L., and Pelton, R. B.: Effects of glutamine on I.Q. scores of mentally deficient children. *Texas Rep Biol Med, 15:*84-90, 1957.
21. Shapiro, A. K.: A contribution to a history of the placebo effect. *Behav Sci, 5:*109-135, 1960.
22. Stone, M. M.: Parental attitudes to retardation. *Amer J Ment Defic, 53:*363-372, 1948.
23. Turkel, H.: Medical treatment of mongolism. In Stur, O. (Ed.) : *Proceedings of the Second International Congress on Mental Retardation, August 14-19, 1961.* Basel, Switzerland, S. Karger, 1963, pp. 409-416.
24. Umbarger, B.: Phenylketonuria—treating the disease and feeding the child. *Amer J Dis Child, 100:*908-913, 1960.
25. Vogel, W., Broverman, D. M., Draguns, J. G., and Klaiber, E. L.: The role of glutamic acid in cognitive behaviors. *Psychol Bull, 65:*367-382, 1966.
26. Waisman, H. A., and Gerritsen, T.: Biochemical and clinical correlations. In Stevens, H. A. and Heber, R. (Eds.) : *Mental retardation: A Review of Research.* Chicago, University of Chicago Press, 1964, pp. 307-347.
27. Wolfensberger, W.: Ethical issues in research with human subjects. *Science, 155:*47-51, 1967.
28. Wolfensberger, W., and Menolascino, F. J.: Basic considerations in evaluating ability of durgs to stimulate cognitive development in retardates. *Amer J Ment Defic, 73:*414-423, 1968.
29. Yannet, H.: Research in the field of mental retardation. *J Pediat, 50* (2) :236-239, 1957.
30. Zimmerman, F. T., Burgemeister, B., and Putnam, T. J.: The effect of glutamic acid upon the mental and physical growth of mongols. *Amer J Psychiat, 105:* 661-668, 1949.

Chapter 15

Prediction of Drug Effect in Personality Disorders*

DONALD F. KLEIN, GILBERT HONIGFELD, AND SYDNEY FELDMAN

ATTEMPTS to predict the effects of psychotropic agents on psychiatric patients have been primarily confined to schizophrenics.[1] Recently, predictive indices on depressives, depressed psychoneurotic outpatients, and anxiety neurotics have been presented.[2,3,4,5] There are few studies of psychotropic agents on character disorders. We present here a preliminary effort at describing clinical predictors of drug response in personality disorders and an approach to developing statistically validated prediction rules.

DEFINITION OF PERSONALITY DISORDER

The American Psychiatric Association Diagnostic and Statistical Manual of 1952, (DSM-I)[6] states that the outstanding characteristics of the personality disorders are "developmental defects or pathological trends in the personality structure, with minimum subjective anxiety, and little or no sense of distress. In most instances the disorder is manifested by a life-long pattern of action or behavior rather than by mental or emotional symptoms." This definition reflects the general impression of the cool, psychopathic, exploitative type of personality disorder. However, it certainly does not fit the category of "emotionally unstable personality disorder," utilized in DSM-I, wherein the predominant symptomatology is labile emotionality.

The 1968 revision of the *Diagnostic Manual,* DSM-II,[7] states, "This group of disorders is characterized by deeply ingrained maladaptive patterns of behavior that are perceptibly different in quality from psychotic and neurotic symptoms. Generally, these are life-long patterns often recognizable by the time of adolescence or earlier." DSM-II emphasizes the life-long pattern of maladaptive behavior that is none-the-less different from psychotic and neurotic states and removes the deemphasis on anxiety and emotional symptoms prominent in DSM-I. Utilizing this definition we shall consider four diagnostic subgroups considered by us[8] to represent distinct types of personality disorder: (a) the histrionic reactions, (b) the emotionally unstable personalities, (c) the passive-aggressive personalities, and (d) the "pseudoneurotic schizophrenics."

*Supported in part by U.S.P.H.S. Grants MH-12273 and MH-14514.

HISTRIONIC REACTION: A SUBGROUP OF THE HYSTERIAS

One patient group causing grave problems in clinical management is comprised of characteristically labile, episodically agitated, erratic, unpredictable, manipulative, tense, and histrionic patients. They are usually rational, relevant, and coherent, although they express occasional paranoid and hallucinatory verbalizations that often lead to a diagnosis of psychosis. They may act panicky and frightened to the point of suicide and several minutes later affably laugh with others. Their therapists readily become emotionally involved and are frequently frustrated and perplexed by their inability to predict or modify the patient's behavior. The patients express great investment in their doctors and psychotherapy, endowing them with miraculous potentialities. They maintain a high degree of interaction with others, being at times sociable, friendly, and supportive, and other times disturbing, hostile, argumentative, and demanding, and yet again pleading for help and direction.

These patients dramatically express their intolerance of medication side effects. Because of their lability, there is much uncertainty as to the effectiveness of medication, so that they tend to receive long treatment courses before drugs are found to be ineffective. However, if the patient responds with somatic complaints, medication is usually terminated promptly.

One clinical feature of predictive value and theoretical import is the marked relationship of their symptoms to environmental impact. Unlike depressed patients who may increase the vigor of their complaints in the presence of psychiatric staff in an attempt to coerce a maximum curative effort from them, but who remain inactive or unproductively agitated when not under staff observation, this group of refractory, hysterical patients may appear in good spirits when apparently unobserved by staff, engage in social games, and gossip pleasantly with others, even shortly after an explosive affective display. The key issue may be histrionic role-playing and symptom imitation. In other words, these patients' symptoms may not be the direct external manifestations of intolerable affective states, but rather may be environmentally oriented, learned, manipulative devices. Agitation, depressive, delusional, and hallucinatory complaints in this group are not the same as similarly labeled phenomena in other patients.

Interestingly, the conversion reactions of the nineteenth century, as described by Charcot, Freud, and others, consisted mainly of pseudoneurological syndromes, such as convulsions, anesthesias, paralyses, blindness, deafness, and dyskinesia. These behavioral syndromes were noted at a time when hysterical patients were housed in hospital wards along with epileptic patients. Hysteroepilepsy may well have been an imitative artifact of exposure.

It is frequently stated that classical grand hysteria is no longer seen, while the diagnosis of schizophrenia has become more and more prevalent, and atypical or pseudoneurotic schizophrenias are widely reported. Since the knowledge of schizophrenic behavior is widespread via books, TV, and movies, and it is common practice to house all patients with emotional disorders together, we believe that hysteroschizophrenics are being produced in much the same fashion as the nineteenth century hysteroepileptic.

The differential diagnosis of hysteroschizophrenia from true schizophrenia presents knotty problems. The major distinguishing feature would seem to be a variant upon the well known hysterical phenomenon, *la belle indifference*. Hysterics may have the most crippling disorders and yet not display appropriate concern or anguished emotional reactions to their infirmities. If their leading motivation is to attain the sick role, one can well understand this phenomenal blandness as resulting from their natural satisfaction with attaining their goal.

An analogous phenomenon occurs in patients with hysteroschizophrenia. Their attainment of the sick role is dependent upon imitation of extreme emotional distress, including psychotic symptomatology. Therefore, in the initial stages of disorder, there is, rather than *la belle indifference,* a histrionic accentuation of numerous affective and psychotic features in a confusing jumble. However, once the patient is adjudged psychiatrically ill, as by hospitalization, one is struck by the marked fluctuations in psychiatric status and by the patient's apparent indifference to the content of his expressed preoccupations and delusions. For instance, a schizophrenic may express the belief that the food is poisoned and promptly give up eating. A hysteroschizophrenic may express the same belief and then eat with good appetite one-half hour later. Similarly, a schizophrenic who expresses suicidal ideation, because he is convinced that his persecutors are about to close in on him, is in an extremely dangerous state and must be kept under constant observation. His affective state remains constant—fear and agitation. A hysteroschizophrenic may express the same delusional content and then, when away from the immediate observation of professional staff, engage in conversation and banter with other patients. Marked fluctuations in symptomatic behavior, depending upon their impact on the environment, is common with hysteroschizophrenics. Furthermore, these patients frequently resort to the use of sedatives, intoxicants, hallucinogens, narcotics, and stimulants, thus further obscuring their status.

These patients have a tendency to become mute under close questioning. This passive-aggressive maneuver is often inaccurately referred to as catatonic or micropsychotic. The diagnosis of histrionic reaction is difficult to defend in the face of skepticism among colleagues as to one's diagnostic acumen. The apparent fluctuations in states of consciousness that occur with this illness should prompt a neurological and electroencephalographic investigation (although in attempting to make the differential diagnosis one must bear in mind for example that petit mal epilepsy can coexist in the same patient with a hysterical character disorder).

This hysterical character disorder grouping was reintroduced into American nosology by DSM-II as "hysterical personality, histrionic personality disorder." However, the category also includes the previous diagnosis "emotionally unstable personality," thus obscuring a valuable distinction.

EMOTIONALLY UNSTABLE PERSONALITY

This is a common and well-recognized syndrome in which the individual reacts with excitability and ineffectiveness when confronted with minor stress. His judgment may be undependable under stress, and his relationship to other people is continually fraught with fluctuating emotional attitudes. DSM-I states that these fluctuating attitudes are due to strong and poorly controlled hostility, guilt, and anxiety. However, the basis for this hypothesis is unclear, and this definition does not emphasize the marked mood lability of these patients. These patients are predominantly female adolescents whose mood disorder consists of short periods of tense, empty unhappiness. accompanied by inactivity, withdrawal, depression, irritability, and sulking, alternating suddenly with impulsiveness, giddiness, low frustration tolerance, rejection of rules, and short-sighted hedonism.

Thus, they resemble a short-period cyclothymic personality. However, the cyclothyme is usually a responsible, mature adult who is attempting to pursue socially acceptable and valued goals. Patients with emotionally unstable personalities on the other hand, are usually young, with a poorly developed conscience and generally immature attitudes, and are frequently irresponsible, hedonistic, extractive, and exploitative. Their marked affective lability is often not immediately noted as core pathology because of their complicated self-presentations. These range from a fragile, immature, dependent image, eliciting protectiveness from the observer, to a hard "wise guy" presentation expressing independence and lack of need for care. The patients are perplexed about their life goals, stating that they do not know who they are, what they are, or what they want to be. They are also confused about issues of dependency, intimacy, and self-assertion, often reacting in a disorganized, flighty, and despairing fashion. There is a pervasive feeling of exclusion from normal life and peer groups, with the conviction of being irreparably bad. They are rational, relevant, and coherent except for periods of giddiness or agitated fearfulness during which their speech and behavior become pressured, scattered, and disorganized. Participation in activities fluctuates considerably, but when involved these patients are often creative, skilled, and original. The major degree of disorganization manifested by the emotionally unstable character disorder (in combination with his frequent habitual use of intoxicants or psychotomimetic substances such as alcohol, dextroamphetamine, marijuana, and LSD) often leads to the appearance of behavior diagnosed as schizophrenic by many psychiatrists. Many emotionally unstable personalities have childhood histories of impulsiveness, hyperactivity, and low frustration tolerance. Others seem to develop this pattern at the time of puberty. Their prognosis is, at present, unclear although their affective swings can generally be moderated by phenothiazines. Preliminary follow-up data suggests that the pathological behavior of many such patients "burns out" during their late twenties. Because of the differential drug response of this group, subsuming them under the "hysterical personality" category as in DSM-II tends to blur a valuable distinction.

PASSIVE - AGGRESSIVE PERSONALITY

This syndrome is defined in DSM-I as consisting of three subtypes, the passive-aggressive, passive-dependent, and aggressive, all believed to be manifestations of the same underlying psychopathology. Unfortunately, the nature of this underlying psychopathology is not specified.

The passive-dependent type, characterized by helplessness, indecisiveness, and clinging dependency, seems to be the final common pathway of a host of affective and cognitive disorders.

The passive-aggressive type is defined by the use of passive sabotaging mechanisms, such as pouting, stubbornness, procrastination, inefficiency, and passive obstructionism in the pursuit of aggressive ends. Again, this behavior would seem to be the final common pathway of many conflicted states wherein the person wishes to behave aggressively and is blocked from doing so by either external circumstances or internal inhibition. In practice, this term is often used for the exploitative, egocentric personality who is not considered extreme enough to be considered sociopathic. These near-sociopaths appear to be attempting to attain a dependent niche without having to accept a subordinate role.

The aggressive type of patient manifests irritability, temper tantrums, and destructive behavior in response to frustration. Again, an aggressive response to frustration appears in association with a wide range of trait constellations and may not warrant syndromal status.

Frequently, it may be difficult to make the differential diagnosis between passive-aggressive personality and emotionally unstable character disorder because during their "high" phase, the emotionally unstable character disorders may be ebullient, over-active, impulsive, and rash, with marked lack of foresight and intolerance of routine and rules. The qualitatively abnormal attitudes and social maneuvers are the most obvious aspects of their pathology and serve to mask their heightened state of affective activation. Therefore, these patients may be incorrectly diagnosed as passive-aggressive character disorders, aggressive type. Since this diagnosis fails to recognize the chronic activation dysregulation, the European term "hyperthymic psychopath" seems more appropriate.

PSEUDONEUROTIC SCHIZOPHRENIC, PSEUDOSCHIZOPHRENIC NEUROSIS, AND PASSIVE - DEPENDENT CHARACTER DISORDER WITH MULTIPLE NEUROTIC AND AFFECTIVE SYMPTOMS

We consider the term "pseudoneurotic schizophrenia" a misnomer applied to extremely severe, passive-dependent character disorders with salient anxious, obsessive-compulsive, and/or hysterical, phobic, and sexually deviant symptomatology. To complicate the phenomenology these patients are particularly prone to the abuse of sedative and stimulant drugs, and in more recent years marijuana and LSD. The heterogeneity of this group is attested to by the fact that all classes of medications have a place in their treatment. The minor tranquilizers are useful under conditions of anticipatory anxiety; the phenothiazines, during agitated depressive states, and the antidepressants, for periods of fearful clinging, withdrawal, and depressive rumination. Although medication may relieve distress, the burden of care falls upon the psychotherapeutic relationship.

The concept of schizophrenia has led to widespread confusion. Kraepelin's original definition of *dementia praecox* was based upon the course of illness. The term was used to distinguish deteriorating patients from other "functional" psychotics such as manic-depressives, who did not deteriorate although they might relapse. In order to make a rational prognosis, Kraepelin isolated certain distinguishing initial clinical features of deteriorated patients and used these to define a syndrome with a specific poor prognosis.

Bleuler, on the other hand, was less impressed with the predictive utility of such initial symptomatology. Rather, he emphasized other clinical features, such as autism and ambivalence, that were assumed to identify a disorder of association considered by him to be the basis of the schizophrenic process. These traits were believed to be discernible even during nonpsychotic periods. These characteristics were not segregated for their prognostic value and indeed did not identify a disorder that necessarily progressed to deterioration. For this reason, even if one were able to apply Bleuler's ill-defined criteria systematically and identify this fundamental psychological defect, thereby diagnosing schizophrenia, one would still be left without any prognostic ability.

This trend to segregate patients on the basis of some inferred psychopathological process and to divorce this categorization from the practical utility of prediction received further emphasis in the recent labels "pseudo-neurotic" or "pseudopsychopathic" schizophrenia. Patients so labeled need not manifest examinational signs of either Kraepelinian or Bleulerian-defined schizophrenia. The reasons for the assumption of a continuum between these states and classically defined schizophrenia are not clear. It is meritorious to make the creative effort necessary to describe a syndrome, but it is unwise for the psychiatric community to accept such syndromes uncritically, without clinical and statistical documentation or practical validation.

Hoch and Polatin,[9] who developed the concept of pseudoneurotic schizophrenia, have stated that these cases are frequently considered psychoneurotic by others; but, since these patients are refractory to exploratory psychotherapy, they argue that there must be a basic difference in psychopathology. Other postulated indicators of a continuum with schizophrenia include "eventual certification and deterioration, an autistic and dereistic life approach, diffuse ambivalence, inappropriate emotional connections and reactions, pan-anxiety, pan-neurosis, omnipotent attitudes, subtle thinking disorders, vague contradictory self-presentations, short-lived psychotic episodes and chaotic sexuality."

Unfortunately, there are no normative data about the uniformity or incidence of these differential clinical signs. Review of their case presentations fails to indicate a basic homogeneity, but rather suggests a heterogeneous collection of treatment-refractory patients. One remembers the wry definition of the "borderline patient" as one who is continually verging on not paying his bills or not showing up for appointments. Although the originators of this concept specifically state that they are not advocating a more refined classification, there is no doubt that the impact of their approach has caused many patients to be labeled "schizophrenic" who would previously have been considered to be suffering from a severe neurosis, affective or character disorder.

One suspects that this diagnosis is used to maintain the belief that exploratory psychotherapy is uniformly effective in psychoneuroses. If a psychoneurotic does not respond to therapy, the method is not at fault, rather the diagnosis is inaccurate. One can avoid even the small loss of self-esteem attended by a missed diagnosis by diagnosing almost all patients who are not grossly psychotic as pseudoneurotic schizophrenics. If they fail to improve, one's diagnostic acumen is supported, and if they do well, one's therapeutic skill is affirmed.

Fish[10] has referred to these patients as "pseudoschizophrenic neurotics." Our experience, both from the point of view of reaction to psychotropic medication, familial and developmental history, as well as follow-up of illness course, leads us to conjecture that many of these patients have suffered from a severe affective disorder in infancy and childhood with a secondary development of neurotic symptoms and character deformations.

It is evident that Bleulerian schizophrenia represents a melange of different psychopathological states. This is confirmed by their diversity in developmental course, response to somatic therapy, and follow-up.

We follow Kraepelin's model in defining schizophrenia as a severe, cryptogenic, potentially psychotic disorder with poor prognosis and a tendency to relapse, with permanent emotional and social deficit. Therefore, we shall consider "pseudoneurotic schizophrenia" as a type of personality disorder.

CLINICAL PREDICTORS

From the theory that the major psychotropic agents work reparatively on activation-affective dysregulation,[8] it follows that conditions not characterized by this type of defect should be refractory to these drugs. This is largely accurate. Inadequate, dyssocial, antisocial, passive-aggressive, and narcissistic personality disorders, perversions, obsessive-compulsive states, mental deficiency, histrionic, conversion, and hypochrondriacal reactions, and chronic, burned-out schizophrenics are all refractory to phenothiazines and imipramine-like drugs. When drugs prove useful in these conditions, it is in the treatment of an intercurrent affective derangement, without alteration of the patient's chronic difficulty. Drug treatment mimics natural course i.e. unremitting chronic symptoms that have been exacerbated by affective flare-ups slowly return to baseline after the affective disorder subsides.

However, some patients with affective-activation disorders may not respond to psychotropic agents; that is, some patients' specific defects elude drug treatment. Under the usual clinical circumstances it is difficult to try methodically one antidepressant or phenothiazine after another in search of a suitable agent, especially since ECT is often effective in many drug-refractor states. However, certain depressives who are refractory to imipramine respond to desmethylimipramine or an MAO inhibitor. It seems likely that these therapeutic specificities are due to different defects in the basic pathophysiology that are not reflected in the manifest symptomatology. Another possibility is variation in detoxification mechanisms leading to different net availability of the drugs at target sites. Careful comparative studies of diagnostically and phenomenally similar patients who respond differentially to drugs may help isolate such basic patho-physiological differences.

With histrionic patients there is no sustained response to medication although a transient initial improvement is common. Since we hypothesize that these patients' symptoms may not be the direct external manifestation of intolerable affective states, but rather environmentally oriented, learned, and manipulative devices, failure of the major psychotropic agents to work in this group is compatible with the theory that these drugs work on a basic activation derangement. The high incidence of somatizing reactions to medication in this group further supports the belief that their emotional difficulties revolve about validating the "sick" role. Everything is grist for the mill, including side effects. Thus, these patients define themselves as mysteriously untreatable and a therapeutic challenge.

Another group of patients comparatively refractory to phenothiazines or imipramine consists of those with chronic anticipatory anxiety. A pharmacodiagnostic observation is the moderate usefulness in these patients of the sedative class of drugs, i.e. alcohol, barbiturates, meprobamate, glutethimide, ethchlorvinyl, diazepam, chlordiazepoxide, etc. The usefulness of these agents is limited by pharmacological tolerance since increasingly large doses are often required to maintain equanimity, and these patients may self-administer these compounds to the point of addiction. This is in sharp contrast to the effects of the phenothiazines and imipramine in severe depressions and schizophrenia where generally, following initial effective treatment, progressively less medication is necessary to maintain remission. Also in sharp contrast is the general uselessness of sedatives and minor tranquilizers in conditions of marked activation-affective dysregulation.

Some theories of phenothiazine effect place heavy emphasis on the central role of alleged "antianxiety" actions. That is, various symptoms, such as hallucinations, delusions, and agitation are seen as secondary responses to "anxiety," and the ameliorative effects of the drug are ascribed to reduction of anxiety. This type of theory has been supported by the reports of supposed specific effects of phenothiazines on conditioned avoidance reactions. The clinical refractoriness of chronically anxious patients to phenothiazines casts doubt on this.

EXPERIMENTAL STUDY OF RELATIONSHIP OF PERSONALITY DISORDER DIAGNOSIS TO DRUG EFFECT

An experimental program was initiated at Hillside Hospital, in 1961, to study the effects of chlorpromazine and imipramine. The subjects of the study were patients at this two hundred-bed, open ward, voluntary psychiatric facility. All patients were considered to have early and acute mental disorders and were treated in individual psychotherapy sessions for varying periods of time before drugs were prescribed. Psychotherapy and intensive milieu therapies continued during drug treatment. Most patients were well-educated and came from middle-class social backgrounds. Hospital stay was independent of ability to pay. All psychotropic drug therapy was initiated by referral of the patient's supervising staff psychiatrist to the research team.

It should be emphasized that all referrals for psychotropic medication were accepted, regardless of diagnosis or symptomatology, since it was hoped to be able to utilize the drug effects as tools for discriminating subgroups of patients; thus, a large heterogeneous group was required. Pretreatment examinations consisted of research psychiatric interviews, behavioral ratings by the patient's psychiatrist and ward personnel, self-ratings of symptoms and attitudes, psychological tests, electroencephalograms, medical examination and physiological tests, including blood pressure response to mecholyl and radioactive iodine uptake.

Subjects were randomly assigned to placebo or one of two fixed increment drug schedules for six weeks. Daily dosage of imipramine for each week was 75 mg, 150 mg, 225 mg, and 300 mg thereafter. Daily dosage of chlorpromazine for each week was 300 mg, 600 mg, 900 mg, and 1,200 mg thereafter. To prevent akinesia, akathisia, and other extrapyramidal disorders each dose of chlorpromazine was combined with 1.25 percent (to a maximum of 15 mg daily) procyclidine. Each medication was dissolved in a highly flavored liquid placebo vehicle, and each patient received a constant 40 cc/day from individually labeled bottles. Maximum dosage was maintained for two weeks, and retesting was conducted during the sixth week of medication.

During the seven weeks of the experimental program, longitudinal clinical observations were maintained. In addition, following the experimental period, all patients were followed throughout their hospital stay so that their clinical response to other interventions could be assessed. To gain information concerning long-term outcome, both for diagnostic clarification and estimates of treatment efficacy, all patients who entered this program were later followed by the research staff through detailed interviews of the patients and informed relatives, two and three years after hospital discharge.

No attempt was made, in this initial study, to make a diagnostic statement prior to the patients' entry into the study. One hundred and forty-four patients completed this first study.

The clinical impression of the author (D.K.) who had interviewed each patient weekly was that diagnostic statements were capable of making valid predictions about treatment effect. Therefore, all patients were again reviewed thoroughly and diagnoses made. Since the diagnoses were made after the drug effect was observed, there is a methodological flaw in this procedure. This could conceivably have influenced the diagnostic statements made, although pains were taken to try to avoid this contamination.

However, to extend the study further, the research design was repeated in 1963, and an additional group of 151 patients was studied. In all, 295 patients completed both drug administration periods. Sixteen patients, who had received at least eighteen days of treatment, were dropped for various reasons related to their psychiatric status. Since they were considered to have a clinically adequate drug trial, they were included in this analysis, for a total sample of 311.

In the second study diagnoses were made prior to the administration of drugs. Comparison of the same diagnostic groups showed no significant differences with regard to treatment outcomes during the first and second parts of the study on any drug. Therefore, it is believed that any retrospective diagnostic bias during the first part of the study was minimal, and in this presentation data from both study periods are pooled.

Our data show that diagnosis is predictive of drug effect, particularly if two aspects of illness that do not usually form part of diagnostic categorization are considered. The first aspect is the degree of retardation or excitation in the initial clinical state.

Each patient, prior to the administration of drugs, was described in terms of the well-substantiated bipolar dimension, retarded depression versus manic excitement. Three categories were delineated: manic, normoactive, and retarded. The retarded patients had long latencies in their responses, psychomotor inhibition, lack of spontaneity, and dearth of thought. The excited patients showed psychomotor acceleration, flight of ideas, low frustration tolerance, inability to maintain a goal set, and occasionally euphoria.

The second significant diagnostic issue is the developmental history of the patient, with special emphasis upon signs of childhood deviancy that are compatible with suspected early minimal brain damage, as discussed elsewhere.[11]

The major outcome measure reported here is a global outcome scale ranging from +5 to 15, where 10 equals no change. The results for the pseudoneurotic group are given in Table 15-I, along with results for sixty schizo-affective and fifty "process" schizophrenics. A significant imipramine effect was found for the pseudoneurotic patients contrasting with the pronounced chlorpromazine effect in the schizo-affective group. This differential drug response strengthens our conviction that the pseudoneurotic group is improperly classified as a schizophrenic subtype.

Among the other personality disorders, analyzed as a total group, chlorpromazine as compared to placebo had a slight beneficial clinical effect that achieved statistical significance. However, as shown in Table 15-II, this chlorpromazine effect was restricted entirely to the emotionally unstable subgroup. No effect due to imipramine was noted.

However, when the character disorders were subdivided according to

TABLE 15-I
MEAN OUTCOME RATINGS FOR "SCHIZOPHRENIC PATIENTS IN EACH
DRUG GROUP

Subdiagnosis	N	Placebo	Imipramine	Chlorpromazine-Procyclidine
Process	50	10.9	10.2	11.3
Schizoaffective	60	10.3	10.9	12.6**
Pseudoneurotic	32	10.6	11.6*	11.0

*Significantly different from placebo (U test, P. < .05, 1-tailed test).
**Significantly different from placebo (U test, P. < .001, 1-tailed test).

their initial activation state, retarded patients on imipramine showed a significant clinical improvement, despite the very small N (Table 15-III). In addition, normoactive patients showed a statistically significant clinical improvement on chlorpromazine.

TABLE 15-II
MEAN OUTCOME RATINGS FOR OTHER CHARACTER DISORDERS IN EACH
DRUG GROUP

Subdiagnosis	N	Placebo	Imipramine	Chlorpromazine-Procyclidine
Hysterical	27	10.6	10.2	10.8
Emotionally Unstable	43	10.7	10.9	12.1*
Passive Aggressive	10	10.0	10.9	10.6
Total:	80	10.6	10.7	11.5*

*Significantly different from placebo (U test, P. < .05, 1-tailed test).

The imipramine finding is an interesting lead, since it may indicate that some psychopathological states considered as characterological reactions are actually retarded depressions in abnormal personalities.

TABLE 15-III
MEAN OUTCOME RATINGS FOR CHARACTER DISORDERS BY ACTIVATION LEVEL

Activation	N	Placebo	Imipramine	Chlorpromazine-Procyclidine
Manic	14	11.2	10.2	11.0
None	59	10.5	10.6	11.7*
Retarded	7	10.0	12.8*	10.0
Total:	80	10.6	10.7	11.5*

*Significantly different from placebo (U test, P. < .05, 1-tailed test).

Decision Tree Systematization

The previous discussion has shown the utility of clinical diagnosis in predicting the response (or nonresponse) of certain classes of personality disorders to chlorpromazine, imipramine, and placebo. However, the unreliability of psychiatric diagnosis is well-known and is one of the primary reasons for the current lack of interest in psychodiagnosis in general. Since the predictive utility of properly done diagnoses is supported by the present investigation, the development of new methods for systematizing the psychiatric diagnostic process to increase both reliability and validity seems justified.

At Hillside we have developed an automated method of psychiatric classification based upon the empirical analysis of cross-sectional psychiatric interview data.[12] The system can be described in brief as a "peak clipping" technique which searches the tails of distributions looking for areas of nonoverlap in which subjects can, with relatively little false positive error, be assigned to diagnostic categories. The trait sets so defined are polythetic in the sense that individual members of the class need not share any traits in common. We have felt that the more traditional model of multiple discriminant function analysis for this purpose was unjustified, primarily on the basis of markedly nonnormal univariate, and heteroscedastic bivariate data distributions. Preliminary work comparing our decision tree method with multiple discriminant function methods suggest that the decision tree method has the virtue of defining a smaller set of clinically salient predictors.

TABLE 15-IV

CROSS-TABULATION OF MACHINE-MADE DECISION TREE

Diagnoses versus Criterion Clinical Diagnoses

Decision Tree Diagnoses	Clinical Diagnoses			
	PNS	EUCD	HCD and PA	Total
PNS	25	4	8	37
EUCD	3	29	4	36
HCD and PA	4	10	24	38
Total	32	43	36	111

Kappa = .55 (p. < .001)

Table 15-IV is a cross tabulation of clinical diagnoses (criterion diagnoses) compared with decision tree program diagnoses. There were 111 patients clinically assigned to the pseudoneurotic, emotionally unstable, and hysterical character disorder groups. The small passive-aggressive character disorder group was combined with the hysterical character disorders for this analysis. The number of corresponding classifications is given in the main diagonal, where it will be seen that there were 78 machine classifications out of 111 which agreed with the criterion diagnoses, a "hit" rate of 70 percent. Classification errors can be seen in the off-diagonal elements and are uniformly low. These findings are highly significant statistically, yielding a kappa of .55, p < .001.

TABLE 15-V

EIGHT ITEMS FOR DISCRIMINATING CHARACTER DISORDERS FROM PSEUDONEUROTICS

Item	Level	True Positive	False Positive
Elated Mood	>6	7	0
Suicidal Preoccupation	>7	6	0
Feelings of Superiority	>7	5	0
Belief in Hallucinations, Voices	>2	10	1
Inaudible Speech	3	5	0
Uninhibited	7	14	2
No Recurring Thoughts	2	15	3
Under-talkative	4	5	1
		—	—
		67	7

TABLE 15-VI

THREE ITEMS FOR DISCRIMINATING EMOTIONALLY UNSTABLE FROM HYSTERICAL AND PASSIVE-AGGRESSIVE CHARACTER DISORDER

Item	Level	TP	FP
Elated mood	5	18	2
Fast reactions	7	5	1
Under-concerned	=1	6	1
		—	—
		29	4

Tables 15-V and 15-VI show the discrete items and cut-off scores for each diagnostic grouping. The item content defining the machine classifications make good clinical sense. Interestingly the method is able to reflect accurately pathologic variations at both ends of conceptually bipolar items. For example, the combined character disorder group is distinguished from pseudoneurotic patients both by elated mood and uninhibited behavior as well as being undertalkative and having inaudible speech (Table 15-V). The point here is that since certain conditions, particularly affective emotionally unstable and hysterical disorders, are characterized by pathology at both the high *and* low ends of bipolar items, a method is needed that does not sacrifice the potential predictive power of deviation in either direction from mean trends. In addition, classification methods based on weighted, summed, or multiplicative formulas fail to reflect the "polythatic" character of much psychopathology, in which members of the same sub-group, as individuals, need not share with other members of the group the same set of pathognomonic traits.

Perhaps the most telling demonstration of the utility of the automated diagnoses is in the actual prediction of drug response. Table 15-VII is a summary of mean global improvement scores by diagnosis and drug group. Within this matrix will be found results for both the criterion clinical diagnoses and the machine-made decision tree diagnoses.

TABLE 15-VII

MEAN DRUG EFFECTS FOR THREE DIAGNOSTIC GROUPS

Comparing Machine versus Clinical Diagnoses

			Plac			Imip			Chlor		
			X	SD	N	X	SD	N	X	SD	N
PNS	Clin	32	10.33	.62	(12)	11.23*	1.58	(13)	10.86	.83	(7)
	DT	37	10.53	.81	(15)	11.07*	1.39	(15)	11.14	.99	(7)
EUCD	Clin	43	10.57	1.64	(14)	10.78	2.48	(18)	12.09*	1.44	(11)
	DT	36	10.73	1.71	(11)	10.27	2.41	(15)	11.60*	1.36	(10)
HCD/ PACD	Clin	36	10.33	1.74	(15)	10.17	1.86	(12)	10.56	.50	(9)
	DT	38	10.43	1.05	(15)	11.42	1.66	(13)	11.00	1.26	(10)

*"t" test significant, P. < .05.

Table 15-VII shows quite close correspondence of drug effect results evaluated by both clinical and decision tree diagnosis. Pseudoneurotic patients were found by both classification methods to respond positively to imipramine treatment, and emotionally unstable character disorder patients classified both clinically and by decision tree methods were found to respond positively to chlorpromazine.

Additional data bearing on the relationship of our method to the more traditional factor-analytic or multiple prediction methods is given by the individual item correlations with global improvement. Of the 105 correlations, only one was significant at the .01 level, and three, at the .05 level. The items were then clustered by item intercorrelations and seven clusters derived. None of the seven cluster scores correlated significantly with global improvement within any of the three drug treatment groups. The point we wish to stress here is that when these same data are used for decision tree analyses, very respectable levels of predictive accuracy were obtained (see Tables 15-V and 15-VII). The predictive information is in the data, but traditional correlational methods may not allow it to emerge.

It should be remembered that in the present analyses decision tree classifications were made entirely on the basis of thirty-five items of cross-sectional psychiatric interview data while clinical diagnoses were made with the benefit of a wide range of historical information on each patient. The decision tree method is not limited to such data, and in future analyses we will add historical data to the predictor item pool. We feel quite certain that this will increase the already respectable level of classificatory accuracy, yielding a still closer correspondence between diagnosis and drug response.

QUALITATIVE OUTCOME PATTERNS

In addition to the global scale, prior to knowledge of drug assignment, the treatment response of each patient was categorized by the research psychiatrist as belonging to one of a series of qualitative outcome patterns. These patterns can be ordered along the global improvement continuum (see Table 15-VIII). They will be described starting with the most favorable pattern and proceeding to the most unfavorable. Each pattern is distinguished by its salient clinical changes.

Denial

This pattern consisted of a complete disappearance of symptomatology, a renewed ability to function normally, and a massive refusal by the patient to admit to any residual functional or social difficulty. The patient spent much time convincing his psychiatrist of the lack of need for further treatment and the immediate necessity for the patient to return to his usual life routines. This response was very unusual among personality disorders. Only one patient with an emotionally unstable disorder showed this outcome on placebo.

Reduction of Episodic Anxiety

This pattern consisted of the loss of sudden panicky episodes; however, a high level of apprehensive anxiety as to the possibility of the recurrence of these episodes was maintained. Therefore, dependent phobic manipulations may continue although the panics have ceased. In other words, the patient may still demand a companion, although he can actually be alone. This response was very unusual among personality disorders. Only one pseudoneurotic schizophrenic patient showed this response while on imipramine.

Cognitive Reorganization

This pattern consisted of a marked decrease in the psychotic attribution of unusual personal symbolic significances to objects and gestures, along with the associated ideas of reference, perplexity, and suspiciousness. Before treatment these patients frequently had psychomotor retardation, or more rarely acceleration, but tended to become normoactive with drug therapy. No personality disorder showed this response on any medication.

Reduction of Anger

This pattern consisted of a marked reduction in angry hyperactivity, and pressure of thought and speech with increased frustration tolerance. This was uncommon, and only one emotionally unstable patient showed this response while on imipramine.

Affective Stability

This pattern consisted of a marked decrease in lability in patients whose mood was continually swinging from giddy exhilaration to morose withdrawal within a few days span. It is important to note that these patients had mood stabilization, since there was a decrease in both the giddy euphoria and depressed withdrawal. This was a common drug response pattern and will be analyzed below.

Reduction of Agitated Depression

This pattern consisted of a marked decrease in agitated motor activity and expressive complaint, associated with an increased ability to spontaneously participate in constructive activities. This pattern will be analysed below.

Mood Elevation

This pattern consisted of a lessening of depressive mood, accompanied by response facilitation, increased spontaneity and activity as well as improved morale, zestfulness, and the ability to undertake tasks. However, considerable residual apprehension and low self-esteem with symptomatic recrudescence under adaptive stress was common. This response pattern will be analyzed below.

Schizoid Compliance

This response pattern consisted of a drug-induced decrement in these patients' fragmented, jumbled, and rambling thinking processes and fearful self-presentation. This was replaced by a passive, fringe of the crowd, compliant, unspontaneous adaptation. The so-called zombie look was most prevalent in this group. No patients with personality disorder showed this response pattern.

No Change

This label was applied to patients who showed no discernible net clinical change. However, these patients may have shown several sharp fluctuations and were not necessarily clinically inactive. This response pattern will be analyzed below.

Manic

This pattern was associated with the onset of a marked psychomotor acceleration involving hyperactivity, insomnia, pressure of thought and speech, and low frustration tolerance. Euphoric and elated attitudes were not particularly salient. Only two patients with personality disorders developed this pattern, both on imipramine. In general, this reaction is more characteristic of affective disorders treated with imipramine.

Somatizing

In this pattern there were marked complaints about intolerable medication side-effects, frequently involving dizziness and lethargy. These symptoms made the continuation of medication a very difficult procedure. Only three patients developed this pattern, all while on chlorpromazine. This response was characteristic of chlorpromazine and cut across diagnostic categories.

Retardation

This pattern consisted of a marked decrease in psychomotor activity with retardation, paucity of thought, and marked increase in response latencies, approximating a severe retarded depression or stupor. Only one emotionally unstable patient, on placebo, demonstrated this pattern.

Anger

This pattern consisted of marked irritability and chronic hostility with both verbal and behavioral manifestations. Psychotic disorganization did not occur. This pattern will be analyzed below.

Agitated Disorganization

In these patients an inappropriate euphoria was followed by the sudden onset of delusional and bizarre ideation associated with hyperactivity and hostility, quite analogous to an acute excited schizophrenic episode. Interestingly, of the four patients to show this exacerbation, two were hysterics on placebo.

Statistical analyses were conducted by Fisher Exact Tests.

"PSEUDONEUROTIC SCHIZOPHRENIA"

Imipramine produced an increased proportion of positive qualitative outcomes when compared with placebo, 69.2 percent (9/13) versus 25.0 percent (3/12), respectively (p 0.03). Although chlorpromazine showed a trend towards beneficial effect, this failed to reach statistical significance. This is amplified below by specific analysis of qualitative outcomes. Compared with placebo neither drug produced a significantly different incidence of negative qualitative outcomes.

In terms of qualitative outcomes, reduction of agitated depression occurred significantly more often in the chlorpromazine-treated group than

Drugs, Development, and Cerebral Function

TABLE 15-VIII
NUMBER OF SUBJECTS IN EACH QUALITATIVE OUTCOME GROUP
(by Drug and Diagnosis)

Qualitative Outcome Group	Pseudo-Neurotics (32)			Emotionally Unstable (43)			Hyster and Pas-Agg (37)		
	Plac	Impr	Chlor	Plac	Impr	Chlor	Plac	Impr	Chlor
Agit. Disorg. x GIS* = 12.9 SD = 2.5		1						1	
Affect Stability x GIS = 12.4 SD = 0.8		1		2	8	9			
Red. Agit. Depr. x GIS = 12.3 SD = 1.2			3					1	
Mood Elevation x GIS = 12.2 SD = 1.1	3	7	1			3	4	3	
Anger x GIS = 12.2 SD = 1.7					4				2
Retardation x GIS = 11.7 SD = 1.2				1					
Somatization x GIS = 11.6 SD = 1.4			1			1			1
Manic x GIS = 11.0 SD = 0.0		1						1	
No Change x GIS = 10.2 SD = 0.7	9	2	2	10	2	1	10	6	8

x GIS = Mean Global Improvement Score (range = 5-15, 10 = no change and 15 = maximum improvement.

in the placebo-treated group, respectively 42.9 percent (3/7) versus 0 percent (0/12) (p < 0.04). This qualitative chlorpromazine effect is not specific to pseudoneurotic schizophrenia since it occurred in 12.9 percent (12/93) of all other chlorpromazine treated diagnostic groups as opposed to 2.3 percent (2/86) of placebo-treated patients in other diagnostic groups (p < 0.02). It should be noted that the specific usefulness of chlorpromazine in producing reduction of agitated depression in this group of pseudo-neurotics was missed in the analysis of the proportion of all positive outcomes.

Mood elevation was the predominant positive effect of imipramine in this diagnostic group, but just failed to reach statistical significance when compared to placebo.

The no-change pattern occurred in only 20.0 percent (4/20) of the drug treated subjects as opposed to 75.0 percent (9/12) of the placebo treated group (p < 0.003).

EMOTIONALLY UNSTABLE CHARACTER DISORDER

Both imipramine and chlorpromazine were associated with more positive qualitative outcomes than placebo. Placebo produced 21.4 percent (3/14) positive outcomes as compared to 66.7 percent (12/18) with imipramine and 81.8 percent (9/11) with chlorpromazine (placebo versus both drugs p = 0.002). Negative outcomes were infrequent in all drug groups and insignificantly different between agents.

Affective stability was produced by both active drugs more frequently than by placebo. Imipramine produced this pattern in 44.4 percent (8/18) of the patients as opposed to 14.3 percent (2/14) of the placebo-treated patients. However, this difference just fails statistical significance. Chlorpromazine produced the affective stability pattern in 81.8 percent (9/11) patients as opposed to 14.3 percent (2/14) of the placebo-treated patients (p < 0.005). The affective stability response is specific for emotionally unstable character disorders treated with active medication as it occurred in 58.6 percent (17/29) of such patients as opposed to 1.8 percent (5/280) of all other patients (p < 0.001).

The anger response occurred in 22.2 percent (4/18) of the imipramine treated emotionally unstable character disorders, as opposed to 0 percent (0/25) of the combined chlorpromazine and placebo group (p = 0). (p = 0.025). The emotionally unstable character disorders were more prone to respond with the anger pattern to imipramine than other patients insofar as 22.2 percent (4/18) of such patients became angry as opposed to 2.2 percent (2/93) of the other patients treated with imipramine (p < 0.01).

HYSTERICAL AND PASSIVE - AGGRESSIVE CHARACTER DISORDERS

This group was outstanding in not showing any differential drug effect. Positive qualitative outcomes, negative qualitative outcomes, and all specific qualitative outcome patterns did not distinguish between placebo, imipramine, and chlorpromazine. Also, the no change pattern occurred far more frequently in the hysterical and passive-aggressive character disorders than in all other diagnostic categorizations, respectively 64.9 percent (24/37) versus 24.6 percent (67/272) (p < 0.001).

Of the eight patients in this group who were treated with active drugs and who manifested clinical change, four showed deleterious effects. Therefore, in general, the treatment of such patients with this regimen of imipramine or chlorpromazine is ill advised.

SUMMARY

Our work in the drug treatment of personality disorders has led to the following conclusions:

1. Drug therapy has a definite, but limited place in the treatment of these conditions.
2. Drug-diagnosis interactions are now clearly established for both global clinical outcome and discrete qualitative outcome categories.
3. The consistently beneficial effects of chlorpromazine in emotionally unstable personalities and imipramine in "pseudoneurotic" patients is contrasted with the lack of drug responsivity in hysterical and passive-aggressive patients.
4. While the present investigation supports the predictive utility of diagnosis, the problem of interjudge unreliability is serious, requiring the development of new, objective diagnostic methods.
5. An empirical, decision-tree method of generating psychiatric diagnoses by computer is described. The method makes no assumptions about univariate or bivariate distribution characteristics, and is consequently free of some of the criticisms leveled at multiple-discriminant function analyses of psychiatric rating scale data.
6. The present data support the validity of these "machine diagnoses," showing drug-diagnosis interactions of a similar magnitude to our criterion, clinical diagnoses.

Future work in this area will include refinements of the objective, diagnostic methods, and extension of the empirical data base to include historical as well as additional cross-sectional predictor items.

REFERENCES

1. Goldberg, S. C.: Prediction of response to antipsychotic drugs. In Efron, D. H. (Ed.) : *Psychopharmacology. A Review of Progress, 1957-1967.* Washington, D.C., Public Health Service Publication, no. 1836, U.S. Government Printing Office, 1968, pp. 1101-1118.
2. Wittenborn, J .R., and May, P. R. A. (Eds.) : *Prediction of Response to Pharmacotherapy.* Springfield, Thomas, 1966.
3. Uhlenhuth, E. H., Rickels, K., Fisher, S., Park, L. C., Lipman, R. S., and Mock, J.: Drug, doctor's verbal attitude and clinic settting in the symptomatic response to pharmacotherapy. *Psychopharmacologia (Berlin), 9:*392-418, 1966.
4. Rickels, K., Cattell, R. B., Weise, C., Gray, B., Yee, R., Mallin, S. and Aaronson, H. C.: Controlled psychopharmacological research in private psychiatric practice. *Psychopharmacologia, 9:*288-306, 1966.

5. Rickels, K., and Downing, R. W.: Drug and placebo-treated neurotic outpatients. Pretreatment levels of manifest anxiety, clinical improvement and side reactions. *Arch Gen Psychiat, 16:*369-372, 1967.

6. American Psychiatric Association: *Diagnostic and Statistical Manual, Mental Disorders.* Washington, D.C., 1952.

7. American Psychiatric Association: *Diagnostic and Statistical Manual, Mental Disorders,* 2nd ed. Washington, D.C., 1968.

8. Klein, D. F. and Davis, J. M.: *Diagnosis and Drug Treatment of Psychiatric Disorders.* Baltimore, Williams and Wilkins, 1969.

9. Hoch, P., and Polatin, P.: Pseudoneurotic forms of schizophrenia. *Psychiat Quart, 23:*148-276, 1949.

10. Fish, F. J.: Outline of psychiatry. Baltimore, Williams and Wilkins, 1964.

11. Pollack, M., Levenstein, S. and Klein, D. F.: A three-year post-hospital follow-up of psychiatric patients: First hospitalization in adolescence vs. adulthood. *Int J Child Psychiat, 33:*224-225, 1966.

12. Honigfeld, G., Klein, D. F., and Feldman, S.: Prediction of psychopharmacologic effect in man: Development and validation of a computerized diagnostic decision tree. *Computers Biomed Res, 2:*350-366, 1969.

PART V

METABOLIC AND BIOCHEMICAL INFLUENCES

Chapter 16

Metabolic and Behavioral Consequences
of Nicotine*

WALTER B. ESSMAN

THE ROLE OF NICOTINE in behavioral studies and in investigations of its
metabolic effects in the central nervous system has been explored at a
relatively superficial level, inasmuch as this agent has not usually been classified among the psychoactive compounds or among the usual series of central
nervous system stimulants. In several respects nicotine bears certain striking
similarities to other central stimulants in that it activates both sympathetic
and parasympathetic ganglia, stimulates skeletal muscle, corotid body receptors, and the supraoptic nucleus of the hypothalamus. When introduced
systemically in sufficient concentration, it leads to onset of convulsions and
produces vasoconstriction through the liberation of norepinephrine present
in the vascular wall, through the direct action on the walls of the blood
vessels. The effect of nicotine and its derivatives in tobacco smoke upon the
central nervous system has been recently summarized (Murphree, 1967).

Evidence concerned with the central action of nicotine has suggested
that its effects are confined to the cholinergic portion of the mesencephalic
activating system; following administration of nicotine to rabbits, EEG activation of hippocampal origin and convulsions at higher doses were observed (Floris et al., 1962). EEG arousal effects and rapid activation produced by subconvulsive doses have indicated that this compound exerts its
central effect rather rapidly.

The metabolic effects of nicotine has implicated several central systems
of possible behavioral relevance; there has been some indication of significant 5-hydroxytryptamine release in rabbit thrombocytes following nicotine
treatment, and it also leads to a significant increase in the urinary excretion
of 5-hydroxyindoleacetic acid following the smoking of five to ten cigarettes
per day (Schuvelein and Werk, 1962). In mice treated with nicotine sulfate
brain levels of 5-hydroxytryptamine were not appreciably altered within one
hour following injection, however nicotine-treated animals showed greater
resistance to the modification of brain serotonin level produced by electroshock (Essman et al., 1968).

Animal studies concerned with the effect of nicotine present several as-

*This work was supported, in part, by a grant from the Council for Tobacco Research—
U.S.A., and Grant HD-03493 from The National Institutes of Health.

273

pects of behavioral findings which have been varied with respect to both of
the species studied, the doses utilized, and the results obtained. The major
point derived is the question of whether the observed central effects of nicotine action is facilitory or actively serves to impair behavior. It is extremely
difficult to evaluate such discrepant studies in view of the fact that dosage,
species, behavioral technique, and the chronocity of treatment has seldom
been consistent from study to study. For example, a dose-dependent increase
in locomotor activity has been observed with nicotine (Bonta, *et al.,* 1960)
whereas rats trained to perform a color discrimination showed a dose-dependent impairment of performance, the duration of which was also dose-related
(Mercier and Desaigne, 1960). Chronic administration of nicotine over a
period of several months resulted in an appreciable decrement in maze performance (Essenberg, 1948, 1954), whereas age-dependent onset of conditioned response elaboration in rats was shown to emerge with nicotine treatment; young adult rats were facilitated to a greater degree by the same dosage of nicotine than were less mature rats, whereas older rats were not affected by similar treatment (Linucher and Michelson, 1965). A number of
studies have reported that nicotine exerts a behaviorally facilitative effect;
this has been observed with respect to conditioned response acquisition by
rats, where again younger rats tended to show a greater facilitative effect
than did older animals (Robustelli, 1966). The age-dependent effect of
nicotine treatment and a dose-dependent facilitation has been observed
utilizing an operant task (Morrison, 1967), and the facilitory effect upon
bar pressing by rats was abolished through prior treatment with physostigmine. A reduced rate of bar pressing was potentiated by physostigmine
given before nicotine treatment and an increased rate of bar pressing was
reduced by a similar drug sequence, providing some evidence thereby for a
central interaction of these possibly cholinergic events (Morrison, 1968).
Shock avoidance conditioning has been enhanced in nicotine-treated mice
(Oliverio, 1967), and a two-pattern choice response mediating shock avoidance was facilitated by nicotine treatment, whereas a more complex five-
pattern choice was not affected (Bovet-Nitti, 1966). The effect of nicotine
in rats has been indicated to lead to superior learning whereas a more
reactive strain of rat showed a greater degree of drug-induced facilitation
than did a nonreactive strain (Garg and Holland, 1968). A strain-dependent
facilitation of shuttle box avoidance behavior by nicotine treatment has
been demonstrated in mice, wherein animals characteristically showing low
initial performance scores showed a greater degree of facilitation while in
another strain with initially high performance scores, the drug effects impaired avoidance behavior (Bovet, *et al.,* 1966). In this study a fifteen-minute interval prevailing between nicotine treatment and the behavioral task,
suggests that what may have been observed as either "facilitatory" or "dis-

ruptive" may merely suggest differences in the time courses for the central action of nicotine as a function of strain.

In previous investigations concerned with the interelationship between the central metabolic effects of nicotine and its effect upon a specific behavioral process, memory consolidation, it has been shown that mice treated with nicotine sulfate prior to training were provided with antagonism toward the amnesia produced by posttraining ECS; this was paralleled by a nicotine-induced reversal of the ECS effect upon brain serotonin level. Whereas in control animals treated with saline, posttraining ECS led to an absence of conditioned response retention in 90 percent of the animals, in mice given nicotine sulfate (1 mg/kg) sixty minutes prior to training, amnesia was shown in only 34 percent of these animals after ECS (Essman *et al.*, 1968). After exploration of the hypothesis that memory consolidation can be interrupted by a variety of agents or events, primary among which is acute electroshock treatment, it was established that nicotine sulfate treatment serves to atenuate the amnestic of ECS; such treatment in mice led to a reduced brain serotonin turnover rate and an increased turnover time. Drug treatment did not affect either monoamine oxidase activity or seizure threshold, whereas, under control conditions electroconvulsive shock led to an increase in brain serotonin level (17%, $p < .01$), a decrease in brain serotonin turnover rate, and an increase in turnover time; nicotine treatment with superimposed electroconvulsive shock treatment led to reversal of these changes in brain serotonin metabolism. Comparable results were observed in this study with other psychoactive and metabolic agents which antagonized the amnestic effect of posttraining electroshock (Essman, 1969 a). In further investigations concerned with the behavioral and biochemical effects of nicotine (Essman, 1969 b), it was established that the antagonistic affect toward electroshock-induced retrograde amnesia can be exerted more rapidly with certain metabolites of nicotine and that the central changes in 5-hydroxytryptamine metabolism followed a regionally specific time course.

The purpose of this presentation is to summarize a series of related biochemical and behavioral findings which may suggest a possible role for nicotine as a potentially important psychoactive agent. In previous studies (Essman, 1969 a) central nervous system stimulants possessing some clinically antidepressant properties acted upon both brain serotonin metabolism and electroconvulsive shock-induced amnesia in a manner similar to that observed with the nicotine.

The behavioral task utilized in our studies of memory consolidation consisted of a single trial passive avoidance conditioning technique (Essman and Alpern, 1964) providing for a stable conditioned avoidance response measured by a change in response latency. It has been previously shown that mice training under these conditions and then given a single, transcorneally administered ECS (10mA, 200 msc) show, upon subsequent testing twenty-four hours later, an absence of retention for the avoidance behavior characteristically observed in mice either given no posttraining electroconvulsive shock or electroconvulsive shock at posttraining times no longer effective in mediation retrograde amnesia. There has been some difference of opinion regarding the duration of the effective posttraining interval within which electroconvulsive shock is capable of interferring with memory consolidation; suggestions have been made that this effective interval is as short as several seconds or as long as several hours, and our experience has indicated that the duration is highly strain-and-species-dependent as is subject to seasonal, diurnal, and temperature variations. In the initial study CF-1s strain male mice, weighing approximately 27 gm, were given a single intraperitoneal (i.p.) of nicotine sulfate in a 0.9 percent saline vehicle in a dose of 1.0 mg/kg. Animals were randomly assigned to twenty different groups of sixty mice each with sixteen of these groups receiving nicotine injections and four groups being treated with an equivalent volume (I.P.) of 0.9 percent of saline. At either fifteen, thirty, forty-five, or sixty minutes following injection of either nicotine or saline, one group of each of these conditions was given a single training trial to establish a passive avoidance response as previously described, and for each of these differing postinjection-training times, electroconvulsive shock was given either ten, twenty, thirty, or sixty seconds following the training trial. The percent incidence of conditioned response retention, based upon a criterion of response latency measured on a testing trial, given twenty-four hours following training, of sixty seconds or more is summarized in Figure 16-1. for each of the experimental conditions. It may be noted that saline-treated animals showed a graded incidence of electroconvulsive shock-induced retrograde amnesia as a function of the time between training and electroconvulsive shock, i.e. the greatest incidence of retrograde amnesia (70%) was shown in those animals with a training-ECS interval of ten seconds, whereas, only 20 percent of the animals given ECS sixty seconds following training showed a retrograde amnesia. It is of interest to note that there is a clear difference between the effects of posttraining nicotine treatment at the fifteen-minute and forty-five-minute conditions, and for those groups of mice treated and given posttraining electroconvulsive shock fifteen minutes following nicotine injection there was a clear and consistent degree of reduced conditioned response retention, differing at each of the training-ECS intervals from both the saline-treated controls and groups receiving nicotine forty-five minutes or more prior to training. These data provide strong evidence for the suggestion that an interval of fifteen minutes between nicotine treatment and the training-ECS sequence is sufficient to potentiate the amnestic effects of ECS. The high incidence of conditioned response reten-

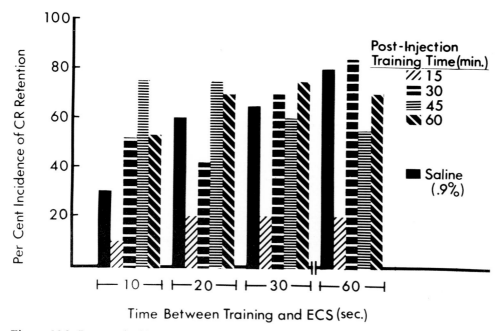

Figure 16-1. Percent incidence of conditioned response retention shown by mice treated with saline or nicotine at differing pretraining times.

tion observed in mice treated with nicotine forty-five minutes, or more, prior to training indicates that, consistent with our previous findings, a significant degree of antagonism toward the amnestic effect of posttraining ECS has been provided. In consideration of the metabolic role played by drug treatment and its central interaction with those circumstances, which in the absence of such drug treatment led to interference with the neural-correlates of the memory consolidation process, the interaction of nicotine treatment and ECS under conditions wherein prior optimal antagonism of the amnestic effects of ECS were observed were then investigated. With the administration of nicotine sulfate (1.0 mg/kg i.p.) forty-five minutes preceding ECS or sham $\overline{(ECS)}$—application of transcorneal electrodes without passage of current—or saline treated under comparable conditions, brain tissue excised ten minutes following ECS treatment was assayed, utilizing a standardized fluorometric procedure for 5-hydroxytryptamine (5-HT) and 5-hydroxyindoleacetic acid (5-HIAA). The results, summarized in Figure 16-2, indicate that saline-treated animals showed a significant elevation in whole brain 5-HT levels with no significant alteration in 5-HIAA content. In nicotine-treated mice electroconvulsive shock did not significantly change the whole brain level of 5-HT, but did elevate brain 5-HIAA significantly beyond that observed under sham-ECS conditions. In consideration

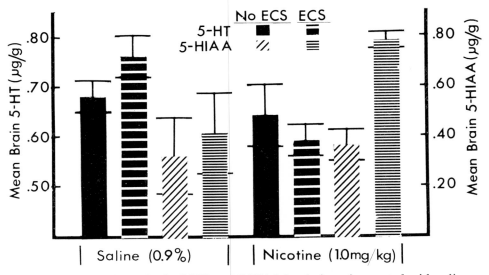

Figure 16-2. Mean (±σ) brain 5-HT and 5-HIAA levels for mice treated with saline or nicotine before ECS or sham-ECS.

of the possibility that the changes in brain levels of 5-HT under conditions of nicotine treatment and/or electroconvulsive shock might bear upon the relationship between the central affects of this interaction and memory consolidation, a study was undertaken to investigate brain 5-HT turnover. It was previously indicated (Essman 1969a) that nicotine treatment affects brain 5-HT turnover and that electroconvulsive shock affected brain 5-HT turnover rate without having appreciable effects upon turnover time. Utilizing conditions described for the previous study and employing a monoamine oxidase inhibitor, tranylcypromine (20 mg/kg), following which tissue samples were obtained at either ten, thirty, or sixty minutes following the drug-ECS sequence, for which it was determined that steadystate 5-HT levels did not differ between treatment conditions, measures of turnover rate and turnover time were derived from rate constants based upon the decrease in brain 5-HIAA levels resulting. In Figure 16-3, the brain 5-HT turnover results are summarized; these indicate that whereas ECS under control conditions leads to an increase in turnover rate, nicotine treatment in the absence of ECS leads to a decreased turnover rate and an increased turnover time. The question of the relationship between the interaction of nicotine at optional times with either ECS or its postictal effects remains to be explored in terms of providing a more firm basis for the apparent dual effect of nicotine upon ECS-induced retrograde amnesia, i.e. the apparent potentiation of the ECS-amnesic effect at fifteen minutes following treatment versus the apparent antagonistic effect when the drug is given forty-five min-

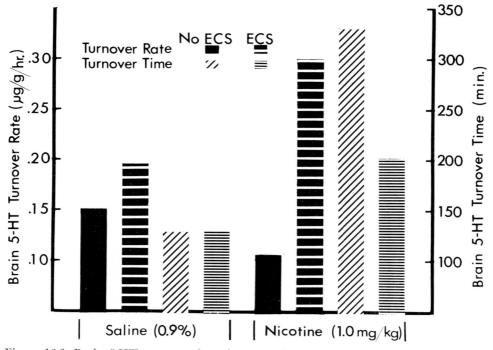

Figure 16-3. Brain 5-HT turnover for mice treated with saline or nicotine before ECS or sham-ECS.

utes prior to ECS. In a subsequent study, levels of 5-HT and 5-HIAA were determined for several regions of the mouse brain for conditions of drug treatment and post-drug ECS, as previously described. ECS or $\overline{\text{ECS}}$ were administered either fifteen minutes or forty-five minutes following (I.P.) injection of nicotine sulfate (1.0 mg/kg) or 0.9 percent saline in an equivalent volume. Ten animals each were utilized for each of the eight times, drug, and ECS conditions. At ten minutes following treatment, a time interval selected largely on the basis of the previous observations of brain amine changes resulting from ECS treatment, brain tissue was excised and carefully dissected to yield samples of olfactory bulbs, cerebral cortex, mesencephalon, diencephalon, and cerebellum. The results of this investigation are summarized in Table 16-I. By forty-five minutes following injection of nicotine a significant elevation in the 5-HT concentration of the cerebral cortex was observed. Under saline treated conditions, as might be anticipated, no alterations in these indole levels resulted. With the administration of ECS, saline-treated animals showed an elevation of 5-HT concentration in the mesencephalon, and in the diencephalon and cerebral cortex by forty-five minutes; in the later case, following saline injection. These findings are

TABLE 16-I

MEAN (±) REGIONAL BRAIN CONCENTRATION OF 5-HYDROXYTRYPTAMINE (5-HT)
AND 5-HYDROXYINDOLEACETIC ACID (5-HIAA) IN MICE GIVEN ECS OR SHAM-ECS
FIFTEEN AND FORTY-FIVE MINUTES FOLLOWING INJECTION (I.P.) WITH NICOTINE SULPHATE OR SALINE

(Concentration Expressed as Micrograms per Grams of Wet Weight of Tissue)

(Number of Samples per Group Equals Ten)

Condition	Olfactory Bulbs		Cerebral Cortex		Mesencephalon		Diencephalon		Cerebellum	
	5-HT	5-HIAA	5-HT	5-HIAA	5-HT	5-HIAA	5-HT	5-HIAA	5-HT	5-HIAA
Nicotine Sulfate (1.0 mg/kg) ECS$_{15}$	—	—	0.42	0.55	0.82	0.45	0.96	0.45	0.05	0.04
			(0.01)	(0.06)	(0.02)	(0.02)	(0.20)	(0.09)	(0.02)	(0.03)
ECS$_{45}$	0.04	—	0.66	0.37	0.64	0.35	0.90	0.45	0.03	0.04
			(0.04)	(0.04)	(0.06)	(0.06)	(0.15)	(0.18)	(0.01)	(0.02)
ECS$_{15}$	0.08	—	0.31*	0.53	0.68*	0.31	0.82	0.33	0.04	0.03
			(0.05)	(0.19)	(0.08)	(0.05)	(0.17)	(0.01)	(0.00)	(0.01)
ECS$_{45}$	0.02	—	0.28	0.38	0.66	0.31	0.50*	0.38	0.03	0.03
			(0.06)	(0.07)	(0.08)	(0.05)	(0.08)	(0.03)	(0.01)	(0.01)
Saline (0.9%) ECS$_{15}$	—	—	0.34	0.33	0.72	0.42	0.86	0.34	0.09	0.04
			(0.02)	(0.01)	(0.04)	(0.07)	(0.16)	(0.02)	(0.01)	(0.03)
ECS$_{45}$	0.02	—	0.36	0.66	0.78	0.90	0.90	0.74	0.06	0.06
			(0.10)	(0.31)	(0.02)	(0.45)	(0.12)	(0.41)	(0.01)	(0.02)
ECS$_{15}$	0.03	—	0.22	0.33	0.94*	0.42	1.00	0.34	0.03	0.04
			(0.02)	(0.01)	(0.02)	(0.07)	(0.11)	(0.02)	(0.01)	(0.03)
ECS$_{45}$	0.04	—	0.72*	0.36	1.06*	0.33	1.08*	0.35	0.09	0.03
			(0.19)	(0.03)	(0.12)	(0.05)	(0.04)	(0.07)	(0.01)	(0.01)

*p < .01.

consistent with our previous observations regarding elevation of whole brain 5-HT level following electroshock. With the administration of nicotine sulfate a significant decrease in 5-HT levels in cerebral cortex followed ECS when given at both fifteen as well as forty-five minutes after injection; similar decrements in 5-HT levels were observed as a result of ECS given fifteen minutes after injection, in the mesencephalon and diencephalon at forty-five minutes after injection. These data support our earlier findings to the extent that the anticipated changes in brain 5-HT levels as a consequence of cerebral electroshock would not only be attenuated by treated with nicotine sulfate, but are in fact reversed. Such reversal has been previously shown to occur in conjunction with central events that account for enhanced memory consolidation through the attenuation of postlearning electroshock-induced retograde amnesia.

In view of the fact that our prior investigations had indicated both metabolic as well as behavioral differences in the affect of nicotine as a function of postinjection time, one apparent hypothesis in dealing with these findings was that the central effects of nicotine could possibly be temporally distinct from the central effects of one or more of its peripherally produced metabolites. In order to consider this hypothesis in a more direct way, mice treated as described previously with nicotine sulfate or saline were compared with other groups of mice treated with 0.25 mg/kg of several nicotine analogs or metabolites; these included nornicotine, (-) cotinine, 3-pyridylacetic acid, myosmine, and anabasine, administered either fifteen or forty-five minutes prior to training and a posttraining ECS following training yielded the results summarized in Table 16-II. The latency difference measures represent the difference between the testing trial latency with a maximum cut off of

TABLE 16-II

MEDIAN LATENCY DIFFERENCE (TESTING-TRAINING) AND PER CENT INCIDENCE OF CONDITIONED RESPONSE RETENTION AFTER ECS FOLLOWING TRAINING AT TWO POSTTREATMENT TIMES

Treatment*	Postinjection Training Time (Min)			
	15		45	
	Latency Diff. (Sec)	*Percent Retention†*	*Latency Diff. (Sec)*	*Percent Retention†*
Saline (0.9%)	4.0	25	11.0	15
Nicotine Sulfate	3.0	10	4.0	75
Nornicotine	>110.0	95	99.5	80
(−) Cotinine	36.0	70	77.0	85
3-Pyridylacetic Acid	32.0	60	33.0	70
Myosmine	18.0	40	35.5	70
Anabasine	>113.0	85	35.0	65

*N/GP = 20; nicotine sulfate dose = 1.00 mg/kg; dose of each of the nicotine metabolites = 0.25 mg/kg.

†$p < .001$.

120 seconds and the training trial latency which usually represented the occurrence of response within approximately ten seconds after introduction to the apparatus. As observed previously, nicotine treatment fifteen minutes prior to the training-ECS sequence led to a greater incidence of ECS induced amnesia than observed for saline treated animals; at fifteen minutes post-injection, however, all of the metabolites or analogs of nicotine showed varying degrees of antagonism toward the amnestic affect of electroconvulsive shock. This was similarly observed for all nicotine metabolite-treated animals at the forty-five-minute sequence; these findings offer further partial support for the view that the central action of nicotine is partially accounted for by the central action of its metabolites and these may, in fact, represent actions of a dual nature. The possibility of this duality may, of course, involve other central biochemical systems aside from the serotonogenic mechanism simply applied to the present model for retrograde amnesia. For example, further investigation of the parallel in 5-HT alterations mediated to those behavioral conditions just described indicated nornicotine, 3-pyridylacetic acid, and (-) cotonine led to differences in 5-HIAA levels at fifteen or forty-five minutes following injection; a regional elevation of 5-HIAA occurred by fifteen minutes after drug treatment and electroshock, whereas when ECS was given forty-five minutes after injection, elevations of 5-HIAA regularly occurred with myosmine and anabasine treatment. In instances wherein the amnestic effect of ECS is antagonized there appears to be a reversal of regional changes observed in brain 5-HIAA levels. When ECS was given to saline-treated animals cortical, mesencephalic, and diencephalic 5-HIAA levels were elevated; a decrease in regional 5-HIAA levels occurred for these compounds which successively antagonized the amnesia produced by ECS—the reduced 5-HIAA content appears consistently to occur in drug treated animals by fifteen minutes following ECS in mesencephalon or by forty-five minutes following ECS in diencephalon. It may be observed that generally the nicotine metabolites lead to a regionally increased 5-HT concentration; this is seen in the mesencephalon by fifteen minutes following injection, accompanied by a decrease cortical 5-HIAA content, whereas such drug treatment led to elevation of cortical 5-HIAA levels by fifteen minutes following injection. Our prior suggestion that dual functions on brain metabolism may relate to behavioral differences in either the time course of nicotine action or in the central uptake of one or more of its peripherally produced metabolites, points to the possibility of the more popular suggestion that nicotine is a drug, the action of which involves cholinergic mechanisms. In addition to the observations that regional alterations in certain brain amines attend electroconvulsive shock, there is also a long standing observation that electrical stimulation and subsequent convulsions produced electrically result in a phasic decrement in brain acetylcholine (ACh) con-

tent (Richter and Crossland, 1949). We have recently confirmed and extended these observations in an experiment in mice; these animals were given a single transcorneal electroconvulsive shock (ECS) following which the cerebral cortex was removed at varying times and assayed for acetylcholine content in the total tissue ("total" ACh), the tissue homognate ("bound" ACh), and in synaptosome fractions derived from such tissue samples (sealed presynaptic nerve endings). The results, summarized in Table 16-III, indicate that total ACh level is depleted to less than half of base line concentration within ten minutes following ECS and by one to two

TABLE 16-III

MEAN ($I\sigma$) ACETYLCHOLINE CONCENTRATION (mM/g) IN MOUSE CEREBRAL CORTEX AS A FUNCTION OF TIME AFTER ELECTROCONVULSIVE SHOCK

Brain Tissue Fraction	Time After ECS (Min)				
	0	10	30	60	120
Total Tissue	16.43	7.26	9.70	15.36	16.53
	(2.3)	(2.4)	(2.3)	(3.2)	(2.2)
Tissue Homogenate	10.00	2.00	5.00	5.00	4.00
	(0.6)	(1.4)	(1.2)	(1.0)	(0.8)
Synaptosomes	1.13	0.90	0.21	0.34	0.53
	(0.16)	(0.30)	(0.05)	(0.07)	(0.10)

hours following the seizure levels are returned to within base line. The "bound" ACh, as reflected by recovery of this amine following homogonization, also shows a clear decrement following those observed in total tissue but not reverting to within base-line variation, even by two hours following ECS. This parallel is again observed for ACh levels in synaptosomes. These data suggest that there is approximately equivalent loss of "free" ACh as a consequence of homogonization, and that the ACh decrement produced by ECS appears to reside in the loss of "bound" material.

In view of the findings considered above and the often suggested view that nicotine is a cholinergic drug, the possible interaction between this compound and the effects of ECS were considered in a study wherein nicotine treatment (1.0 mg/kg) was given (I.P.) to mice forty-five minutes preceding a single ECS; fifteen minutes following this sequence cortical tissue was removed and assayed for acetylcholine. Appropriate controls consisting either of saline treatment and/or sham ECS were included. In Table 16-IV the mean acetylcholine content of several fractions of mouse cerebral cortex are shown for each of the treatment conditions; the total tissue, tissue homogonate, and vesicles showed differences which easily reached levels of statistical significance. These differences, which are summarized in Table 16-V and interpreted to reflect "total," "bound," and the vesicular acetyl-

TABLE 16-IV

MEAN (I_σ) ACETYLCHOLINE CONTENT OF SEVERAL FRACTIONS OF MOUSE
CEREBRAL CORTEX AFTER SEVERAL TREATMENT CONDITIONS

Condition	*Acetylcholine Content (mM/g)*		
	Total Tissue	*Tissue Homogenate*	*Vesicles**
Nicotine — *ECS*	8.06 (0.49)	1.22 (0.07)	370 (22.20)
Nicotine — ECS	15.00 (1.00)	9.20 (0.61)	610 (36.60)
Saline — *ECS*	16.43 (2.30)	10.00 (1.40)	1130 (158.20)
Saline — ECS	7.26 (2.40)	2.00 (0.66)	900 (297.00)

*Concentration expressed as PM/g.

choline changes and also summarize the parallel results obtained for acetylcholinestrase. It may be noted that whereas both nicotine treatment as well
as ECS individually deplete "total" and "bound" ACh levels by approximately the same magnitude, there is a greater decrement in vesicular acetylcholine levels among the nicotine-treated mice than for the ECS-treated animals; correspondingly, synaptosomal-and vesicular-associated acetylcholinestrase activity was considerably higher following nicotine treatment. The
effects of ECS given to nicotine-treated animals as compared to comparable
treatment given to mice injected with saline indicates that whereas the total
and "bound" acetylcholine levels is increased, vesicular acetylcholine content is reduced, and there is correspondingly an elevation in acetylcholinesterase activity. Whereas ECS tends to reduce acetylcholine levels and increases acetylcholinesterase activity in the presence of nicotine, it is apparent
that nicotine serves to attenuate the magnitude of acetylcholine decrement
produced in "total" level and "bound" level of this amine in mouse cerebral
cortex.

TABLE 16-V

PERCENT CHANGE IN ACETYLCHOLINE CONCENTRATION FOR TOTAL CEREBRAL
CORTEX, CORTEX HOMOGENATES, AND CHOLINERGIC SYNAPTIC VESICLES
(With Acetycholinesterase Changes for Synaptosomes [SYN] and Synaptic Vesicles)

Treatment	*Percent Change in Concentration or Activity**				
	Acetylcholine			*Acetylcholinesterase*	
	Total	*"Bound"*	*Vesicular*	*Syn.*	*Ves.*
Nicotine	↓ 51	↓ 87	↓67	↑130	↑ 78
ECS	↓ 55	↓ 80	↓25	↑ 47	↑ 36
Nicotine + ECS (N)	↑106	↑360	↓50	↑ 12	↑101
Nicotine + ECS (E)	↑ 86	↑736	↑64	↓ 27	↓ 39

*All differences indicated reached statistical significance ($p < .02$) Nicotine dosage = 1.0
mg/kg, I.P., forty-five minutes pretreatment, and all values were obtained for tissue available
fifteen minutes after treatment.

In view of the possibility that cholinergic mechanisms may be involved
in the action of nicotine upon memory consolidation, a study was initiated

in which pharmacological alterations $\overset{+}{N}$ functional groups contributing to nicotine effects were considered. It has been noted that the $\overset{+}{N}$ effects are increased by trimethylamine and that these effects are decreased triethylamine; the addition of N-methly or N-ethyl functional groups should therefore provide for modification of the central nervous system, which is not possible with quartenary ammonium compounds that are too polar to penetrate the blood-brain barrier. It might therefore be predicted that if a mechanism of action involving cholinergic mediation relates the interaction of ECS and nicotine to memory consolidation process, differences in the effect of nicotine may depend upon the extent to which nicotonic action is either potentiated or inhibited by the addition of $\overset{+}{N}$ functional groups. Mice were treated either with saline, triethylamine (TEA)-2.5 mg/kg, or trymethylamine (TMA)-2.5 mg/kg; thirty minutes following this initial injection animals were given either saline 0.9 percent (I.P.), or nicotine sulfate (1.0 mg/kg I.P.) forty-five minutes following the second injection animals were trained to acquire the passive avoidance response previously described, and this was then followed with either ECS or sham ECS. A single testing trial was given twenty-four hours following training trial with response latency taken as an indication of retention or amnesia for the conditioned avoidance response. The results are summarized in Table 16-VI. Since it might be expected that

TABLE 16-VI

MEDIAN RESPONSE LATENCY DIFFERENCE (SEC) BETWEEN TESTING AND TRAINING TRIAL AND PERCENT INCIDENCE OF CONDITIONED RESPONSE RETENTION FOR MICE

(Pretreated with either Saline [0.9%] Triethylamine [TEA-2.5 mg/kg] or Trimethylamine [TMA-2.5 mg/kg] and then Given Either Saline or Nicotine Sulfate [1.0 mg/kg])

Treatment Condition	ECS		ECS	
	Median Resp. Latency Diff.	*% Incidence of CR Retention*	*Median Latency Diff.*	*% Incidence of CR Retention*
Saline — Saline	23.0	20	111.0	100
Saline — Nicotine	115.0	60	116.0	100
TEA — Saline	31.0	40	113.0	80
TEA — Saline	18.0	30	110.0	100
TMA — Saline	43.0	60	109.0	90
TMA — Nicotine	— 1.0	10	35.0	50

TMA should increase the nicotine effects, one could expect possible potentiation of the ECS-induced amnesia normally induced by nicotine sulfate treatment alone. Whereas 80 percent of control treated mice showed retrograde amnesia when given ECS, only 40 percent of nicotine treated animals showed retrograde amnesia. Although essentially the same mangitude of antagonism for the amnesic effect may be noted for saline-treated animals pretreated with TMA, nicotine treated animals pretreated with TMA showed a 90 percent incidence of retrograde amnesia. Even in the absence of posttraining ECS, potentiation of the nicotinic effect by TMA treatment resulted in a reduced incidence of conditioned response acquisition. Decreased nicotinic effects, as predicted by pretreatment with TEA apparently occurred in view of the reduced degree of a nicotine-induced antagonistic effect. It is apparent that TEA alone had a relatively greater antagonistic effect than did the TEA-nicotine combination; however, since this latter combination in the absence of ECS did not modify the degree of conditioned response acquisition, it is more likely that TEA interacts with the ECS effect, whereas the TMA interacts more directly with the behavioral effect of nicotine.

The studies and results summarized in this paper represent a series of attempts to interrelate the neurochemical events associated with the action of a centrally active compound, nicotine, with a central process, memory consolidation, probably relevant to the former. What appears to have emerged throughout these investigations are a series of complex interactions, indicating and implicating multiple chemical systems possibly involved at different levels in the mediation of intracellular and synaptic events which are related to the process of memory consolidation. Another observation that may be made is to reinforce the suggestion made earlier that nicotine, as well as some of its metabolites and analogs, behave very much like other compounds having psychoactive properties. There appear to be striking similarities in both the biochemical and behavioral effects of nicotine to the effect of compounds which, without acting as MAO inhibitors, serve an antidepressant role clinically. Such a role for nicotine may be strongly indicated and further investigations of this possibility appears to be warranted.

REFERENCES

1. Bonta, I. L., Delver, A., Simons, L., and deVos, C. J.: A newly developed motility apparatus and its applicability in two pharmacological designs. *Arch Int. Pharmacodyn, 129*:381-394, 1960.
2. Bovet, D., Bovet-Nitti, F., and Oliverio, A.: Effects of nicotine on avoidance conditioning in inbred strains of mice. *Psychopharmacologia, 10*:1-5, 1966.
3. Bovet-Nitti, F.: Facilitation of simultaneous visual discrimination by nicotine in the rat. *Psychopharmacologia, 10*:59-66, 1966.
4. Essenberg, J. M.: The effect of nicotine on maze learning ability of albino rats. *Fed Proc, 7*:31-32, 1948.
5. Essenberg, J. M.: The effect of nicotine on maze behavior of albino rats. *J Psychol, 37*:291-295, 1954.
6. Essman, W. B.: Alterations in brain serotonin metabilism mediating enhanced memory consolidation. In Cerletti, A., and Bové, F. J. (Eds.): *The Present Status of Psychotropic Drugs.* Amsterdam, Excerpts Medica, 1969a., pp. 305-306.
7. Essman, W. B.: Mediation of memory consolidation: Behavioral and biochemical

effects of nicotine and nicotine metabolites. *Proceedings of the 4th International Congress of Pharmacology, Basel*, 1969b, p. 289.

8. Essman, W. B., and Alpern, H.: Single trial learning: Methodology and results with mice. *Psychol Rep, 14:*731-740, 1964.

9. Essman, W. B., Golod, M. I., and Stenberg, M.: Alterations in the behavioral and biochemical effects of electroconvulsive shock with nicotine. *Psychonom Sci, 12:*107-108, 1968.

10. Floris, V., Morocutti, G., and Ayala, G. F.: Azione della nicotina sulla attivitá biolettrica della corteccia del talamo e dell' ippocampo nel cooniglio. *Boll Soc Ital Biol Sper, 38:*407-410, 1962.

11. Garg, M., and Holland, H. C.: Consolidation and maze learning: a further study of post-trial injections of a stimulant drug (nicotine). *Int J Neuropharmacol, 7:*55-59, 1968.

12. Linucher, M. N., and Michelson, M. J.: Action of nicotine on the rate of elaboration of food motor conditioned reflexes in rats of different ages. *Activ Nerv Sup, 7:*25-30, 1965.

13. Mercier, J., and Dessaigne, S.: Determination de l' accountumance experimentale par une methode psychologique. *Ann Pharm Franc, 18:*502-518, 1960.

14. Morrison, C. F.: Effects of nicotine on operant behaviour of rats. *Int J Neuropharmacol, 6:*229-240, 1967.

15. Morrison, C. F.: The modification by physostigmine of some effects of nicotine on bar-pressing behaviour of rats. *Brit J Pharmacol, 32:*28-33, 1968.

16. Murpree, H. B. (Ed.): The effects of nicotine and smoking on the central nervous system. *Ann NY Acad Sci, 142:*1-333, 1967.

17. Robustelli, F.: Azione della nicotina sur condezionamento di saluaguardia di ratti di un mese. *Rend Sci Mat Nat, 40:*490-497, 1966.

Chapter 17

Biogenic Amines of the Central Nervous System and Their Possible Involvement in Emotion and Learning*

SEYMOUR S. KETY

MOTIONS MAY BE SEEN as adaptive states of a generalized nature involving the brain as well as the autonomic and endocrine systems in response to a significant change in the environment, and serving to bring about or facilitate appropriate behavior. Some basic emotions are arousal, pleasure, fear, and rage; and their counterpart behaviors are to attend, to approach, to avoid, or to attack. There is a body of suggestive evidence that some of the biogenic amines play crucial roles at various points in bringing about these states.

BIOGENIC AMINES IN THE CENTRAL NERVOUS SYSTEM

Although there is much to be learned regarding the mechanisms of release and action of neurotransmitters at peripheral synapses, a transmitter function appears well-established for norepinephrine, as is its peripheral involvement along with epinephrine in emotional expression. In the brain, however, no biogenic amine has been conclusively shown to be a transmitter, nor even to be specifically associated with a particular behavioral or affective state. The evidence is indirect and inferential but sufficiently extensive and consistent, nevertheless, to permit the formulation of hypotheses that central as well as peripheral actions of biogenic amines mediate arousal and emotion.

By means of the characteristic fluorescence of their condensation products after reaction with formalin vapor (Eränkö, 1955) serotonin and catecholamines have been demonstrated throughout the brain and spinal cord, concentrated in the presynaptic varicosities along the terminal axons of particular neurons (Hillarp *et al.*, 1966). Their cell-bodies themselves appear to be clustered in the brain stem; the serotonin-containing neurons, in the midline raphé nuclei, and those containing catecholamines, more laterally disposed with a high density in the locus ceruleus. Axons from those amine-containing neurons pass downward into the spinal cord and upward

*Adapted from a chapter in *The Neurosciences:* Second Study Program (F. O. Schmitt, Editor-in-Chief). New York, New York, The Rockefeller University Press, 1970.

by way of the medial forebrain bundle to innervate most of the brain (Fuxe, 1965). There are especially high densities of their terminals in the various nuclei of the hypothalamus, but the entire cerebral cortex and even the cerebellar cortex contain many very fine fibers with the characteristic serotonin or catecholamine fluorescence which is intensified after treatment with monoamine oxidase inhibitors and diminishes following reserpine (Dahlström and Fuxe, 1965) or medial forebrain bundle lesions. Although dopamine and norepinephrine cannot be distinguished by histofluorescence, complementary chemical studies indicate that most of the catecholamine in the telencephalon is norepinephrine, except for the important dopamine-containing nigrostriatal tract (Anden *et al.*, 1966). Sufficient attention has been given to norepinephrine in the brain and its possible relationship to mood to permit using that amine as an example of the group without suggesting that it has a predominant or exclusive role.

The early studies relied upon the total content of norepinephrine in the brain or its concentration in particular regions. Thus Barchas and Freedman (1963) showed a decrease in this amine in the brain along with an increase in serotonin in rats forced to swim to exhaustion. Maynert and Levi (1964) found a 40 percent decrease in norepinephrine in the brainstem after thirty minutes of foot shocks. Reis and Gunne (1965) induced rage in cats by stimulating the amygdala and demonstrated a highly significant decrease in the norepinephrine levels of the telencephalon. More recent studies (Reis and Fuxe, 1969) have confirmed the relationship between induced rage and norepinephrine levels in the brain and have adduced further evidence for the crucial involvement of this amine in that form of behavior by augmenting and inhibiting the manifestations of rage by drugs which respectively potentiate and block the pharmacologic actions of norepinephrine at receptors in the periphery.

Closer to the dynamic relationships involved in synthesis and release is the examination of the turnover of norepinephrine in the brain. If synthesis is coupled to release in the central nervous system as it appears to be in the periphery, simple levels of the endogenous amine would reflect only disparities between the two processes and not the magnitude of either. On the other hand, the disappearance of labeled amine from a pool into which it had been introduced would be affected by alterations in its rate of release, even though these were completely compensated by corresponding changes in synthesis. Although norepinephrine does not cross the blood:brain barrier (Weil-Malherbe *et al.*, 1961) the tritium-labeled amine is rapidly distributed to various parts of the brain after intraventricular (Glowinski and Axelrod, 1966) or intracisternal (Schanberg *et al.*, 1967) injection and concentrated at presynaptic endings, largely of norepinephrine-containing neurons (Descarries and Droz, 1969). The disappearance of the labeled amine from the brain does not follow a monoexponential curve, suggesting the presence of two or more compartments with different rates of turnover. Its initial slope, however, should approximate the average turnover rate, and the decrements over standard periods of time have been used for qualitative comparison of turnover rates between experimental and control groups of animals (Thierry *et al.,* 1968). An alternative method of examining turnover rate is afforded by following the curve of disappearance of the endogenous amine after blocking its synthesis by means of α-methyltyrosine (Costa and Neff, 1966). Although this technique does not require the use of exogenous material and obviates questions regarding the specificity of the material the turnover of which is being examined, it requires the assumption that turnover rate is independent of endogenous levels and would not be expected to reflect changes in rate of turnover brought about by changes in synthesis, since the latter process is blocked.

In addition to yielding valuable information on the effects of drugs on norepinephrine metabolism (Glowinski and Axelrod, 1966; Schanberg *et al.,* 1967), the rate of turnover has also been examined in some behavioral states where it has been found to be more sensitive and informative than study of endogenous levels alone. In foot shock of milder form than that used previously, it was possible to demonstrate a significant increase in turnover throughout the brain and spinal cord with no systematic change in endogenous levels of the amine (Thierry *et al.,* 1968). This suggested an augmented synthesis coupled with release which has been demonstrated more directly in the periphery (Alousi and Weiner, 1966; Sedvall *et al.,* 1968). Repeated exposure to such stress over a period of three days was associated with a significant elevation of endogenous levels of the amine, further supporting the hypothesis that synthesis was stimulated and compatible with an induction of the rate-limiting enzyme.

The turnover of norepinephrine was found to be substantially increased after one week of a regimen of twice daily electroconvulsive shocks and twenty-four hours after the last shock at a time when the behavior of the animals was quite normal (Kety *et al.,* 1967). This, coupled with a significant elevation in endogenous norepinephrine, implied a persistent increase in synthesis of the amine. An increase in tyrosine hydroxylase levels in the brain was demonstrated in animals twenty-four hours after the same regimen of electroconvulsive shocks (Musacchio *et al.,* 1969). The drugs effective in relieving clinical depression (amphetamine, monoamine oxidase inhibitors, imipramine) all affect norepinephrine turnover or metabolism in the brain in ways which would be expected to increase the activity of that amine at central synapses, while drugs causing depression have an opposite effect (Kety, 1967). The finding that electroconvulsive shock, which is probably the most effective treatment for depression, could also increase the availability of norepinephrine at synapses in the brain, in this instance by increasing its synthesis, is also compatible with the possibility that a deficiency of that amine may exist in the brain in states of depression.

Pharmacological tools in conjunction with a form of appetitive behavior have been used to adduce evidence that norepinephrine may be involved in the "reward" system in the brain. Stein (1964) has examined the effects of various drugs on the self-stimulating behavior in rats described by Olds and Milner (1954) and has found that imipramine or amphetamine will significantly increase such activity, while reserpine will suppress it. The effects of amphetamine are greatly diminished following reserpine (Stein, 1964) or α-methyltyrosine (Crow, 1969). The most parsimonious explanation of all these observations is that this form of appetitive behavior requires the intervention of one of the catecholamines. The conditional avoidance response is another form of behavior which can be blocked by drugs (Rech *et al.,* 1966) which deplete catecholamine stores in the brain or by lesions in the posterolateral hypothalamic midbrain junction or medial forebrain bundle (Sheard *et al.,* 1967) which result in a loss of serotonin and norepinephrinè from much of the telencephalon. The effects of catecholamine-depleting drugs are rather specific since they can be demonstrated while escape behavior is unaffected. Depletion of serotonin alone is apparently insufficient to affect conditioned avoidance (Tenen, 1967).

Correlations of turnover rates of biogenic amines with behavioral states or the ability of drugs which affect amines in the brain to alter behavior offer evidence which is compatible with hypotheses that one or another amine is involved in a particular form of behavior. Such evidence hardly constitutes proof, however, since alternative explanations of the various findings must usually be entertained. Better evidence would be the demonstration of the release of a particular putative transmitter in the brain in constant association with a specific type of behavior as has been achieved for acetylcholine, norepinephrine, and gamma-aminobutyric acid at particular peripheral synapses. Brain slices. (Baldessarini and Kopin, 1967) have been shown to release norepinephrine or other amines (Katz *et al.,* 1968) when stimulated with electric current or potassium ion or when exposed to low concentrations of certain drugs. Lithium ion administered *in vivo* or added *in vitro* appears to block the stimulated release of norepinephrine or serotonin from brain slices, suggesting that lithium ion, rather specifically effective in treating mania, may act by inhibiting the release of biogenic amines.

Although a release of norepinephrine from the brain *in vivo* has been reported in association with appetitive stimulation (Stein and Wise, 1967), the specificity of the release was not established; in other experiments neuronal activation has been found to release not only norepinephrine but also urea and inulin (Chase and Kopin, 1968). On the other hand, d-amphetamine has been found to release norepinephrine and its methylated metabolite, but not inulin, from the brain (Carr and Moore, 1969).

The ability of acetylcholine or norepinephrine applied locally on "receptor" regions of a postsynaptic structure to elicit a response that closely mimics the effect of neurostimulation, functionally, electrically, and pharmacologically, constitutes what is probably the best evidence that these substances are neurotransmitters at certain peripheral synapses. For that reason the effects of putative transmitters applied locally in the brain have been of considerable interest. When norepinephrine is injected into the ventricles, or intravenously in animals with a poorly developed blood:brain barrier, the effect produced is not arousal, but in practically every instance, some form of somnolence (Mandell and Spooner, 1968). The microinjection of this amine in the region of individual cells while their electrical activity is being recorded (Salmoiraghi and Bloom, 1964) usually produces an inhibition of spontaneous activity. These observations do not necessarily argue against an important involvement of norepinephrine in arousal, since neither the dose nor the site of application are controlled in the first type of experiment, while an inhibition of random and spontaneous activity throughout the brain may constitute a characteristic feature of arousal with a facilitation of only small, sharply focused, and specifically activated regions, which may have gone undetected in the recording of unit activity.

On the other hand, the elicitation of particular forms of behavior following more specific administration of the amine would suggest its involvement in similar types of natural activity. A number of such observations have been reported. Wise and Stein (1969) suppressed self-stimulation (through electrodes in the medial forebrain bundle of rats) by the administration of diethyldithiocarbamate (disulfiram) which blocks dopamine β-hydroxylase and depletes the brain of norepinephrine but not of dopamine. In such animals, the appetitive behavior could be restored by intraventricular injection of l-norepinephrine (5μg) but not by the dextro-isomer, or by dopamine or serotonin.

Slangen and Miller (1969) have carried out a series of well-designed experiments which strongly suggest the involvement of norepinephrine in a type of feeding behavior. By implanting fine cannulae into the perifornical region at the posterior portion of the anterior hypothalamus, they were able to test the effects of various substances on a region where electrical stimulation is known to induce eating in a previously satiated rat. Small doses of l-norepinephrine (20μmM) were found promptly to elicit the same type of behavior while serotonin had no effect. Dopamine induced no immediate change in behavior but a delayed and weak eating response, compatible with its conversion to norepinephrine. This region responded to other pharmacological agents as do norepinephrine alpha receptors in the periphery.

Phentolamine, which blocks alpha receptors, antagonized the norepineph-rine response, while a beta receptor stimulant (isoproterenol) or antagonist (propranolol) had no effects *per se* or on the norepinephrine response. The norepinephrine-induced behavior was potentiated eightfold by previous treatment of the animal with desipramine. An effect was also obtained from tetrabenazine, which releases norepinephrine and other amines from storage depots, provided monoamine oxidase and previously been blocked by niali-mide. It is difficult to avoid the interpretation that this behavior is mediated by the release of norepinephrine acting on specific adrenergic receptors in this region.

Even the intraventricular administration of norepinephrine need not always lead to generalized sedation. Segal and Mandell (1969) have observ-ed activation and improved performance on a continuous avoidance task in animals receiving a constant infusion of low concentrations of norepineph-rine; the activated behavior gave way to sedation with higher concentration.

In summary, the evidence appears to be quite god, but hardly conclu-sive, that norepinephrine and other amines play important roles in the mediation of various emotional and behavioral states. Norepinephrine ap-pears especially to be implicated in arousal, aggression, and certain appeti-tive behaviors, although some observations (Seiden and Peterson, 1968; Creveling *et al.*, 1968) are more compatible with an important role for dopamine. The best evidence for the involvement of serotonin appears to be in the production of sleep (Jouvet, 1969). No simplistic hypothesis, how-ever, is compatible with all of the observations, and it appears to be quite futile to attempt to account for particular emotional state in terms of the activity of one or more biogenic amines. It seems more likely that these amines may function separately or in concert at crucial nodes of the com-plex neuronal networks which underlie emotional states. Although this in-terplay may represent some of the common features and primitive qualities of various affects, the special characteristics of each of these states are prob-ably derived from those extensions of the networks which represent apper-ceptive and cognitive factors based upon the experience of the individual. A possibility which deserves some exposition and exploration is that an im-portant adaptive role of the biogenic amines is to favor the elaboration of such networks in the learning process and the association of cognitive with appropriate affective elements.

POSSIBLE ROLE OF BIOGENIC AMINES IN MEMORY AND LEARNING

The peripheral autonomic and humoral components of affective states have well-recognized functions in the anticipation, facilitation, and mainte-nance of a variety of adaptive responses. Neither the central components of these states nor their functions have been as well defined, but it is possible that they subserve even more important adaptations—reinforcing significant inputs, suppressing irrelevant ones, evoking or facilitating responses which in the experience of the species or the individual have the greatest survival value, and so influencing the neuronal processes involved in memory as to permit the development, reinforcement, and maintenance of the most appropriate responses.

Most of the earlier hypotheses concerning the neural mechanisms involved in memory emphasized repeated activation of a synapse as a necessary antecedent to some sustained alteration in its function, but failed to consider what may be the crucial importance of contingency with affective states in inducing such persistent changes. In 1963, Young emphasized the importance of the outcome of an act for memory in the octopus and designated the anatomical pathways and physiological processes whereby this interaction could occur. Szilard (1964) proposed a contingency model of learning in which an interaction between specific complementary proteins between synaptic membranes was the basis of alterations in synaptic efficacy. The hypothesis developed by Roberts (1966) linked arousal and memory with the hypothalamic-pituitary neuroendocrine system. A concept which stressed the adaptive association between affect and memory emerged from the 1966 Intensive Study Program (Livingston, 1967). The dependence of learning on attention, and on reward or punishment appears well established at the behavioral level, and there is obvious adaptive advantage in a mechanism which consolidates not all experience equally but only those experiences which are significant for survival (Kety, 1965).

It is not difficult to see how, as a result of selective pressure, some rudimentary adaptive responses to certain prevalent exogenous stimuli could become genetically endowed—crude aversive behavior to noxious stimuli (loud noise, pain, extremes of heat and cold) or appetitive behavior (approach, sucking, swallowing) to stimuli associated with suckling (warmth, nipple in proximity of the mouth, milk in the pharynx). Each response would include a primitive motor pattern, appropriate autonomic, endocrine and metabolic changes, and a state of arousal common to them all.

Now it is necessary to make some assumptions which, although plausible, are far from established on the basis of existing evidence: (a) that the aroused state induced by novel stimuli or by stimuli genetically recognized as significant is pervasive and affects synapses throughout the central nervous system, suppressing most, but permitting or even accentuating activity in those which are transmitting the novel or significant stimuli; (b) that this state, through one or more of its components favors the development of persistent facilitatory changes in all synapses which are currently in a state of excitation or have recently been active; (c) that there is a fairly random network of synapses with sufficient complexity that pathways exist and can be reinforced between many other neurons and the relatively few which are involved in mediating the primitive and genetically endowed adaptive responses.

A nervous system so constructed would have the remarkable capability of responding not only on the basis of a genetically determined input and response code, but of developing a much more elaborate and adaptive neuronal network or state between input and response, but now on the basis of its idiosyncratic experiences.

Thus, the animal so equipped might wander into a new territory and experience some form of pain, responding with reflexive avoidance movements and an appropriate affective state. In addition, however, his state of arousal which would have risen to a higher level during his exploration of unfamiliar surroundings would have tended to accentuate all the novel sensory inputs from a number of modalities associated with the new experiences. The powerful affective state and intense arousal induced by the pain, in addition to its classical autonomic and endocrine concomitants in the periphery, may also act centrally to induce some persistant chemical change in all recently active synapses, but especially in those associated with the novel sensory experiences of the unfamiliar territory, the activity of which the state of arousal had accentuated. With many repetitions of that sequence and by a process of algebraic summation such as that employed in the computer of average transients, those inputs and activated pathways, in short that state of neuronal excitation which preceded and was repeatedly associated with the pain, would be translated into a chemical change of greater magnitude and therefore longer duration than that of random activity. In that way presentation of some of the sensory stimuli peculiar to the new territory could eventually evoke the particular affective state, the heightened arousal, the peripheral autonomic and metabolic responses and the aversive behavior without the intervention of the painful stimulus, and a conditioned avoidance and emotional response would have been established. Thus, what was originally an inborn response only to pain would have been cognitively elaborated on the basis of idiosyncratic experience, anticipating and avoiding or preparing for the noxious stimulus in a remarkable new type of adaptation.

It is possible to suggest certain anatomical pathways and neurochemical mechanisms which may satisfy some of the requirements of this hypothetical process or which seem to merit further investigation from that point of view. If protein synthesis is crucially involved in the consolidation of the memory trace, as much recent work appears strongly to suggest, then the hypothesis outlined above would imply that some chemical components of arousal should be able to facilitate synaptic protein synthesis contingent upon neuronal activity wherever it occurs throughout the brain.

The author has previously developed a highly speculative model of a neuronal process whereby this could be achieved (Figure 17-1). This assumed a population of neurons containing and releasing norepinephrine or another amine in affective states, in this instance arousal and pain, with widely distributed axons, not only to the neurons which mediate the peripheral autonomic and endocrine concomitants, but also feeding back onto central synapses generally, and thus including those whose activity was coincident with or closely antecedent to the pain. It was speculated that the amine released might affect protein synthesis so as to facilitate consolidation at synapses recently activated and still reverberating or otherwise sustaining some differentiating change. Kandel and Spencer (1968) have recently reviewed the evidence for various persistent neuronal changes following activation.

Since that time a number of observations have been made which lend some credence to that hypothesis and suggest one or more sites where such amine-stimulated consolidation could occur. Scheibel and Scheibel (1967) have described multibranched axons of cells in the brain stem which make synapses with thousands of neurons up and down the neuraxis. They have also described in greater detail the architectonics of the "unspecific afferents" to the cerebral cortex with evidence that these long climbing axons of cells, some of which are in the brain-stem reticular system, weave about the apical dendrites of pyramidal cells with an extremely loose axodendritic association in contrast to the vast number of well-defined synapses established by the terminals of the "specific afferents" (Figure 17-2). In 1968, Fuxe, Hamberger, and Hökfelt described the terminations of the norepinephrine-containing axons in the cortex, pointing out the similarities in their distribution to that of the unspecific afferents of Scheibel and Scheibel.

If some of the unspecific afferents are indeed "adrenergic" or "aminergic" terminals invading the millions of sensory-sensory and sensory-motor synapses of the cortex, they would provide a remarkably effective mechanism whereby amines released in arousal could affect a crucial population of synapses throughout the brain. The hippocampal and cerebellar cortex are also characterized by "climbing fibers" some of which are norepinephrine-containing (Anden *et al.*, 1967; Blackstad *et al.*, 1967), and one group has come close to establishing a transmitter role for that amine between the terminals of certain climbing fibers and Purkinje cells (Siggins *et al.*, 1969). There is even some evidence that axons from the same adrenergic neurons in the brain stem may be distributed to cerebral, hippocampal, and cerebellar cortex as well as to hypothalamus and other areas. Marr (1969) has proposed a novel theory of the cerebellar cortex which implies a "learning" of patterns

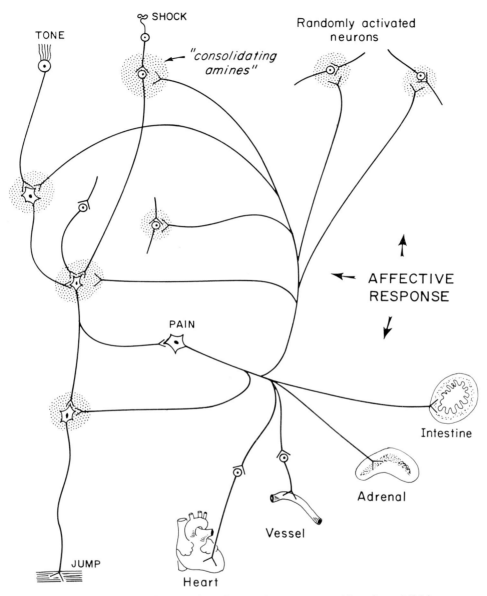

Figure 17-1. An oversimplified model of neural systems capable of establishing a conditioned reflex. It includes a genetically-endowed primary reflex mediating aversive movements in response to pain and indicates how the adrenergic system within the brain could participate in the establishment of more complex and adaptive networks based upon contingent inputs.

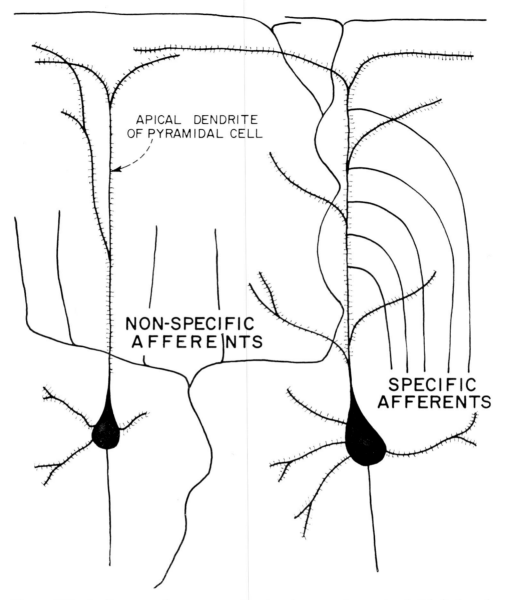

Figure 17-2. A diagrammatic representation based upon the work of Scheibel and Scheibel of the specific and the nonspecific afferents to cortical pyramidal cells. Fuxe, Hamberger, and Hökfelt have mentioned the similarities between the latter and adrenergic nerve endings in the cerebral cortex. It is suggested that the adrenergic endings, stimulated during an affective response, may serve to consolidate synaptic changes at specific afferent endings activated in temporal association with the affective state.

of motor activity by that structure. It is possible that by similar and simultaneous processes in these three cortices the state of arousal may serve concurrently to reinforce and consolidate the significant sensory patterns, the affective associations and the motor programs necessary in the learning of a new adaptive response. It is of interest that Phillips and Olds (1969) have described single units in the midbrain which fire not in response to a stimulus but to its significance in terms of the previous experience of the animal.

Just as the peripheral expressions of arousal and affect are mediated by both neurogenic and endocrine processes, it is possible that the central components employ humoral as well as neural modes. There is a great tendency for these apical dendrites and their afferents in a remarkably similar fashion in the cerebrum, hippocampus, and cerebellum to seek the cortical surface; indeed, the cortical convolutions which increase that surface severalfold must have some adaptive function. Developmental history and the geometrical requirements of the circuity have been invoked to explain this phenomenon, but it is also possible that the position of these structures in close proximity to the cerebrospinal fluid serves another adaptive function. The constant flow of this medium from the ventricles over the whole cortical surface on its way to arachnoid villi offers a means of superfusing the cortex with substances derived from the blood stream at the choroid plexus or intracerebrally secreted by various stations along its path. It is noteworthy that ^{3}H-norepinephrine injected into one ventricle or into the cisterna magna rapidly penetrates the superficial layers of the brain; since the amines do not easily pass the blood-brain barrier and would not readily be removed by the capillaries, such a mechanism would further assure the widespread distribution of any which may be released from endings near the cortical surface. Acetylcholine (Collier and Mitchell, 1967) and prostaglandins (Ramwell and Shaw, 1966) have been shown to be released at the cortex by neuronal activity, and it is likely that other substances are released and may be broadcast by this process.

Secretions of the hypothalamus, trophic hormones of the pituitary, and the steroid hormones of the adrenal cortex, some of which are regularly secreted in states of arousal and stress, may thus have additional access to this rich population of synapses. Many of these substances have, in one system or another, displayed a capacity to stimulate the synthesis of RNA or of a protein. The steroid hormones and ACTH clearly affect conditioning (Levine, 1969), and in addition to their well-establshed abilities to induce enzymes in other tissues, one of them has recently been found to restore tryptophan hydroxylase activity in the midbrain of the adrenalectomized rat (Azmitia and McEwen, 1969). It is tempting to speculate upon the possible trophic actions of such stress-related hormones on cortical synapses.

A substantial number of recent observations are compatible with this model, and in some cases the hypothesis helps to explain some inconsistencies. RNA and protein synthesis have both been found to be stimulated at sites of increased neuronal activity (Glassman, 1969; Berry, 1969), but inconsistently so, perhaps because the crucial contingent factor of arousal has not been held constant (Altman and Das, 1966). Conversely, Roberts and Flexner (1969) have pointed out that the increased protein synthesis demonstrated by some experiments during learning is considerably greater than would be required by the newly established neuronal patterns, unless a generalized facilitation of synthesis of new protein occurred which then decayed except for that in the repeatedly reinforced patterns.

The hypothesis would predict that drugs which release or enhance norepinephrine in the brain or exert its neuronal effects would favor consolidation and facilitate memory. Amphetamine and caffeine appear capable of producing such effects (Bignami *et al.*, 1965; Oliverio, 1968), and recently a more specific ability of amphetamine or foot-shock to counteract the suppression of consolidation brought about by cyclohexamide has been reported (Barondes and Cohen, 1968).

Conversely, lesions or drugs which deplete or block norepinephrine in the brain should retard consolidation and prevent acquisition. Although there are many reports on the ability of such drugs (reserpine, α-methyl tyrosine) to block the established conditioned-avoidance response, there is little information on their effects during acquisition. Recently, however, W. B. Essman (personal communication) has found a significant impairment in acquisition, following α-methyl tyrosine, which was most severe when the brain levels of norepinephrine were lowest. Lesions of the medial forebrain bundle which would be expected to deplete the telencephalon of norepinephrine and serotonin, appeared in one study (Sheard *et al.*, 1967) to depress acquisition. Conversely, stimulation of this region has been used as a means of positive reinforcement in conditioning curarized animals (Trowill, 1967).

The suggestion that the release of norepinephrine may favor consolidation of learning by stimulating protein synthesis is made more tenable by recently acquired information on the possible action of cyclic AMP in the brain. This substance, present in surprisingly high concentration in the central nervous system as is adenyl cyclase, the enzyme which brings about its synthesis, is crucially involved in enzyme induction and protein synthesis in a wide variety of bacterial and mammalian cells and appears to increase the activity of a protein kinase in brain (Miyamoto *et al.*, 1969). Evidence is accumulating that cyclic AMP may mediate the effects of norepinephrine on central neurons (Siggins *et al.*, 1969) as it is believed to do for actions of catecholamines and other hormones on liver, muscle, and other peripheral tissues. It is interesting that the stimulation of protein kinase by cyclic AMP can be markedly potentiated by magnesium or potassium ions and inhibited by calcium which suggests means whereby an effect of adrenergic stimulation could be differently exerted on recently active and inactive synapses.

Earlier hypotheses which assigned an important role to central norepinephrine and other biogenic amines in mediating emotional states have stimulated considerable research. It is possible that these speculations regarding their possible function in the biochemical process which underlie memory and learning may be of some heuristic value.

One must expect, of course, that the true biochemical substrates of learning will be considerably more complicated than any simplistic model and entirely different pathways and processes may be involved. I believe however that the biochemical system which accounts for learning will also have to explain how a value system, at first very primitive and based entirely on genetically transmitted criteria derived from racial experience, learns from the experience of the individual, becoming more differentiated and discriminating, capable of tolerating greater delays to outcome, susceptible to more subtle grades of affect than crude pleasure and pain, and in a species capable of symbolic conceptualization, sensitive to imagined, predicted or planned outcomes in addition to those actually perceived.

REFERENCES

1. Alousi, A., and Weiner, N.: The regulation of norepinephrine synthesis in sympathetic nerves: Effect of nerve stimulation, cocaine, and cathecholamine-releasing agents. *Proc Nat Acad Sci, 56:*1491-1496, 1966.
2. Altman, J., and Das, G. D.: Behavioral manipulations and protein metabolism of the brain: Effects of motor exercise on the utilization of leucine-H³. *Physiol Behav, 1:*105-108, 1966.
3. Anden, N. E., Fuxe, K., and Ungerstedt, U.: Monoamine pathways to the cerebellar and cerebral cortex. *Experientia (Basel), 23:*838-839, 1967.
4. Anden, N.-E., Fuxe, K., Hamberger, B., and Hokfelt, T.: A quantitative study on the nigro-neostriatal dopamine neuron system in rat. *Acta Physiol Scand, 67:*306-312, 1966.
5. Azmitia, E. C., Jr., and McEwen, B. S.: Corticosterone regulation of tryptophan hydroxylase in midbrain of the rat. *Science, 166:*1274-1276, 1969.
6. Baldessarini, R. J., and Kopin, I. J.: The effect of drugs on the release of norepinephrine-H³ from central nervous system tissues by electrical stimulation *in vitro*. *J Pharmacol Exp Ther, 156:*31-38, 1967.
7. Barchas, J. D., and Freedman, D.: Response to physiological stress, *Biochem Pharmacol, 12:*1232-1235, 1963.
8. Barondes, S. H., and Cohen, H. D.: Arousal and the conversion of "short-term" to "long-term" memory. *Proc Nat Acad Sci, 61:*923-929, 1968.
9. Berry, R. W.: Ribonucleic acid metabolism of a single neuron: correlation with electrical activity. *Science, 166:*1021-1023, 1969.
10. Bignami, G., Robustelli, F., Janku, I., and Bovet, D.: Psychopharmacologie, *CR Acad Sci Paris, 260:*4273-4278, 1965.

11. Blackstad, T., Fuxe, K., and Hökfelt, T.: Noradrenaline nerve terminals in the hippocampal region of the rat and the guinea pig. *Z Zellforsch, 76*:463-473, 1967.
12. Carr, L. A., and Moore, K. E.: Norepinephrine: Release from brain by d-amphetamine in vivo. *Science, 164*:322-323, 1969.
13. Chase, T. N., and Kopin, I. J.: Stimulus-induced release of substances from olfactory bulb using the push-pull cannula. *Nature, 217*:466-467, 1968.
14. Collier, B., and Mitchell, J. F.: The central release of acetylcholine during consciousness and after brain lesions. *J Physiol, 188*:83-98, 1967.
15. Costa, E., and Neff, N. H.: Isotopic and nonisotopic measurements of catecholamine biosynthesis. In Costa, E., Cote, L., and Yahr, M. D. (Eds.): *Biochemistry and Pharmacology of the Basal Ganglia.* New York, Raven Press, 1966.
16. Creveling, C. R., Daly, J., Tokuyama, T., and Witkop, B.: The combined use of -methyltyrosine and threo-dihydroxyphenyl-serine-selective reduction of dopamine levels in the central nervous system. *Biochem Pharmacol, 17*:65-70, 1968.
17. Crow, T. J.: Mode of enhancement of self stimulation in rats by methamphetamine. *Nature, 224*:709-710, 1969.
18. Dahlström, A., and Fuxe, K.: Evidence for the existence of monoamine neurons in the central nervous system. II. Experimentally induced changes in the intraneuronal amine levels of bulbospinal neuron systems. *Acta Physiol Scand, 64*:1-36, 1965.
19. Descarries, L., and Droz, B.: Intraneuronal distribution of exogenous norepinephrine in the central nervous system of the rat. *J Cell Biol*, vol. 44 (in press).
20. Eränkö, O.: The histochemical demonstration of noradrenaline in the adrenal medulla of rats and mice. *J Histochem Cytochem, 4*:11, 1955.
21. Von Euler, U. S.: *Noradrenaline.* Springfield, Thomas, 1956.
22. Fuxe, K.: Evidence for the existence of monoamine neurons in the central nervous system. IV. The distribution of monoamine nerve terminals in the central nervous system. *Acta Physiol Scand, 64*:39-85, 1965.
23. Fuxe, K., Hamberger, B., and Hökfelt, T.: Distribution of noradrenaline nerve terminals in cortical areas of the rat. *Brain Res, 8*:125-131, 1968.
24. Glassman, E.: The biochemistry of learning: an evaluation of the rate of RNA and protein. *Ann Rev Biochem, 38*:605-646, 1969.
25. Glowinski, J., and Axelrod, J.: Effects of drugs on the disposition of H^3-norepinephrine in the rat brain. *Pharmacol Rev, 18*:775-785, 1966.
26. Hillarp, N. A., Fuxe, K., and Dahlström, A.: Demonstration and mapping of the central neurons containing dopamine, noradrenaline, and 5-hydroxytryptamine and their reactions to psychopharmaca. *Pharmacol Rev, 18*:727-741, 1966.
27. Jouvet, M.: Biogenic amines and the states of sleep. *Science, 163*:32-41, 1969.
28. Kandel, E. R., and Spencer, W. A.: Cellular neurophysiological approaches in the study of learning. *Physiol Rev, 48*:65-134, 1968.
29. Katz, R. I., Chase, T. N., and Kopin, I. J.: Evoked release of norepinephrine and serotonin from brain slices: Inhibition by lithium. *Science, 162*:466-467, 1968.
30. Kety, S. S.: The incorporation of experience into the central nervous system. In de Ajuriaguerra, J. (Ed.): Désafférentation experimentale et clinique. Geneva, Georg et Cie, 1965, pp. 251-256.
31. Kety, S. S., Javoy, F., Thierry, A.-M., Joulou, L., and Glowinski, J.: A sustained effect of electroconvulsive shock on the turnover of norepinephrine in the central nervous system of the rat. *Proc Nat Acad Sci, 58*:1249-1254, 1967.
32. Kety, S. S.: The central physiological and pharmacological effects of the biogenic

amines and their correlations with behavior. In Quarton, G. C., Melenchuk, T., and Schmitt, F. O. (Eds.): *The Neurosciences, A Study Program.* New York, Rockefeller University Press, pp. 441-451, 1967.

33. Levine, S.: Hormones and conditioning. In Arnold, W. (Ed.): *Nebraska Symposium on Motivation.* Lincoln, University of Nebraska Press, 1969.

34. Livingston, R. B.: Reinforcement. In Quarton, G. C., Melenchuk, T., and Schmitt, F. O. (Eds.): *The Neurosciences, a Study Program.* New York, Rockefeller University Press, pp. 568-577.

35. Mandell, A. J., and Spooner, C. E.: Psychochemical research studies in man. *Science, 162*:1442-1453, 1968.

36. Marr, D.: A theory of cerebellar cortex. *J Physiol, 202*:437-470, 1969.

37. Maynert, E. W., and Levi, R.: Stress induced release of brain norepinephrine and its inhibition by drugs. *J. Pharmacol Exp Ther, 143*:90-95, 1964.

38. Miyamoto, E., Kuo, J. F., and Greengard, P.: Cyclic nucleotide-dependent protein kinesis. III. Purification and properties of adenosine 3'5'-monophosphate-dependent protein kinase from bovine brain. *J Biol Chem, 244*:6395-6402, 1969.

39. Musacchio, J. M., Julou, L., Kety, S. S., and Glowinski, J.: Increase in rat brain tyrosine hydroxylase activity produced by electroconvulsive shock. *Proc Nat Acad Sci, 63*:1117-1119, 1969.

40. Olds, J., and Milner, P.: Positive reinforcement produced by electrical stimulation of septal area and other regions of rat brain. *J Comp Physiol Psychol, 47*:419-427, 1954.

41. Oliverio, A.: Neurohumoral systems and learning. In *Psychopharmacology; a review of progress 1957-1967.* USPHS Publication No. 1836, U. S. Government Printing Office, pp. 867-878.

42. Phillips, M. I., and Olds, J.: Unit activity: Motivation-dependent responses from midbrain neurons. *Science, 165*:1269-1271, 1969.

43. Ramwell, P. W., and Shaw, J. E.: Spontaneous and evoked release of prostaglandins from cerebral cortex of anesthetized cats. *Amer J Physiol, 211*:125-134, 1966.

44. Rech, R. H., Borys, H. K., and Moore, K. E.: Alterations in behavior and brain catecholamine levels in rats treated with α-methyltyrosine. *J Pharmacol Exp Ther, 153*:412-419, 1966.

45. Reis, D. J., and Fuxe, K.: Brain norepinephrine: Evidence that neuronal release is essential for sham rage behavior following brainstem transection in cat. *Proc Nat Acad Sci, 64*:108-112, 1969.

46. Reis, D. J., and Gunne, L.-M.: Brain catecholamines: Relation to the defense reaction evoked by amygdaloid stimulation cat. *Science, 149*:450-451, 1965.

47. Roberts, E.: Models for correlative thinking about brain, behavior, and biochemistry. *Brain Res, 2*:109-144, 1966.

48. Roberts, R. B., and Flexner, L. B.: The biochemical basis of long-term memory. *Quart Rev Biophys, 2*:135-173, 1969.

49. Rosenfeld, J. P., Rudell, A. P., and Fox, S. S.: Operant control of neural events in humans. *Science, 165*:821-823, 1969.

50. Salmoiraghi, G. C., and Bloom, F. E.: Pharmacology of individual neurons. *Science, 144*:493-499, 1964.

51. Schanberg, S. M., Schildkraut, J. J., and Kopin, I. J.: The effects of psychoactive drugs on norepinephrine-H[3] metabolism in brain. *Biochem Pharmacol, 16*:393-399, 1967.

52. Scheibel, M. E., and Scheibel, A. B.: Structural organization of nonspecific thalamic nuclei and their projection toward cortex. *Brain Res, 6*:60-94.

53. Sedvall, G. C., Weise, V. K., and Kopin, I. J.: The rate of norepinephrine synthesis measured *in vivo* during short intervals; influence of adrenergic nerve impulse activity. *J Pharmacol Exp Ther, 159:*274-282, 1968.

54. Segal, D. S., and Mandell, A. J.: Behavioral activation of rats during intraventricular infusion of norepinephrine. *Proc Nat Acad Sci,* (in press).

55. Seiden, L. S., and Peterson, D. D.: Reversal of the reserpine-induced suppression of the conditional avoidance response by l-dopa. *J Pharmacol Exp Ther, 159:*422-428, 1968.

56. Sheard, M. H., Appel, J. B., and Freedman, D. X.: The effect of central nervous system lesions on brain monoamines and behavior. *J Psychiat Res, 5:*237-242, 1967.

57. Shimizu, H., Creveling, C. R., and Daly, J.: Factors affecting cyclic AMP formation in brain: Use of slices pre-labelled by incubation with adenine-^{14}C. *Trans Amer Soc Neurochem, 1:*67, 1970.

58. Siggins, G. R., Hoffer, B. J., and Bloom, F. E.: Cyclic adenosine monophosphate: Possible mediator for norepinephrine effects of cerebellar Purkinje cells. *Science, 165:*1018-1020, 1969.

59. Slangen, J. L., and Miller, N. E.: Pharmacological tests for the function of hypothalamic norepinephrine in eating behavior. *Physiol Behav, 4:*543-552, 1969.

60. Stein, L.: Self-stimulation of the brain and the central stimulant action of amphetamine. *Fed Proc, 23:*836-850, 1964.

61. Stein, L., and Wise, G. D.: Release of hypothalamic norepinephrine by rewarding electrical stimulation or amphetamine in the unanesthetized rat. *Fed Proc, 26:*651, 1967.

62. Szilard, L.: On memory and recall. *Proc Nat Acad Sci, 51:*1092-1099, 1964.

63. Tenen, S. S.: The effects of p-chlorophenylalanine, a serotonin depletor, on avoidance acquisition, pain sensitivity and related behavior in the rat. *Psychopharmacologia, 10:*204-219, 1967.

64. Thierry, A. -M., Javoy, F., Glowinski, J., and Kety, S. S.: Effects of stress on the metabolism of norepinephrine, dopamine and serotonin in the central nervous system of the rat. I. Modifications of norepinephrine turnover. *J Pharmacol Exp Ther, 163:*163-171, 1968.

65. Trowill, J. A.: Instrumental conditioning of the heart rate in the curarized rat. *J Comp Physiol Psychol, 63:*7-11, 1967.

66. Weil-Malherbe, H., Whitby, L. G., and Axelrod, J.: The blood-brain barrier for catecholamines in different regions of the brain. In Kety, S. S., and Elkes, J. (Ed.): *Regional Neuro-Chemistry.* Oxford, Pergamon Press, pp. 284-292.

67. Wise, C. D., and Stein, L.: Facilitation of brain self-stimulation by central administration of norepinephrine. *Science, 163:*299-301, 1969.

68. Young, J. Z.: Some essentials of neural memory systems. Paired centres that regulate and address the signals of the results of action. *Nature, 198:*626-630, 1963.

Chapter 18

Further Characterization of Acetylcholine Pools in Brain

LOUIS A. BARKER, M. J. DOWDALL, AND V. P. WHITTAKER

INTRODUCTION

HISTORICALLY, acetylcholine was the first chemical transmitter to be identified (Loewi and Navratil, 1924). The role of acetylcholine as the chemical mediator at parasympathetic nerve endings, autonomic ganglia, and neuromuscular junctions is generally accepted. Ample evidence is now available for accepting acetylcholine as one of the central transmitter agents (Crossland, 1960; Mitchell, 1963). The form in which acetylcholine exists in brain and other nervous tissue has been the subject of extensive investigation and review (Gaddum, 1935; Feldberg, 1945; Hebb, 1963; Michaelson, 1967; Whittaker, 1968, 1969 a, b).

ACETYLCHOLINE POOLS IN BRAIN

Early investigators recognized that acetylcholine did not exist in tissue as the freely diffusible ester, but was in some form bound to the cell or some cellular granule (Gaddum, 1935; Mann et al., 1938, 1939; Feldberg, 1945). Several investigators had shown that acetylcholine remains largely in the particulate fraction when brain tissue is mechanically disrupted in aqueous solutions. The particulate acetylcholine was shown to be resistant to cholinesterases and pharmacologically inactive (Mann et al., 1938, 1939; Feldberg, 1945). If, however, a cholinesterase inhibitor such as eserine were added to the solution, acetylcholine was found in the supernatant. Observations such as these lead to concept of acetylcholine existing in brain in two forms: free and bound, the former being readily extractable into neutral eserinized isotonic saline solutions, and the latter, only extracted if the particulate material were treated with an organic solvent or extracted at an acidic pH.

The existence of a free pool of acetylcholine in brain was difficult to reconcile with the known activity of cholinesterases. Feldberg (1945) rejected the notion of free acetylcholine and proposed that all of the acetylcholine present in brain was bound, being synthesized in that form. However, the concept of free and bound acetylcholine was generally accepted and provided a working model on which to explain the action of various drugs and physiological treatments on the levels of brain acetylcholine (Welsh and

Hyde, 1943). More recent work by Chakrin and Whittaker (1969) and Beani *et al.* (1969) has provided good evidence that free acetylcholine does exist in the neuron and that its most probable location is in the cytoplasm of cell bodies and axons. The argument that free acetylcholine cannot exist because of the presence of cholinesterase is overcome by the electron microscopic observations on the localization of cholinesterases in neurons (Lewis and Shute, 1966; Brzin *et al.,* 1966; Duffy *et al.,* 1967). These show that the enzyme is localized, in the cell body, within the lumen of the endoplasmic reticulum, while in the axon and terminals it is found only on the external cell membrane. It thus appears that, functionally, the active site of the enzyme is always extracellular and not readily available to intracellular acetylcholine.

BOUND ACETYLCHOLINE

Bodian (1942) suggested that mitochondria might be the binding site for acetylcholine. This suggestion was reinforced by the observation of Hebb and Smallman (1956) that the mitochondrial fraction isolated from brain homogenates contained 70 percent of the choline acetyltransferase activity. Like acetylcholine, full activity of the enzyme was not obtained until the particulate material was treated with an organic solvent or other nondenaturing procedures which would disrupt membranes. During this time, synaptic vesicles were observed by electron microscopists. The idea that synaptic vesicles might contain transmitter substances seems to have occurred to at least four groups of investigators (DeRobertis and Bennett, 1955; del Castillo and Katz, 1955; Palay, 1954; Fernandez-Moran, 1956). However, only indirect experimental evidence was available to support this idea. This was provided by del Castillo and Katz (1954) who had demonstrated the quantal release of transmitter, acetylcholine, at the neuromuscular junction. The vesicles were thought to be the morphological counterpart of the quanta or packets of acetylcholine.

The first biochemical investigations on the localization of bound acetylcholine were performed by Hebb and Whittaker (1958). The distribution of bound acetylcholine in sucrose homogenates of brain tissue was found to parallel that of choline acetyltransferase, about 70 percent of the bound acetylcholine, and choline acetyltransferase sedimented with the mitochondrial (P_2) fraction. Further fractionation of the P_2 fraction, by means of density gradient centrifugation, showed that bound acetylcholine and choline acetyltransferase were contained in particles (P_2B) that had an equilibrium density intermediate between that of myelin and mitochondria.

Further investigations by Whittaker (1959) and Gray and Whittaker (1962) showed by electronmicroscopic examination that these particles were nerve endings. Evidently, during homogenization, the nerve endings were sheared away from the axon and postsynaptic attachments and the broken ends sealed by a process similar to that which occurs during the formation of microsomes. These particles have been termed "synaptosomes" (Whittaker, *et al.,* 1964; for a review of the synaptosome see Whittaker, 1969 b) .

Whittaker *et al.* (1963, 1964) further characterized bound acetylcholine in the synaptosome as existing in two pools: labile or readily releasable, and stable-bound acetylcholine. The labile pool is released by hypotonic rupture, whereas the stable pool is not. When the P_2 or P_2B fraction was subjected to osmotic rupture and further fractionated by means of density gradient centrifugation, the stable bound acetylcholine was found to exhibit a bimodal distribution. The lightest particles (D) containing bound acetylcholine, having a density equal to that of 0.4 M sucrose, were shown to be synaptic vesicles. The heavier particles (H) , banding in 1.1 M sucrose were shown to be partially disrupted synaptosomes, which retained vesicles and mitochondria. If eserine were included at the osmotic rupture stage, the labile-bound acetylcholine was preserved and isolated at the top of the density gradient along with cytoplasmic constituents, such as lactate-dehydrogenase and K^+ ion. These observations provided the first biochemical evidence that a transmitter substance, acetylcholine, is bound to synaptic vesicles.

Studies such as those cited above, on the distribution of endogenous acetylcholine combined with a morphologic and biochemical evaluation of the subcellular fractions, have given rise to the hypothesis that three forms of acetylcholine exists in brain: free, stable-bound, and labile-bound (Whittaker *et al.,* 1964) . These are summarized in Table 18-I.

TABLE 18-I
Compartments of Brain Acetycholine (ACh)

	Type of ACh	Fraction	Presumed location
(I)	Free ACh	S_3 from eserinized homogenate	Cell sap from cell bodies or disrupted synaptosomes
(II)	Bound ACh:	P_2 or B from uneserinized homogenate	Synaptosomes
	(a) "labile"	0 from eserinized P_2 or B	Synaptosomal cytoplasm
	(b) "stable"	(1) D from uneserinized P_2 or B	Synaptic vesicles
		(2) H from same	Synaptic vesicles in partially disrupted synaptosomes

An important feature of the three-pool hypothesis is that it provides an excellent model on which to base a biochemical evaluation of the vesicle hypothesis of synaptic transmission. Stated succinctly, acetylcholine that is released from nerve endings during synaptic transmission is derived from synaptic vesicles. Naturally, this would not be realistic unless the three pool hypothesis could be shown to be a feasible model as opposed to a redistribution artifact.

Tests of the Three Pool Hypothesis

The three pool hypothesis was tested by Chakrin and Whittaker (1969) in an investigation of the subcellular distribution of [N-Me-^{3}H] acetylcholine ([^{3}H]-acetylcholine) synthesized by brain tissue *in vivo* in barbituate-anesthetized guinea pigs. The specific radioactivities of the various forms of acetylcholine isolated (see Scheme 1) from tissue excised one hour after the intracerebral administration of [^{3}H]-choline were significantly different. Labile-bound (synaptosome cytoplasm) had the highest, stable-bound (vesicular, D) ; acetylcholine, the next highest, and free (cell body and axonal cytoplasm) acetylcholine had the lowest specific activity. It is most unlikely that these results would have obtained from the redistribution of a single pool during fractionation.

Having satisfied the requirement that the initial premise of three pools was tenable, further work by Whittaker and Chakrin, in conjunction with Dr. J. M. Mitchell (cited by Whittaker, 1969 a) was done in an effort to determine the subcellular site of acetylcholine released on stimulation. In these experiments, the exposed occipital cortex of the rabbit was infiltrated with [^{3}H]-choline, and the acetylcholine released during rest and stimulation of the lateral geniculate body was collected in an "Oborin" cup. The levels and specific activity of the released acetylcholine were determined. Immediately after stimulation and about one hour after the initial administration of [^{3}H]-choline, the brain tissue in the vicinity of the cup was excised, subjected to subcellular fractionation, and the specific activities of synaptosomal cytoplasmic and vesicular acetylcholine determined. It was found that acetylcholine released on stimulation had a specific activity approaching that calculated for the synaptosomal cytoplasmic pool and greater than that of the vesicular pool. These results show, in agreement with the findings of Collier (1969) , that newly synthesized transmitter is preferentially released. However the results are not readily compatible with the vesicle hypothesis and suggest that the released transmitter is derived from a pool other than the stable-bound vesicular pool as represented by fraction D.

This conclusion is only valid if there is a rapid equilibrium between acetylcholine released in the tissue and acetylcholine that diffuses into the cup. One must ask whether or not the specific radioactivity of the cup acetylcholine at time t is the same as a given tissue compartment at time t, or is it that of the compartment at time t-x? Evaluation of these experiments are further complicated because the animals used were anesthetized with barbiturates and eserine was used to stabilize the released acetylcholine. Barbiturates, on one hand, have been shown to decrease the turnover of brain acetylcholine (Schuberth *et al.*, 1969), increase free and labile-bound acetylcholine (Beani *et al.*, 1969), as well as decrease the mean quantum content in spinal monosynaptic pathways (Weakly, 1969). Eserine, on the other hand, can inhibit the synaptosomal choline transport system (Marchbanks, 1969; Diamond and Kennedy, 1969), as well as inhibit the uptake of acetylcholine by brain slices (Schuberth and Sundwall, 1967; Liang and Quastel, 1969).

We decided to further investigate choline metabolism at nerve endings *in vivo*. In view of the above criticisms an experimental procedure which would circumvent these objections was adopted. Thus, conscious rather than anesthetized guinea pigs were used, and subsequent isolation of subcellular particles was carried out in the absence of eserine. Using this approach it was hoped that a base line pattern of choline metabolism would be established on which the effect of various drugs and metabolic states could be evaluated. Since choline is a precursor to the main membrane lipid, phosphatidylcholine, as well as acetylcholine, we could also provide an answer to the question: Does any relationship exist between the turnover of acetylcholine and the turnover of lipid in vesicle and nerve ending membrane such as might be expected if vesicles must be formed afresh to be charged with acetylcholine?

In these experiments, [³H]-choline has been administered intraventricularly (I.V.T.) into conscious guinea pigs under local anesthesia. At various times following the I.V.T. injection the animals were killed, cerebral corticies removed, scraped free of white matter, and subjected to a subcellular fractionation procedure which combined the methods of Gray and Whittaker (1962) and Whittaker *et al.* (1964) (see Scheme 1). Acetylcholine was extracted from the particulate fractions by the method of Hebb and Whittaker (1958), and a small portion of the extract was used for the determination of acetylcholine by bioassay on the guinea pig ileum. The remainder of the extract was processed as shown in Scheme 2 for the separation of acetylcholine from other radioactive choline metabolites (Fonnum, 1969). Overall recoveries are on the order of 85 percent. Control experiments show that the material in the acetylcholine band is not significantly contaminated with other radioactive material, the separation of choline from acetylcholine being 99.8 percent.

The metabolic fate of choline at the nerve ending is shown in Figure 18-1. It is seen that choline is readily taken up by the nerve ending *in vivo* and fairly quickly converted to acetylcholine and phosphorylcholine. After a lag of about ten minutes, phosphatidylcholine is labeled in detectable amounts. The incorporation of [³H]-choline into synaptosomal phospholipid continues to increase throughout the periods investigated (up to 60 min). Studies on the time course of lipid-choline (M. J. Dowdall, unpublished

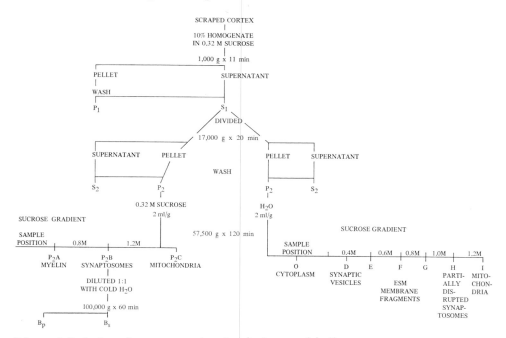

Scheme 1. Isolation of synaptosomal and vesicular acetylcholine.

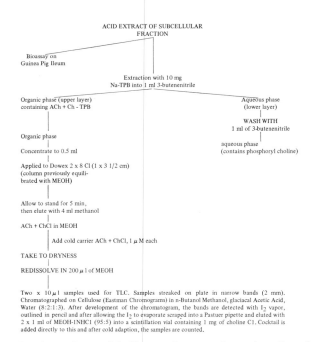

Scheme 2. Determination of acetylcholine and separation of radioactive acetylcholine from other radioactive products of choline metabolism.

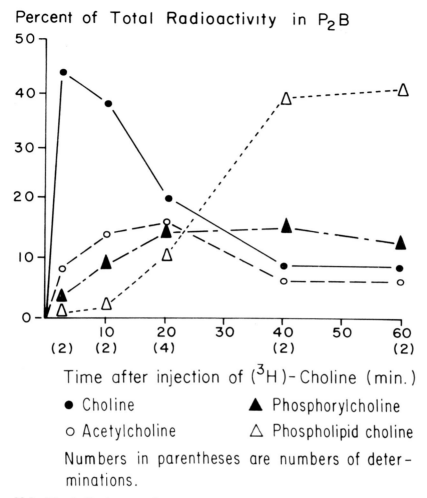

Figure 18-1. Metabolic fate at the nerve ending of intraventricularly injected [³H]-choline.

observations) and acetylcholine labeling in nerve ending organelles (See Fig. 18-2) demonstrate that the turnover of vesicular acetylcholine is much more rapid than that of vesicular membrane (fraction D). Also, no readily apparent relationship between membrane turnover and acetylcholine turn-over is found. If the acetylcholine in fraction D is the transmitter pool this indicates that synaptic vesicles probably maintain their structural integrity during the process of synaptic transmission, or if structural changes occur, they are of a transient physical nature.

Time course studies (Fig. 18-2) on the incorporation of [³H]-choline into various acetylcholine pools shows that incorporation into the synapto-

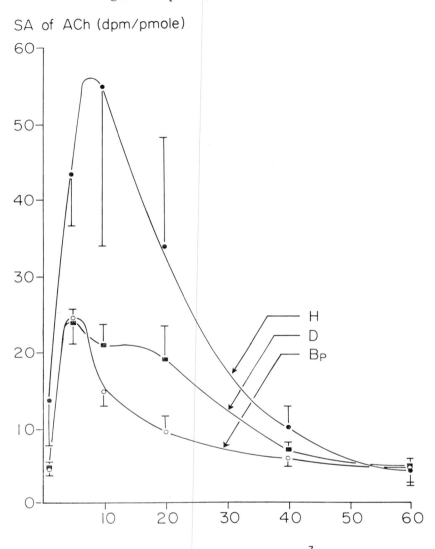

Figure 18-2. Turnover of acetylcholine in synaptosomes (B_p) vesicles (D) and partially disrupted synaptosomes containing vesicles and mitochondria (H). The values are mean ± S.E.M. for at least three experiments.

some, Bp, is maximal at five minutes, whereas incorporation into fraction D suggests two maxima, a peak between five and ten minutes and a shoulder ten and twenty minutes, the latter suggesting a second peak. It is seen that during the early times after [³H]-choline administration, marked differences exist between the specific radioactivities of acetylcholine present in the various pools, but that at forty and sixty minutes all of the synaptosomal pools appear to be in isotopic equilibrium.

It should be noted that the omission of eserine during subcellular fractionation precluded direct measurement of the labile-bound pool. However, preliminary results of experiments in which the specific radioactivity of the labile pool has been estimated (based on the amounts and specific radioactivities of acetylcholine in fractions P_2 and P_2W), we find that at five and ten minutes, the calculated specific radioactivity of labile-bound acetylcholine is essentially the same as that present in fraction D.

The shape of the incorporation curve for fraction D is quite interesting in that a peak and shoulder are observed. Presumably this represents either an intraterminal heterogeneity of vesicular incorporation of acetlycholine or reutilization of released transmitter.

The preponderance of evidence derived from *in vitro* studies shows that synaptic vesicles as isolated in fraction D are heterogeneous with respect to their ability to bind or retain acetylcholine. In studies on the release of endogenous acetylcholine from isolated synaptic vesicles, Barker (1968) showed that there are at least two populations of vesicular acetylcholine. Guth *et al.* (1970) have shown that at least three populations of vesicles are isolated in fraction D and that these differ in their abilities to take up and retain added acetylcholine. These differences, however, may be a result of different sucrose concentrations at the various layers in the D band (P. S. Guth, personal communication). More direct evidence for the heterogeneity of acetylcholine in synaptic vesicles has been obtained by Marchbanks and Israël (1970). Marchbanks and Israël showed that when tissue chops from the electric organ of Torpedo are incubated with labeled choline, vesicular acetylcholine becomes labeled. The passage of a labeled vesicle preparation through a Sephadex gel removes acetylcholine of a high specific radioactivity, leaving relatively colder acetylcholine still bound to the vesicles. In double labeling experiments (Marchbanks and Israël, personal communication), it was shown that the most recently added acetylcholine is the one which comes off first. Thus, it is quite clear that vesicular acetylcholine is heterogeneous. It remans to be shown whether this heterogeneity is due to differences between individual vesicles or due to different acetylcholine pools within vesicles.

Our observations that the specific radioactivity of acetylcholine in fraction D is always greater than or equal to that to synaptosomal (B_p) acetylcholine was quite unexpected in view of the results of Chakrin and Whittaker (1969). A comparison of the specific radioactivities of synaptosomal acetylcholine at various stages of the isolation procedure (Table 18-II) indicates the existence of a small rapidly turning over pool of acetylcholine which escaped notice in experiments involving only the measurement of endogenous acetylcholine. This pool is rapidly lost when synaptosomes (fraction B) are sedimented (fraction B_p). The release of this "hot" acetylcholine pool does not seem to require osmotic lysis, since it occurs when sedimentation is brought about without dilution of fraction B and without detectable release of the soluble cytoplasmic marker lactate dehydrogenase.

The presence or absence of this "hot" acetylcholine in the synaptosome preparation is sufficient to determine whether or not the specific radioactivity of synaptosomal acetylcholine is higher (fraction B) or lower (fraction B_p) than that of vesicular acetylcholine.

The subcellular localization of the fraction of acetylcholine has not yet been established, but on the basis of specific radioactivies it appears to be associated with fraction H (see Fig. 18-3A and Table 18-II).

TABLE 18-II

THE SPECIFIC RADIOACTIVITY OF SYNAPTOSOMAL ACETYLCHOLINE AT VARIOUS STAGES OF ISOLATION

Figures are from a typical experiment in which subcellular fractions were isolated from the cortices of animals exposed to [³H]-choline for ten minutes.

Fraction	Acetylcholine		
	Concentration (n Mole/gm) ± S.D.	S.A.* (dpm/pMole) ± S.D.†	S.A. of Lost Pool (dpm/pMole)
Homogenate	12.60 ± 4.30	14.40 ± 1.0	
P_2	6.15 ± 0.40	14.2 ± 0.8	
P_2B	3.65 ± 0.01	16.8 ± 0.8	
P_2Bp	3.50 ± 0.01	12.8 ± 0.8	100
D	1.00 ± 0.01	13.9 ± 0.3	

*S.A., Specific Radioactivity.
†S.D., Standard Deviation.

Of particular interest is our observation that the specific radioactivity of acetylcholine in fraction H is always greater, although more variable, than that of fraction D or B_p at the early time after [³H]-choline administration. A plot of the specific radioactivity against the amount of endogenous acetylcholine in the fraction (Fig. 18-3A) shows that at ten and twenty minutes a marked reciprocal relationship exists which is not seen in fraction D (Fig. 18-3B). Thus, the variability in the specific radioactivity in fraction H is due to its heterogeneous composition. Apparently there is a very small hot pool and a larger variable pool of less highly labeled acetylcholine, and the proportion of the two pools in the fraction varies. It is quite likely that these two pools differ in their subcellular localization: The less highly labeled pool might be associated with vesicles of the type in fraction D, or alternatively be associated with cytoplasm remaining entrapped in the partially disrupted synaptosomes; the smaller more highly labeled pool might represent a population of metabolically active vesicles sticking to the

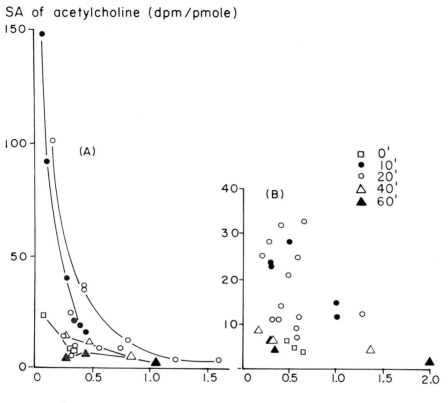

Figure 18-3. Relationship between specific radioactivity and amount of endogenous acetylcholine in (a) fraction H and (b) fraction D.

external membrane. The specific radioactivity of fraction H would then vary with the extent of the osmotic rupture of the synaptosomes.

It is clear that there exists in fraction H a metabolically unique pool of acetylcholine. It is not quite as clear why this uniqueness exists. If one assumes that mixing of [³H]-choline or newly synthesized acetylcholine is rapid compared to the labeling of bound pools, then D and H represent two distinctly different rather than apparently different pools of stable-bound acetylcholine. However, the recent results of Collier (1969) and March-banks and Israël (1970) strongly suggest that the assumption of rapid mixing is not valid. Instead, mixing appears to be rate limiting. Viewed in this manner, H-acetylcholine and presumably the small hot pool in fraction B simply represent the most recently formed and stored acetylcholine. The differences between D and H can then be explained on the localization within the nerve ending of different populations of synaptic vesicles: One population (H) is in close association with the presynaptic membrane, thereby spatially linked to the choline transport system and thus having first contact with newly synthesized acetylcholine, and the other (D) is predominantely in regions of the nerve ending distal to the presynaptic membrane.

Implicit in this interpretation is the hypothesis that H-acetylcholine represents the primary transmitter pool and that D-acetylcholine is a secondary-mobilizable pool in equilibrium with H. Such a hypothesis is consistent with the observations: (a) Newly synthesized transmitter is preferentially released (Collier, 1969) and has a higher specific radioactivity than vesicular (D) acetylcholine (Mitchell, cited above). (b) Procedures that accelerate transmitter release at neuromuscular junctions of the rat diaphragm result in the decrease of in the size of a specific population of vesicles that exist in relationship to the presynaptic membrane (Hubbard and Kwanbunbumpen, 1968). (c) Transmitter release continues in the presence of blockade of transmitter synthesis (MacIntosh, 1963).

Our results are consistent with the two compartment model (vesicular and cytoplasmic) for synaptosomal acetylcholine when viewed in light of the above hypothesis. They do show that the acetylcholine pools in brain and especially nerve-endings are not as simple as once thought. Indeed our present interpretation of the data is probably an over simplification, but does provide a working model on which to base new experiments as well as a new basis for the mode of action of presynaptically acting drugs.

ACKNOWLEDGMENTS

We should like to express our gratitude to Mr. W. Bear, Mrs. S. Brassel, and Miss F. Macdonald for skilled assistance. The work was supported, in part, by the N. Y. S. Department of Mental Hygiene, and by grants (to V. P. Whittaker) from the U. K. Medical and Science Research Councils and the U.S.P.H.S. (NINDS-postdoctoral fellowship to L.A.B.).

This investigation was conducted at the Department of Neurochemistry, New York State Institute for Research in Mental Retardation, Staten Island, N. Y. during the senior author's tenure as a NINDS postdoctoral fellow.

REFERENCES

1. Barker, L. A.: *Studies On Factors Affecting The Release of Acetylcholine From Isolated Synaptic Vesicles*. A Dissertation submitted to The Graduate School, Tulane University, New Orleans, 1968.
2. Beani, L., Bianchi, C., Megazzini, P., Ballotti, L., and Bernard, G.: Drug induced changes in free, labile and stable acetylcholine of guinea-pig brain. *Biochem Pharmacol, 18:*1315-1324, 1969.
3. Bodian, D.: Cytological aspects of synaptic function. *Physiol Rev, 22:*146-169, 1942.

4. Brzin, M., Tennyson, V. M., and Duffy, P. E.: Acetylcholinesterase in frog sympathetic and dorsal root ganglia. *J Cell Biol, 31:*215-242, 1966.

5. Chakrin, L. W., and Whittaker, V. P.: The subcellular distribution of [N-Me-³H] acetylcholine synthesized by brain *in vivo. Biochem J, 113:*97-107, 1969.

6. Collier, B.: The preferential release of newly synthesized transmitter by a sympathetic ganglion. *J Physiol, 205:*341-352, 1969.

7. Crossland, J.: Chemical transmission in the central nervous system. *J Pharm Pharmacol, 12:*1-36, 1960.

8. del Castillo, J., and Katz, B.: Quantal components of the end plate potential. *J Physiol, 124:*560-573, 1954.

9. DeRobertis, E., and Bennett, H. S.: Some features of the submicroscopic morphology of synapses in frog and earthworm. *J Biophys Biochem Cytol, 1:*47-58, 1955.

10. Diamond, I., and Kennedy, E. P.: Carrier-mediated transport of choline into synaptic nerve endings. *J Biol Chem, 244:*3258-3263, 1969.

11. Duffy, P. E., Tennyson, V. M., and Brzin, M.: Cholinesterase in adult and embryonic hypothalamus.*Arch Neurology, 16:*385-403, 1967.

12. Feldberg, W.: Present views on the mode of action of acetylcholine in the central nervous system. *Physiol Rev, 25:*596-642, 1945.

13. Fernandez-Moran, H.: Electron microscopy of nervous tissue. In Richter, D. (Ed.) : In *Metabolism Of The Nervous System.* London, Pergamon Press, 1956, pp. 1-34.

14. Fonnum, F.: Isolation of choline esters from aqueous solutions by extraction with sodium tetraphenylboron in organic solvents. *Biochem J., 113:*291-298, 1969.

15. Gaddum, J. H.: Choline and allied substances. *Ann Rev Biochem, 4:*311-330, 1935.

16. Gray, E. G., and Whittaker, V. P.: The isolation of nerve endings from brain: An electron-microscopic study of cell fragments derived by homogenization and centrifugation. *J Anat, 96:*79-88, 1962.

17. Guth, P. S., Stockwell, M., and Williams, T. H.: The subfractionation of whittaker's synaptic vesicle fraction-D. *The Pharmacologist,* 1970 (in press) .

18. Hebb, C.: Formation, storage, and liberation of acetylcholine. In Koelle, G. B. (Ed) : *Handbuch Des Experimentellen Pharmakologie,* Band XV. Berlin, Springer-Verlag, 1963, pp. 56-88.

19. Hebb, C. O., and Smallman, B. N.: Intracellular distribution of choline acetylase. *J Physiol, 134:*385-392, 1956.

20. Hebb, C. O., and Whittaker, V. P.: Intracellular distribution of acetylcholine and choline acetylase. *J Physiol, 142:*187-196, 1958.

21. Hubbard, J. L., and Kwanbunbumpen, S.: Evidence for the vesicle hypothesis. *J. Physiol, 194:*407-420, 1968.

22. Lewis, P. R., and Shute, C. C. D.: The distribution of cholinesterase in cholinergic neurons demonstrated with the electron microscope. *J Cell Sci, 1:*381-390, 1966.

23. Liang, C. C., and Quastel, J. H.: Effects of drugs on the uptake of acetylcholine in rat brain cortex slices. *Biochem Pharmacol, 18:*1187-1194, 1969.

24. Loewi, O., and Navratil, E.: Über humorale Übertragbarheit der Herznewenwirkung. X. Mitteilung. Über das Schickral des Vagusstoffs. *Pflügers Archiv Ges Physiol, 214:*678-688, 1924.

25. MacIntosh, F. C.: Synthesis and storage of acetycholine in nervous tissue. *Canad J Biochem Physiol, 41:*2555-2571, 1963.

26. Mann, P. J. G., Tennenbaum, M., and Quastel, J. H.: On the mechanism of acetylcholine formation *in vitro. Biochem J, 32:*243-261, 1938.

27. Mann, P. J. G., Tennenbaum, M., and Quastel, J. H.: Acetylcholine metabolism in the central nervous system. The effects of potassium and other cations on acetylcholine liberation. *Biochem J., 33*:822-835, 1939.

28. Marchbanks, R. M.: The uptake of [^{14}C]-choline into synaptosomes *in vitro*. *Biochem J, 110*:533-541, 1968.

29. Marchbanks, R. M., and Israël, M. *J Neurochem, 18*:439, 1971.

30. Michaelson, I. A.: The subcellular distribution of acetylcholine, choline acetyltransferase and acetylcholinesterase in nerve tissue. *Ann NY Acad Sci, 144*:387-410, 1967.

31. Mitchell, J. F.: The spontaneous and evoked release of acetylcholine from cerebral cortex. *J Physiol, 165*:98-116, 1963.

32. Palay, S. L.: Elctron microscopic study of the cytoplasm of neurons. *Anat Rec, 118*:336, 1954.

33. Schuberth, J., and Sundwall, A.: Effect of some drugs on the uptake of acetylcholine in cortex slices of mouse brain. *J Neurochem, 14*:807-812, 1967.

34. Schuberth, J., Sparf, B., and Sundwall, A.: A technique for the study of acetylcholine turnover in mouse brain *in vivo*. *J Neurochem, 16*:695-700, 1969.

35. Weakly, J. N.: Effect of barbiturates on 'quantal' synaptic transmission in spinal motoneurones. *J Physiol, 204*:63-77, 1969.

36. Welsh, J. H., and Hyde, J. E.: Acetylcholine level of rat cerebral cortex under conditions of anoxia and hypoglycemta. *J Neurophysiol, 6*:329-336, 1943.

37. Whittaker, V. P.: The isolation and characterization of acetylcholine containing particles from brain. *Biochem J, 72*:694-706, 1959.

38. Whittaker, V. P.: The subcellular frationation of nervous tissue. In Bourne, G. H. (Ed.) : *Structure And Function Of Nervous Tissue*, vol. III, *Biochemistry and Disease*. New York, Academic Press, 1968, pp. 1-24.

39. Whittaker, V. P.: The nature of the acetylcholine pools in brain tissue. *Progr. Brain Res, 31*:211-222, 1969a.

40. Whittaker, V. P.: The Synaptosome. In Lajtha, A. (Ed.) : *Handbook of Neurochemistry*, vol. II. New York, London, Plenum Press, 1969b, pp. 327-364.

41. Whittaker, V. P., Michaelson, I. A., and Kirkland, R. J. A.: The separation of synaptic vesicles from disrupted nerve-ending particles. *Biochem Pharmacol, 12*: 300-302, 1963.

42. Whittaker, V. P., Michaelson, I. A., and Kirkland, R. J. A.: The separation of synaptic vesicles from nerve-ending particles (synaptosomes) . *Biochem J, 90*:293-305, 1964.

Chapter 19

The Effect of Catecholamines on Protein Synthesis in Embryonic Cells*

RAYMOND U. SEALE, KENNEAL Y. C. CHUN, AND JOHN T. WILLSON

ELLS UNDERGOING differentiation synthesize specific proteins different from those formed by other cells. The role of messenger RNA in determining the types of proteins formed and in regulating the rates of synthesis of specific proteins is now widely accepted (Watson, 1965). Information concerning the extent to which external conditions interact with a potentially uniform genetic system to direct or alter the formation of a specific protein is necessary for a better understanding of the mechanisms of differentiation. Since the structure, function, mode of synthesis, and genetic regulation of hemoglobin are better understood than for most other proteins (Wilt, 1967), hemoglobin synthesis represents a system suitable for the study of such developmental interactions.

We have been studying the effects of exogenous catecholamines on hemoglobin formation in the early developing chick blastoderm *in vitro*. The events of hemoglobin synthesis are detectable during the first forty-eight hours of incubation. At this time, the primary embryonic erythroblasts are the only generation of developing red cells present (Lucas and Jamroz, 1961). These primary erythroblasts are derived from yolk sac mesodermal precursor cells. The homogeneity and common origin of this red cell population greatly simplify the analysis of drug action on hemoglobin and its formation. Further, the chemical events in the initial synthesis of hemoglobin in chick blastoderms have been critically analyzed by O'Brien (1961 a), Wilt (1967), and Wainwright and Wainwright (1966 and 1967). Since only dopamine and no other catecholamine is found in the forty-eight-hour blastoderm, and then only occasionally, the catecholamine synthesizing system appears to be activated late during this period of incubation (Ignarro and Shideman, 1968).

In the studies reported here, chick blastoderms of Hamburger-Hamilton (1952) stage 6 or 7 (head fold or 1-somite stages, respectively) were explanted with the endodermal surface downward into a watch glass containing Spratt's (1960) semisolid, Ringer-Agar-egg extract media. In the experimental series, varying concentrations of catecholamines ranging between

*Supported in part by a grant from the Milheim Foundation for Cancer Research and in part by U.S.P.H.S. grant FR-05357.

319

$50\mu g/ml$ and $500\mu g/ml$ of medium were added at $50\mu g$ increments; control blastoderms were cultured on identical media without catecholamines. After twenty-four hours incubation at 38 degrees Centigrade, the blastoderms were examined with a dissecting microscope and evaluated as to the organizational development of the embryo proper and the amount of visible hemoglobin in the area vasculosa.

Hemoglobin synthesis in treated and control blastoderms was evaluated qualitatively in a manner previously described by O'Brien (1961 a). This evaluation was accomplished by direct microscopy of the living blastoderms and histochemically with 3, 3'-dimethoxybenzidine in the presence of hydrogen peroxide (O'Brien, 1961 b). Furthermore, hemoglobin synthesis was estimated quantitatively by the methods of Crosby and Furth (1956). In control and dopamine treated blastoderms a given blood sample for quantitation consisted of pooled blood cells of five to ten blastoderms. Cell counts were done on each pooled sample and a known volume of the same cell suspension analyzed colormetrically using the benzidine procedure. The hemoglobin concentration of each group was expressed as the mean corpuscular hemoglobin (MCH).

We have found that dopamine can reduce the amount of hemoglobin formed by early blastoderms grown *in vitro* without a disruption in embryonic organization (Seale and Prasad, 1969 a; Prasad and Seale, 1969). This ability to reduce hemoglobin formation without causing disorganization of the embroy appears to be specific for dopamine and is not characteristic of other catecholamines (Seale and Prasad, 1969 b). At the highest concentration $(500\mu g/ml)$, epinephrine and norepinephrine were lethal to the developing blastoderms, while concentrations of $150\mu g/ml$ or lower did not effect hemoglobin formation or embryonic development. Both of these catecholamines in concentrations of $300\mu g/ml$ were able to cause a reduction in total blastodermal hemoglobin, but this reduction was accompanied by a high incidence of grossly abnormal embryos.

The catecholamine catabolite homovanillic acid and the biogenic amine 5-hydroxytryptamine did not inhibit hemoglobin synthesis in the developing chick blastoderm. It should be noted, however, that L-dopa, the precursor of dopamine, also reduced total blastodermal hemoglobin. The reduction of hemoglobin formation by L-dopa may be a result of the conversion of L-dopa to dopamine since dopa decarboxylase, which catalyzes the conversion of dopa to dopamine, is present at the primitive streak stage of the chick blastoderm (Ignarro and Shideman, 1968). In preliminary studies with tyrosine hemoglobin synthesis was not inhibited (Chun and Seale, unpublished).

Recently we have shown that the diminution of hemoglobin in dopamine-treated chick blastoderms is in part a reflection of a lower mean corpuscular hemoglobin (Chun and Seale, 1970). The quantitative measurements of hemoglobin concentrations of primary embryonic erythroblast cell suspensions are presented in Table 19-I. A decrease in MCH was first noted

TABLE 19-I

MEAN CORPUSCULAR HEMOGLOBIN VALUES OF CELL SUSPENSIONS OF PRIMARY ERYTHROCYTES

Control	D_{50}	D_{100}	D_{150}	D_{200}	D_{250}	D_{300}	D_{350}	D_{400}	D_{500}
.154	.141	.157	.144	.172	.127	.140	.112	.121	.062
.141	.167	.136	.106	.176	.129	.112	.125	.118	.095
.181		.149	.110	.167	.090	,106	.105	.120	
.207		.181		.188		.100		.124	.079
.137		.151		.128				.074	.080
.166				.111					
.134				.150					
.169									
.145									
.159	.154	.155	.120	.156	.115*	.115†	.114*	.111†	.076†

MCH expressed as milligrams × 10⁻⁷.
Significant at p 0.01.
†Significant at p 0.005.

in samples from blastoderms exposed to 150μg of dopamine/ml, however, at the next dosage level (200μg/ml) the mean MCH of the erythroblast suspension reverted to levels comparable to controls. This reversal in quantitative measurements of hemoglobin occurred in the same experimental group which, qualitatively, appeared to have visible hemoglobin approaching that of controls. The MCH level of cell suspensions of erythroblasts treated with 250μg of dopamine/ml or greater were significantly less ($P < .01$) than the MCH level of control erythroblasts (analyzed by the Student t-Test). At all higher concentrations of dopamine, significant reductions in MCH were observed. There is considerable variation about the mean MCH's in control and experimental groups, however the mean MCH's show that experimental groups treated with higher concentrations of dopamine had appreciably lower MCH levels than control blastoderms. In fact, at 500μg/ml the MCH level was approximately half that of controls.

Since the most dramatic inhibition of hemoglobin was present in blastoderms treated with 500μg/ml, serial sections of the area vasculosae of blastoderms from this group and the control group were studied. Cell counts indicated that there were fewer primary embryonic erythroblasts in blastoderms exposed to high levels of dopamine than in controls. The area of highest cell density showed a mean cell count of 277 cells/mm/section for control embryos as compared to 155 cells/mm/section for the experimental group.

Although the mechanism of dopamine reduction of blastodermal hemoglobin is unknown, it is indicative that this effect is manifested at the level of hemoglobin synthesis and at the level of differentiation of precursor cells to embryonic erythroblasts. Since the embryos used in the present study are of the head fold stage or older, dopamine may be acting on the latter part of transcription or subsequent processes in hemoglobin synthesis (i.e. translation). Studies by Wilt (1965) showed that inspite of the obvious block of heavy RNA synthesis by actinomycin, the sRNA (soluble or transfer RNA) fraction continues to incorporate uridine C 14 for up to twelve hours after application of the metabolic inhibitor. Studies employing 8-azaquanine showed that this drug blocks hemoglobin synthesis up to the 7-somite stage (O'Brien, 1961 a; Hell, 1964; and Wilt, 1965). It was observed that this analogue was incorporated into the slow sedimenting fraction of RNA, probably sRNA (Wilt, 1965). It has been proposed that the sRNA containing this analogue is defective in function and interferes with the translation phase in the synthesis of hemoglobin as well as other proteins (Chantrene and LeClerq-Calinguert, 1963; see also Wilt, 1965).

The antibiotic proflavine has been shown to suppress hemoglobin formation as well as the accumulation of small RNA molecules. This inhibition can be overcome by adding sRNA from *E. coli* (Wainwright and Wainwright, 1967). The data from these studies (Wilt, 1965; Wainwright, 1967) suggested that an essential prerequisite for normal onset of hemoglobin formation between the 1-6 somite stages is the synthesis of sufficient amounts of functional sRNA. Dopamine potentially could be operating as an inhibitor of synthesis or function of this soluble RNA.

Clinical evidence of hemolysis of adult erythrocytes in patients receiving α-methyldopa (AldoMET®), an analogue of L-dopa, was reported by Carstairs (1968). This hemolysis was characterized by a positive, direct Coomb's test, IgG type (Lo Bugleo *et al.*, 1967), and may result in clinically detectable anemia in some individuals soon after treatment with methyldopa (Buchanan *et al.*, 1966) or in other cases after a relatively long period of treatment (Hamilton, 1968). It was suggested by Wurzel and Silverman (1968) that it is methyldopamine, a metabolic product of methyldopa, rather than methyldopa itself which may be responsible for the sensitization reaction that produces the positive direct Coomb's test. Since the early chick embryo is not immunologically competent (Billingham *et al.*, 1956) and therefore incapable of producing antibodies, drug-induced changes in blastodermal hemoglobin could not be produced by an autoimmune response to sensitized embryonic erythroblast.

Whether dopamine has an effect on DNA synthesis, mitosis, or cell proliferation needs to be investigated directly. Since heme insertion in the growing globin chain may regulate the rate of hemoglobin synthesis (Winslow and Ingram, 1966) and heme and iron were able to increase the polyribosomal size and rate of globin formation (Conconi and Marks, 1966), the effect of dopamine on these constituents of the hemoglobin molecule must be elucidated.

REFERENCES

1. Billingham, R. E., Brent, L., and Medawar, P. B.: *Trans Roy Soc, 239*:357, 1956.
2. Buchanan, J. B., Rush, B., and deGruchy, G. C.: *Med J Aust, 2*:700, 1966.
3. Carstairs, K.: *Proc Roy Soc Med, 61*:1309, 1968.
4. Chun, K. Y. C., and Seale, R. U.: *Anat Rec, 166*:290, 1970.
5. Conconi, F., and Marks, P. A.: *Fed Proc, 25*:581, 1966.
6. Crosby, W. H., and Furth, F. W.: *Blood, 11*:380, 1956.
7. Hamburger, V., and Hamilton, H. L.: *J Morph, 88*:49, 1952.
8. Hamilton, M.: *Postgrad Med J, 44*:66, 1968.
9. Hell, A.: *J Embryol Exp Morph, 12*:621, 1964.
10. Ignarro, L. J., and Shideman, F. E.: *J Pharmacol Exp Ther, 159*:38, 1968.
11. LoBuglio, A. F., and Jandl, J. H.: *New Eng J Med, 276*:658, 1967.
12. Lucas, A. M., and Jamroz, C.: *Atlas of Avian Hematology.* Agriculture Monograph 25, United States Department of Agriculture, Washington, D.C., 1961.
13. O'Brien, B. R. A.: *J Embryol Exp Morph, 8*:202, 1961a.
14. O'Brien, B. R. A.: *Stain Techn, 36*:57, 1961b.
15. Prasad, K. N., and Seale, R. U.: *Proc Soc Exp Biol Med, 131*:1308, 1969.
16. Seale, R. U., and Prasad, K. N.: *Anat Rec, 163*:259, 1969a.
17. Seale, R. U., and Prasad, K. N.: *J Colo Wyo Acad Sci, 6*:65, 1969b.
18. Spratt, N. T., Jr., and Haas, H.: *J Exp Zool, 144*:139, 1960.
19. Wainwright, S. D., and Wainwright, L. K.: *Canad J Biochem, 44*:1543, 1966.
20. Wainwright, S. D., and Wainwright, L. K.: *Canad J Biochem, 45*:1483-1493, 1967.
21. Watson, J. D.: *Molecular Biology of the Gene.* New York, Benjamin, 1965.
22. Wilt, F. H.: *J Molec Biol, 12*:231, 1965.
23. Wilt, F. H.: *The control of embryonic hemoglobin synthesis.* In Abercrombie, M., and Brachet, J. (Eds.): *Advances in Morphogenesis.* New York, Academic Press, 1967.
24. Winslow, R. M., and Ingram, V. M.: *J Biol Chem, 241*:1144, 1966.
25. Wurzel, H. A., and Silverman, J. L.: *Transfusion, 8*:84, 1968.

Chapter 20

Intermolecular Interactions of
5-Hydroxytryptamine*

ROBERT BITTMAN

T HE INTERACTION of various types of small molecules with nucleic acids
has generated considerable interest. The binding of certain antibiotics,
hormones, dyes, and carcinogens to nucleic acids has been studied in efforts
to gain information about biological regulatory mechanisms, to correlate
the known biological effects of these compounds with their nucleic acid
interactions, and to probe the function and secondary structure of the
nucleic acids.

The present study reports on the interaction of the biogenic amine
5-hydroxytryptamine (5-HT, serotonin) with nucleic acids. In previous
reports an interdependent relationship between 5-HT and RNA levels in
the brain has been noted (Bittman and Essman, 1970; Bittman, Essman, and
Golod, 1969; Essman, 1968). For example, negative correlations between
RNA and 5-HT levels in various regions of the brain have been found from
electroconvulsive shock treatment and tetracyanopropene administration,
and decreases in brain protein level and in estimated single cell RNA content have been measured following intracranial administration of 5-HT
and intraperitoneal administration of 5-hydroxytryptophan (5-HTP). It
was therefore of interest to examine the physical properties of the 5-HT-
nucleic acid complex (es). Furthermore, the interactions of other indoles,
such as LSD and mitomycin, with DNA has received attention recently
(Yielding and Sterglanz, 1968; Wagner, 1969; Iyer and Szybalski, 1963,
1964; Cohen and Crothers, 1970). For these reasons experiments have been
conducted in this laboratory to characterize the nature of the forces which
stabilize the complex and to learn about the strength, specificity, and possible significance of the interaction.

The interaction of the drug with nucleotides and nucleic acids was
studied by absorption, fluorescence, and circular dichroism spectroscopy,
and by equilibrium dialysis, viscometry, ultracentrifugation, and thermal
denaturation. These techniques have been used successfully to characterize
the binding constants, number of binding sites and types of complexes

*This research was supported in part by grants from the American Cancer Society (#T-
433A), City University of New York Graduate Division, and Queens College Biomedical Sciences Committee.

formed by other small molecules with macromolecules. Application of these techniques to the 5-HT-nucleic acid complex leads to the conclusions that 5-HT (a) binds to bases, nucleosides, and nucleotides, with an apparent specificity for cytidine, (b) binds to nucleic acids, including RNA, tRNA, DNA and polynucleotides, (c) does not cause appreciable distortion of the DNA helix, and (d) is bound by coulombic interaction with contributions from hydrogen bonding.

The change in the absorption spectrum of 5-HT on interaction with 5'-deoxycytidine monophosphate is shown in Figure 20-1, in which the complex reveals a slight hyperchromicity relative to the isolated components. In most examples of ligand-intermolecular interactions reported in the literature the absorption spectrum of the ligand in the visible is monitored as a function of varying concentrations of the macromolecule, which generally only absorbs in the ultraviolet. However, when both compounds absorb in the same region of the spectrum, as in the case with 5-HT and nucleotides, accurate and detailed measurements are difficult to make.

The excitation and emission spectrum of 5-HT in the presence and absence of RNA are shown in Figure 20-2. The narrowing of the bandwidth in the excitation spectrum on binding probably largely results from the strong absorption of RNA at short wavelengths; however, a different pattern of vibrational levels corresponding to a decrease in the change of shape occurring upon excitation for the excited states of the bound 5-HT molecule compared to free 5-HT, or a decrease in anharmonicity for the bound 5-HT molecule compared with free 5-HT may also contribute to the observed narrowing. On binding there is a quenching of the emission of 5-HT. The quenching has been used to study the binding, qualitatively and quantitatively, of 5-HT, 5-methoxytryptamine, 5-hydroxy-N-acetyltryptamine, and 5-methoxy-N-acetyltryptamine to nucleosides, nucleotides, and nucleic acids using an excitation wavelength at which the absorption of the nucleic acid and nucleotides is minimal (Table 20-I). There appears to be little binding to adenosine and uridine monophosphates, whereas the quenching observed with cytidine and deoxycytidine monophosphates is striking. Similar results were obtained with 5-methoxytryptamine. The N-acetyl derivatives, which have much lower pKα values, underwent less quenching, suggesting that coulombic forces involving the aralkylammonium moiety are of importance in the binding of 5-HT and 5-methoxytryptamine to neucleotides and nucleic acids. Measurements of fluorescence quenching in DMSO have also indicated that there is not appreciable interaction of 5-HT with uridine, deoxyuridine, adenosine, and deoxyadenosine, whereas there is very appreciable interaction with deoxycytidine and ribocytidine.

The quenching of fluorescence of 5-HT was studied as a function of the concentration of deoxycytidine monophosphate in 0.01 M sodium phosphate

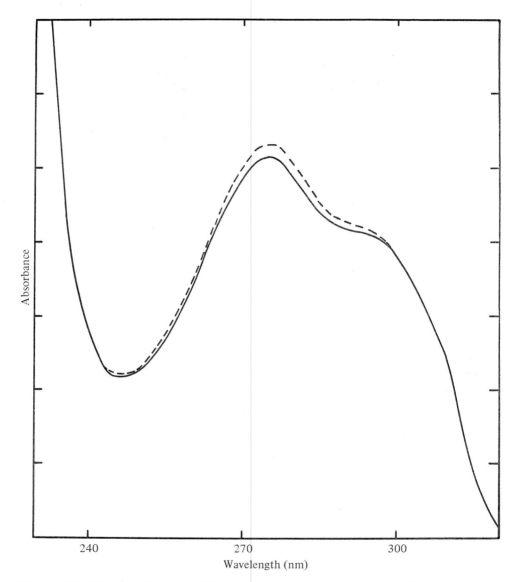

Figure 20-1. Effect of 5'-deoxycytidine monophosphate on the absorption spectrum of 5-HT. Solutions were made in 0.05 M sodium acetate buffer (pH 3.9) and contained 9.0×10^{-5} M 5-HT. The concentration of dCMP was 4.2×10^{-1}—, 5-HT and dCMP separately; - - -, 5-HT in contact with dCMP.

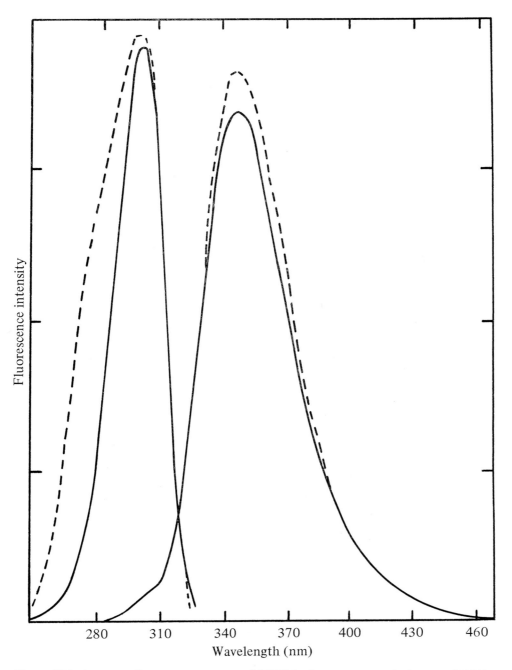

Figure 20-2. Apparent fluorescence spectra of 5-HT in the presence and absence of RNA. The excitation spectrum was taken with λ em 342 nm. The emission spectrum was taken with λ ex 303 nm. Solutions were made in 0.01 M sodium phosphate (pH 7.0) and contained 1.5×10^{-5} M 5-HT. The concentration of RNA was $500 \mu g/ml$. —, 5-HT + RNA; --- 5-HT in absence of RNA. The fluorescence intensity is in arbitrary units.

TABLE 20-I

BINDING TO NUCLEIC ACIDS AND NUCLEOTIDES

	% Quenching	
Nucleic Acids*	5-HT†	5-OMeT‡
DNA	27	—
tRNA	39	22
RNA	30	18
Polyuridylic acid	9	14
Polyguanylic acid	34	35
Nucleotides§		
AMP	7	4
dAMP	7	4
UMP	7	7
GMP	17	8
dGMP	20	9
CMP	49	25
dCMP	58	34

*500 μg/ml.

†3.8 $\times$ 10^{-6} M, λ_{ex}304, λ_{em}342 nm, 0.05 M sodium acetate, pH 3.9.

‡5-Methoxytryptamine, 1.0 $\times$ 10^{-5} M, λ_{ex}310, λ_{em}342 nm, 0.05 M sodium acetate, pH 3.9.

§12.5 $\times$ 10^{-4} M.

buffer and of cytidine in DMSO (Fig. 20-3). The concentrations of free and bound 5-HT were calculated from each point of the fluorescence titration curve. The data were treated according to the method of Scatchard (1949):

$$\frac{r}{c} = Kn - Kr$$

where r is the concentration of 5-HT bound per nucleotide, n is the number of binding sites per nucleotide, c is the concentration of free 5-HT, and K is the intrinsic association constant = [occupied sites]/[unoccupied sites] · [free 5-HT]. A plot of r/c *versus* r should give a straight line with a slope of −K and an intercept on the r-axis of n if there is no difference between the possible binding sites. Curvature has generally been interpreted as indicative of heterogeneity of binding sites in which the different sites are characterized by different intrinsic association constants. Figure 20-3 shows binding isotherms obtained from the fluorescence titration curve by plotting the data according to the Scatchard relationship. It is possible to treat the results by assuming two types of sites or an interaction between the sites and to obtain different n and K values for each class of sites. These values are shown in Table 20-II. Curvature may be due to electrostatic interaction between sites, leading to aggregation; for the binding of 5-HT to dCMP the strong binding is characterized by K_1 with 1 5-HT per 10 dCMP molecules, and the weak binding of K_2 with 1 5-HT per 5 dCMP molecules. For cytidine in DMSO the simplified resolution of the Scatchard curve into two components suggests the formation of both 1:1 and 2:1 complexes between

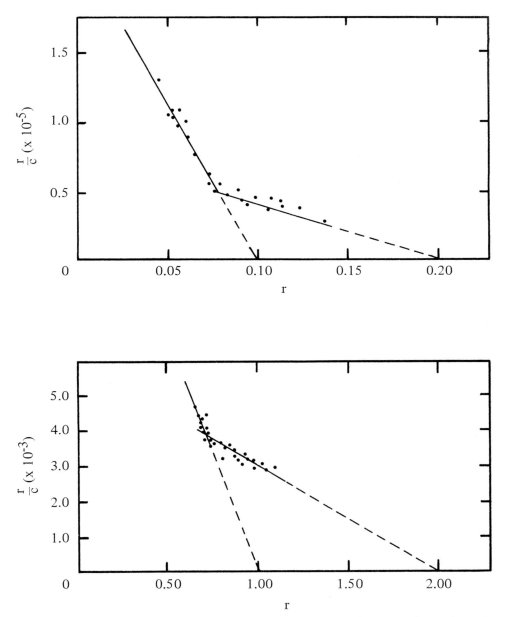

Figure 20-3. Binding isotherms. *Top:* Scatchard plot of the binding of 5-HT to 5'-deoxycytidine monophosphate in 0.01 M sodium phosphate (pH 7.0). *Bottom:* Scatchard plot of the binding of 5-HT to cytidine in DMSO. Measurements of fluorescence quenching were made at 342 nm, using λ ex 310 nm.

TABLE 20-II
EQUILIBRIUM CONSTANTS AND NUMBERS OF BINDING SITES*

	5-HT + dCMP†	5-HT + Cytidine‡
n_1	0.10	1.0
K_1	2.5×10^6 (M⁻¹)	1.3×10^4 (M⁻¹)
n_2	0.20	2.0
K_2	4.4×10^5 (M⁻¹)	2.8×10^3 (M⁻¹)

*These values are calculated assuming that the break in the binding isotherms corresponds to two classes of equilibria.

†The buffer was 0.01 M sodium phosphate, pH 7.0.

‡The solvent was DMSO.

5-HT and cytidine. Since indoles are good electron donors and are known to form charge transfer complexes (Foster and Hanson, 1964; Green and Malrieu, 1965; Snyder and Merril, 1965; Foster and Fyfe, 1966), and since cytidine is expected to be an electron acceptor (Pullman and Pullman, 1960), it is conceivable that a charge transfer complex may be formed between 5-HT and cytidine (although we find no direct evidence in favor of its formation from absorption and fluorescence spectroscopy). Furthermore, a charge transfer mechanism has been invoked to explain some cases of the quenching of fluorescence, including the quenching of acridines by nucleic acids via a hydrogen-bonding interaction (Mataga and Tsuno, 1957; Orgel, 1954; Majumdar and Basu, 1960; Tubbs, Ditmars and Van Winkle, 1964).

Binding parameters were also obtained from equilibrium dialysis studies with ¹⁴C-5-HT carried out for twenty-four hours or longer in lucite cells separated by membranes prepared from Visking dialysis tubing. Table 20-III shows the influence of ionic strength on the binding of 5-HT to RNA. The interaction is clearly electrostatic, as would be expected since the negatively charged phosphate groups can interact ionically with the positively charged 5-HT ion. Although these long-range ionic forces are not highly selective, they enhance the approach of 5-HT to the nucleic acid to short distances where specific hydrogen bond, charge transfer, and van der Waals forces can exert their effects (see below).

The 5-HT-DNA complex has been investigated by a variety of methods in efforts to learn about the mechanism of the interaction. Studies of the binding of dyes and antibiotics to DNA, although complicated by the

TABLE 20-III
BINDING OF 5-HT TO RNA: INFLUENCE OF IONIC STRENGTH

Ionic strength (M)	nK (M⁻¹) *
0.012	1.6×10^4
0.312	4.1×10^3

*Calculated from equilibrium dialysis assuming that the number of unliganded binding sites is large relative to the number of occupied binding sites.

heterogeneity of DNA, generally have concluded that various factors may be important in determining specific interactions, such as the conformation of the nucleic acid, the number of strands, the mode of base stacking and orientation of the (deoxy) ribose, the pitch and sense of the helix, the number of base pairs per turn, and the orientation of the base pairs with respect to the helical axis. In many examples of the interaction of planar molecules with DNA the strong binding process has been interpreted in terms of intercalation. In this process the planar molecule slips into the helix between and parallel to the successive planes of base pairs, causing an extension of the helix and a change in the pitch (Lerman, 1961). A necessary but insufficient condition for proof of an intercalation mechanism is the observation of an increase in viscosity and a decrease in sedimentation coefficient of DNA on interaction with the dye or drug because of the increased rigidity and decreased mass per unit length of the macromolecule, respectively, expected for the process of intercalation. The results of hydrodynamic studies conducted with DNA and 5-HT are reported in Table 20-IV. In contrast with the appreciable increase in viscosity observed on interaction of anthracyclines and acridines with DNA (Kersten, Kersten, and Szybalski, 1966), a slight decrease in viscosity and a very small increase in sedimentation coefficient are observed for the DNA-5-HT complex compared to free DNA.

TABLE 20-IV
SEDIMENTATION AND VISCOSITY DATA FOR DNA AND DNA + 5-HT

Sample	*Ratio*[*]	$S°_{20,w}$[†] Svedberg units	[n][‡] (dl./g)
DNA	—	16.1	36.5
DNA + 5-HT	2.2	16.5	
DNA + 5-HT	6.6		36.0
DNA + 5-HT	3.3		34.7

[*]Ratio = (DNA-P) / (5-HT).

[†]The buffer was 0.07 M sodium phosphate, 0.13 M sodium chloride, 0.007 M Na_2EDTA, pH 7.0. The concentration of 5-HT was 4.2×10^{-5}M. Rotor speed was 50,740 rev/min.

[‡]The buffer was 0.01 M sodium phosphate, 0.17 M sodium chloride, pH 7.0 at 26.0°. The concentrations of 5-HT were 1.9×10^{-5} and 3.8×10^{-5}M.

These results are clearly inconsistent with a mechanism of intercalation and furthermore suggest that 5-HT does not cause DNA to undergo appreciable conformational change. In confirmation of this finding, it is found that the thermal denaturation profiles of DNA and DNA + 5-HT (at a ratio of [DNA-P]/[5-HT] = 1.7) are virtually identical.

Detailed studies of optical activity have provided important insights into subtle structural changes occurring in biological macromolecules. Optical rotatory dispersion and circular dichroism spectroscopy are potentially

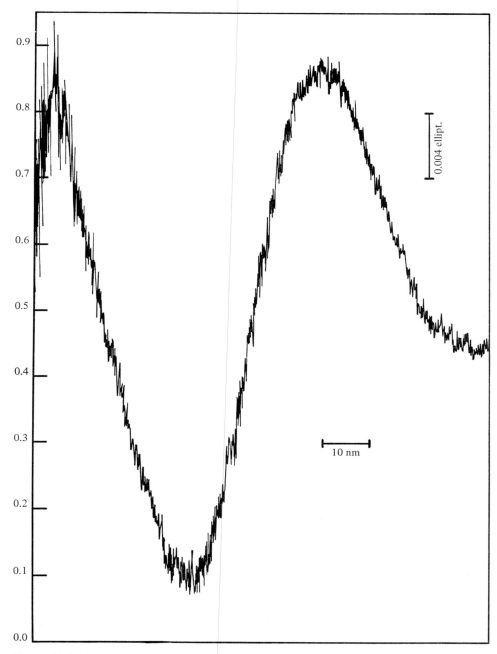

Figure 20-4. Photograph of a typical CD spectrum of denatured DNA + 5-HT obtained on a Cary 60 spectropolarimeter with circular dichroism attachment.

sensitive techniques for examining the conformations of DNA, RNA, and polynucleotides in solution (Yang and Samejima, 1967; Beychok, 1966; Tinoco and Cantor, 1970). As mentioned earlier, the interaction of dyes with nucleic acids often shifts the wavelength of the visible absorption maximum of the dye, and in several examples Cotton effects are induced in the visible absorption band of the dyes (Yang and Samejina, 1967). To gain further insights into the properties of the 5-HT-nucleic acid complex ultraviolet CD spectra were run. A photograph of an experimentally obtained CD spectrum of denatured DNA is shown in Figure 20-4, from which the molar ellipticity and difference in extinction coefficients ($E_L - E_R$) between left and right circularly polarized light can be calculated provided that the molarity and pathlength are known. Figure 20-5 shows the CD spectra of native DNA isolated from and in contact with 5-HT. The positive dichroism of DNA in the 260-305 nm region is diminished in the DNA-5-HT complex, but the negative dichroism is unaffected. This suggests that 5-HT, although symmetric in the free state, acquires asymmetry on binding to DNA; the negative dichroism acquired by 5-HT closely mimics the absorption spectrum of 5-HT (Fig. 20-6). Furthermore, the CD spectrum of tRNA[phe], which is shifted to shorter wavelengths relative to that of DNA (Fig. 20-7), does not undergo a shift in the positive ellipticity band (even though it forms a complex with 5-HT under these conditions). This is probably because of the lack of coincidence between the λ maxima of the 5-HT absorption band and the tRNA positive ellipticity band. Therefore, it is concluded that DNA does not undergo a significant conformational change on interaction with 5-HT, a conclusion which is in agreement with the hydrodynamic properties discussed earlier.

In 1.0 M sodium chloride the positive ellipticities of DNA and DNA-5-HT are identical, and the negative ellipticities are nearly the same (Fig. 20-7); therefore, the interaction appears to be electrostatic in nature, in agreement with the results from equilibrium dialysis studies.

With formaldehyde-treated DNA the difference in the CD spectrum isolated from and in contact with 5-HT is clearly diminished (Fig. 20-8) compared with native DNA ($\pm$ 5-HT, Fig. 20-5). A reasonable explanation is that less 5-HT is bound to formaldehyde-treated DNA than to native DNA. Since reaction of nucleic acids with formaldehyde gives products in which exocyclic amino groups are hydroxymethylated (Grossman, Levine, and Allison, 1961; Stollar and Gross, 1962), amino groups are implicated in the binding process; in addition, denaturation leading to an opening of the secondary structure probably also plays a role.

Figure 20-9 shows that the CD spectrum of heat-denatured DNA + 5-HT has a somewhat greater positive ellipticity band than that of heat-denatured DNA itself, suggesting that the mechanism of interaction with denatured DNA may be different from that with native DNA.

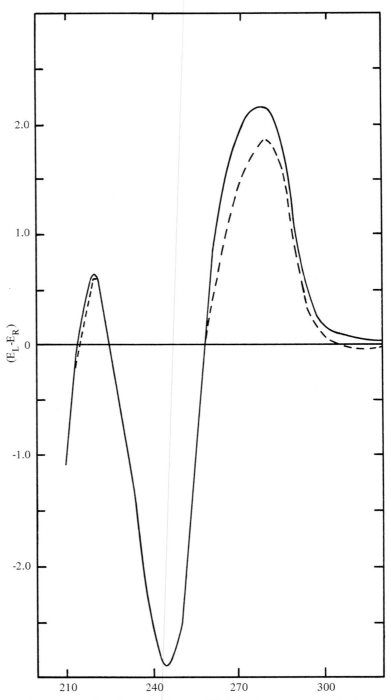

Figure 20-5. CD spectra of native calf thymus DNA in the presence and absence of 5-HT obtained in a tandem cell consisting of two compartments, each having a 1-cm pathlength. Solutions were made in 0.01 M sodium phosphate (pH 7.0) and contained 2.1 $\times$ 10^{-4} M DNA-P. The concentration of 5-HT was 4.1 $\times$ 10^{-5} M. —, DNA and 5-HT in separate compartments; - - -, DNA + 5-HT.

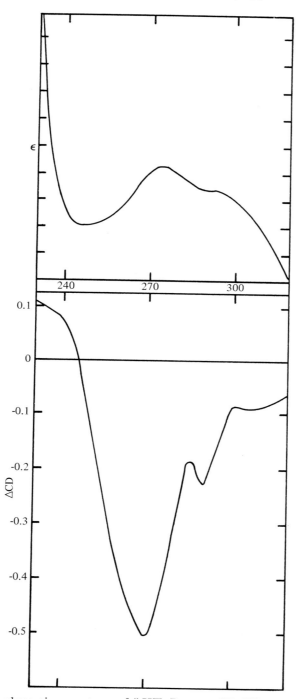

Figure 20-6. Top: absorption spectrum of 5-HT. Bottom: CD difference spectra obtained from subtraction of curves of Figure 20-5.

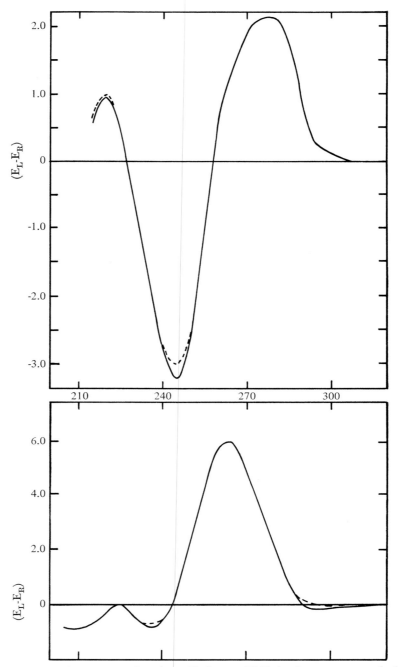

Figure 20-7. Top: CD spectra of native calf thymus DNA in the presence and absence of 5-HT in solutions containing 0.01 M sodium phosphate and 1.0 M sodium chloride (pH 7.0). The conditions were as in Figure 20-5. The concentrations were 2.5×10^{-4} M DNA-P, 4.1×10^{-5} M 5-HT. —, DNA and 5-HT in separate compartments; - - -, DNA + 5-HT. Bottom: CD spectra of Phe tRNA in the presence and absence of 5-HT in 0.01 M sodium phosphate (pH 7.0). The concentrations were 1.5×10^{-4} M tRNA-P, 4.1×10^{-5} M 5-HT. —, tRNA and 5-HT in separate compartments; - - -, tRNA + 5-HT.

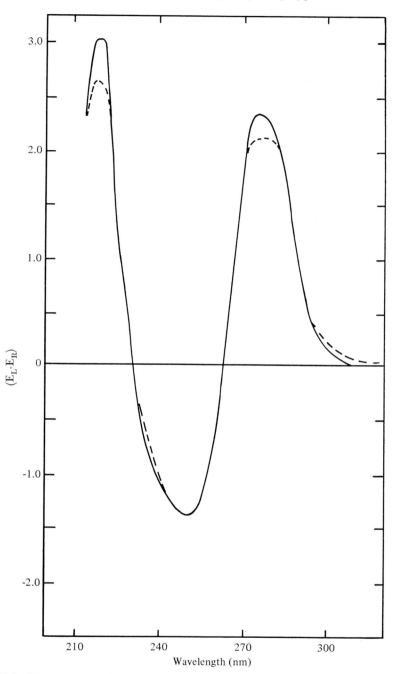

Figure 20-8. CD spectra of formaldehyde-treated calf thymus DNA in the presence and absence of 5-HT. The conditions were as in Figure 20-5. The concentrations were 1.1 × 10^{-4} M DNA-P (assuming ϵ_{260} 9350 M^{-1} cm^{-1}) , 4.1 × 10^{-5} M 5-HT. —, DNA and 5-HT in separate compartments; - - -, DNA + 5-HT.

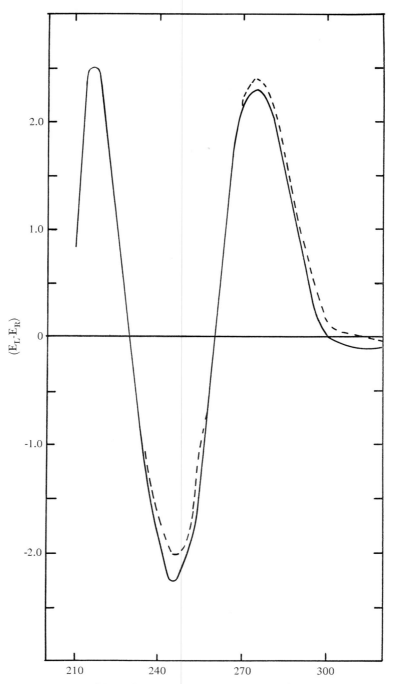

Figure 20-9. CD spectra of heat-denatured calf thymus DNA in the presence and absence of 5-HT. The conditions and concentrations were identical to those in Figure 20-5.

It is concluded from these studies that 5-HT forms a complex with DNA which involves electrostatic interactions between the aralkylammonium moiety of 5-HT and the negatively charged phosphate groups of DNA and does not involve intercalation or significant distortion of the helix. Symthies and Antun (1969) conclude from model building studies that 5-HT interacts with RNA and DNA by intercalation. However, the evidence presented in this work refutes their proposal. Consideration of space-filling (Corey-Pauling-Koltun) models of the 5-HT-DNA interaction is presented here which is consistent with the results obtained from the spectral, equilibrium dialysis, and hydrodynamic studies. The principal determinants of biological specificity, namely coulombic interactions and stereospecific hydrogen bonding, are invoked as the predominant forces controlling the interaction of 5-HT with DNA with possible contributions from apolar binding. It is proposed that the function of the carbon skeleton of 5-HT is to provide the correct location of the functional groups which allow for specific interactions with the macromolecule. Figure 20-10 shows a model of 5-HT; its side chain may assume several conformations (Kier, 1968).

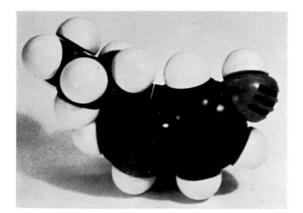

Figure 20-10. View of space-filling model of the 5-HT molecule.

Since 5-methoxytryptamine binds to nucleotides and nucleic acids (Table 20-I), it is assumed that the oxygen atom at the 5-position of 5-HT may serve as an electron pair donor to accept a hydrogen bond. Figure 20-11 shows 5-HT in the minor groove of DNA. The 2-amino group of guanine donates a proton to form a hydrogen bond to the oxygen atom of 5-HT; the indole proton of 5-HT is hydrogen-bonded to a furanose oxygen; and the aralkylammonium moiety of 5-HT is located adjacent to the oxygen atom of a phosphodiester linkage (and between two negatively charged phosphate groups). Figure 20-12 shows another model of the 5-HT-DNA complex,

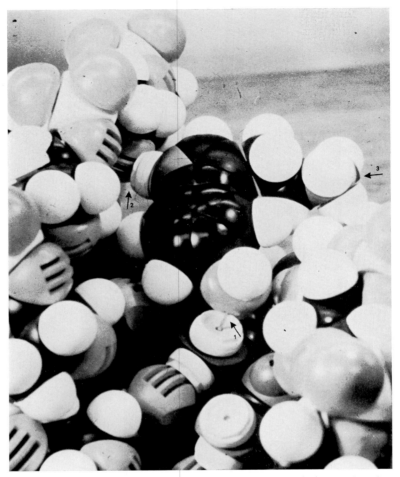

Figures 20-11, 20-12, and 20-13—views of space-filling models of 5-HT and a short section of the DNA helix illustrating possible modes of binding. See text for details. The arrows indicate proposed interaction sites, and the numbers refer to the order in which they are described in the text.

again with 5-HT lying in the minor groove. Again, the 2-amino group of guanine donates a proton to the oxygen of 5-HT; the indole proton of 5-HT forms a hydrogen bond to a phosphodiester oxygen; and the aralkylammonium moiety of 5-HT is adjacent to a phosphodiester oxygen atom. Each of these models predicts that (a) hydroxymethylation of DNA would result in diminished binding (see Fig. 20-8) since the 2-amino group of guanine in DNA reacts with formaldehyde, (b) polyguanylic acid would be expected to react with 5-HT (see Table 20-I), (c) a 5-methoxyl group would not cause serious interference compared to a 5-hydroxyl group (see Table 20-I), and

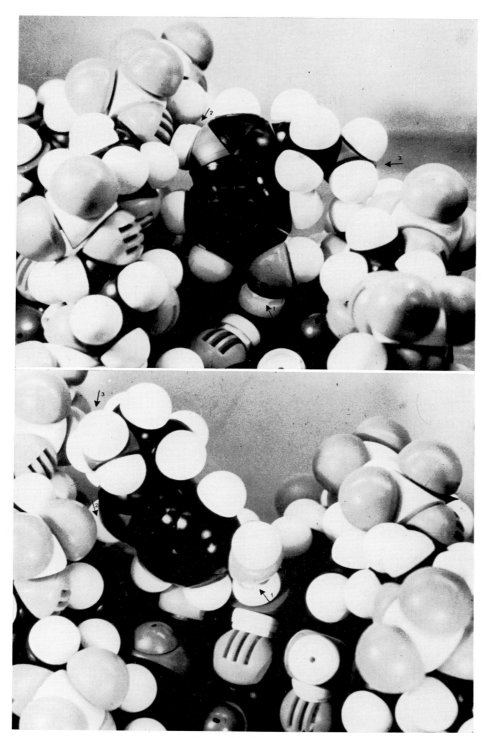

Figure 20-12 *(top)*.
Figure 20-13 *(bottom)*.

(d) substitution at various positions in the indole ring should interfere. Figure 20-13 shows a model of 5-HT in the major groove with the N-H of cytosine donating a proton to form a hydrogen bond with the oxygen atom of 5-HT; the indole proton of 5-HT forms a hydrogen bond to N-7 of guanine and the aralkylammonium moiety lies adjacent to a phosphate group. Several other models may be proposed and precise definition of the binding site(s) is probably not possible even after extensive studies with derivatives of 5-HT.

Finally, it is of interest to speculate about the functional significance, if any, of the 5-HT-nucleic acid complex in the brain. It remains to be shown if the complex has any relevance to the major pharmacological sites of action of the amine and its relationship to other drugs, such as LSD, mescaline, and reserpine. In view of reports of the presence of RNA at presynaptic and postsynaptic membranes (Austin and Morgan, 1967; Kogan and Zaguskin, 1966; Radin, Kishimoto, Agranoff, and Burton, 1967; Von Hungen, Mahler, and Moore, 1968), it may be conjectured that after 5-HT is transferred from vesicular storage sites, its release from the presynaptic membrane may be partially controlled by the presence or absence of the 5-HT-nucleic acid complex because of permeability phenomena and competition with lipoprotein complexes occurring at the membrane level. Thus, perhaps the complex may be considered to exert control on the availability of free 5-HT associated with the presynaptic membrane pool, which may in turn be indirectly related to its release from its vesicular storage sites.

REFERENCES

1. Austin, L., and Morgan, I. G.: *J Nurochem, 14*:377, 1967.
2. Beychok, S.: *Science, 154*:1288, 1966.
3. Bittman, R., and Essman, W. B.: Second Annual Winter Conference on Brain Research, Aspen, Colorado, 1970.
4. Bittma, R., Essman, W. B., and Golod, M.: (1969). *Abstr Amer Chem Soc,* Div. Biol. Chem., New York, paper 330.
5. Cohen, R. J., and Crothers, D. M.: *Biochemistry, 9*:2533, 1970.
6. Essman, W. B.: *Physiol Behav, 3*:527, 1968.
7. Foster, R., and Fyfe, C. A.: *J Chem Soc (B):* 926, 1966.
8. Foster, R., and Hanson, A. W.: *Trans Faraday Soc, 60*:2189, 1964.
9. Green, J. P., and Malrieu, J. P.: *Proc Nat Acad Sci, 54*:659, 1965.
10. Grossman, L., Levine, S. S., and Allison, W. S.: *J Molec Biol, 3*:47, 1961.
11. Iyer, V. N., and Szybalski, W.: *Proc Nat Acad Sci, 50*:355, 1963.
12. Iyer, V. N., and Szybalski, W.: *Science, 145*:55, 1964.
13. Kersten, M., Kersten, H., and Szybalski, W.: *Biochemistry, 5*:236, 1966.
14. Kier, L. B.: *J Pharm Sci, 57*:1188, 1968.
15. Kogan, A. B., and Zaguskin, S. L.: *Fed Proc,* vol. T191, 1966.
16. Lerman, L. S.: *J Molec Biol, 3*:18, 1961.
17. Majumdar, D. K., and Basu, S.: *J Chem Phys, 33*:1199, 1960.
18. Mataga, N., and Tsuno, S.: *Bull Chem Soc (Japan), 30*:711, 1957.

19. Orgel, L. E.: *Quart Rev (London)*, *8*:422, 1954.
20. Pullman, B., and Pullman, A.: *Rev Mod Phys*, *32*:428, 1960.
21. Radin, N. S., Kishimoto, Y., Agranoff, B. W., and Burton, R. M.: *Fed Proc, 26:* 676, 1967.
22. Scatchard, G.: *Ann NY Acad Sci*, *51*:660, 1949.
23. Smythies, J. R., and Antun, F.: *Nature*, *223*:1061, 1969.
24. Snyder, S. H., and Merril, C. R.: *Proc Nat Acad Sci*, *54*:258, 1965.
25. Stollar, D., and Grossman, L.: *J Molec Biol*, *4*:31, 1962.
26. Tinoco, Jr., I., and Cantor, C. R.: In Glick, D. (Ed) : *Methods of Biochemical Analysis.* New York, John Wiley and Sons, 1970, vol. 18, p. 81.
27. Tubbs, R. K., Ditmars, Jr., W. E., and Van Winkle, Q.: *J Molec Biol*, *9*:545, 1964.
28. Von Hungen, K., Mahler, H. R., and Moore, W. J.: *J Biol Chem*, *243*:1415, 1968.
29. Wagner, T. E.: *Nature*, *222*:1170, 1969.
30. Yang, J. T. and Samejima, T.: In Davidson, J. N., and Cohn, W. E. (Ed.) : *Progress in Nucleic Acid Research.* New York, Academic Press, 1967, vol. 9, p. 223.
31. Yielding, K. L., and Sterglanz, H.: *Proc Soc Exp Biol Med*, *128*:196, 1968.

Chapter 21

The Effects of Diphenylhydantoin*
on Cognitive Functions in Man†

W. LYNN SMITH AND JACK B. LOWREY

INTRODUCTION

DIPHENYLHYDANTOIN (Dilantin®, Parke, Davis & Company) has been the anticonvulsant drug of choice for the control of seizures over the past thirty years. An increasing number of research studies have been conducted over the past few years, however, indicating a wide range of beneficial effects attributed to the drug. In addition to its main use, a sizeable body of research knowledge has been accumulated demonstrating the therapeutic usefulness of diphenylhydantoin (DPH) in a variety of physical conditions ranging from cardiac and metabolic disorders to neuromuscular, thought, mood and behavior disorders. A comprehensive annotated bibliography of DPH studies on its pharmacology, physiology, and effective usefulness has just appeared, selectively summarizing most of the DPH research conducted to date.[1]

Behavioral studies involving DPH have run the gamut from behavioral problem children,[2-5] to actual delinquents,[6,7] and to those children with emotional and learning problems.[8-12] Regarding intellectual functions, two recent controlled studies by Haward have appeared on an adult population.[13,14] One involved neurotic outpatients and the other, normal subjects in a simulated air control tower setting, indicating respectively, that DPH assists concentration when impairment in cognitive functions stems from ruminative preoccupation with irrelevant content and improves concentration under conditions of fatigue—impaired efficiency.

A rather interesting parallel to Haward's studies are those conducted by Smith[15-17] on a similar drug but different group, that is, minimal brain dysfunction. These studies involved children with a syndrome of learning deficit, autonomic dysfunction and 14-6 Hz positive spike EEGs, treated with ethosuximide, a *petit mal* anticonvulsant. Findings in the drug-placebo crossover study series revealed large statistical significance in raising verbal symbolic functions while on ethosuximide. The above cited studies on two types of anticonvulsants in adult neurotic and clinically normal subjects,

*Supplied as Dilantin® by Parke, Davis and Co., Detroit, Michigan.
†This study supported by the Dreyfus Medical Foundation, New York, New York.

as well as children with learning deficit and borderline EEGs, all responded to the drugs with increased concentration.

PURPOSE

The purpose and next logical step in this study sequence on anti-convulsant action and concentration, is to study a group of cortically normal subjects in a general, rather than a specialized complex situation under drug-placebo conditions. Rather than use perceptual or vigilance tests as previously reported by Haward, the approach for this study is to use standardized intelligence tests with alternate forms to examine changes in basic intellectual functions (should they occur) which can be attributed to the drug. Further, these intellectual tests have been used in previous studies as sensitive measures of psychoactive and cerebral vasodilating drugs.[19,20]

METHOD

Subjects and Conditions

Twenty volunteers, nine male and eleven female, of whom four were already taking Dilantin as a mental "normalizer," were given base-line intelligence tests after an initial placebo period, followed by two retests in a double-blind presentation of drug and placebo conditions. Half were started on the drug after the base-line testing while the other half started on placebo. After a three week period the subjects were tested and crossed over to the remaining condition. After the last three week phase they received their final testing.

Instructions

Instructions given to prospective volunteers were simply that they would have a trial period on Dilantin as previous research indicated that the drug may increase intellectual function.

Procedure

According to Parke, Davis & Company studies,[22] a three-week drying out period should be allowed those four subjects already on DPH before the drug (experimental) and placebo (control) conditions are started. In order to bridge this transitional drying-out period, the so-called "Florida design" was used; that is, for the first three weeks before the cross over study started all subjects were placed on placebo, known to the testing psychologists but unknown to the subjects, and then the subjects were tested after that period for their base-line intellectual measurement. This approach gave an interesting check on the later placebo condition. Additional tests, as IPAT

Anxiety Scales, and psychophysical assessments as Critical Flicker Fusion and Raven Coloured Progressive Matrices, were administered to account for emotional or threshold influences (if any), should intellectual changes not be apparent.

Selection of Tests

A standardized intelligence test assesses specific mental abilities, especially in the subtests of the Wechsler Intelligence Scale series, with alternate forms, tests of specific areas such as *memory*, recent and remote, measured by Digit Span and Information subtests; *judgment* by the Comprehension subtest; *abstraction* through similarities; *spatial configuration* with block design; *temporal-sequential*, picture arrangement, and so on. Additionally, the Wechsler series yields verbal symbolic and visual spatial scores as well as a general I.Q. score. The weighted scores of these subtests as well as I.Q. scores are directly comparable one with the other so differences between conditions can be directly measured.

In order to fulfill the three testing sessions following each of the three conditions, the writers were fully aware that the three Wechsler forms selected were not exactly equivalent and equally free from practice effects, one to another. However, with all the inherent test/retest flaws of the Wechsler Scales, they remain the only alternate form possibilities of a high powered intellectual scale. Nevertheless, practice effect in repeated measures needs to be discussed. It might be noted that the crossover design equalizes practice effects for both conditions.

Regarding the Wechsler Scales, the Form I (one), developed in 1939, led to the eventual Form II (two) (1946), and still later the WAIS (three) (1955) was made by revising and lengthening the Form I. The similarities among the forms are noted later. Reported studies of negligible practice effect are mainly between (one) and (two) and some on (two) to (one), although one study indicated that the (two) to (one) sequence practice effect is greater. As to (one) and (three), Guertin, *et al.*,[18] summarized studies and concluded that an average or higher intelligence samples, higher scores appear in Block Design, Digit Symbol, Performance IQ, and Full Scale IQ for the Form I. Nothing is reported in the literature for use as guide lines regarding combinations of the forms in the various test/retest/ retest sequences in the present study. Most writers agree on slight expected practice effect in Performance in all forms of the Wechsler while Verbal subtests are almost free from practice effect. As Vocabulary in the Form (one) and (two) are overlapping in the Verbal Scale and items duplicated in (one) and (three) in the Object Assembly subtests in the Performance Scale these subtests were omitted with the latter part being prorated to yield a Performance Scale IQ score.

Selection of Subjects

Twenty Ss of various ages (16 to 50 with M age 29), sex, with different education (10 to 20 years with M 14 years) and intelligence levels [79-132 (Verbal I.Q.) 81-124 (Performance I.Q. and 77-130 (Full Scale I.Q.) with M117 (Verbal I.Q.), 118 (Performance I.Q.) and 115 (Full Scale I.Q.)] volunteered for this study. Most were general hospital employees from housekeeping, secretarial, business, nursing, and professional staff. The assumption was made that this population was not either psychotic, grossly neurotic, or with a history of acting-out character disorders, of serious head injury, seizures, or alterations in consciousness.

As a check against cortical abnormality 14 of the 20 selected Ss were given EEGs (70%). All EEG protocols had sleep and hyperventilation portions as well as bipolar, transverse montage and monopolar montage, connecting occipital, posterior and mid-temporal and central leads to the opposite ear in order to detect diencephalic disturbances.

Test Drugs and Dose

DPH (Dilantin) in 100 mg capsules and placebos were supplied by Parke, Davis & Company. The hospital chief pharmacist dispersed medication (following recapsuling from #3 to #2 gray opaque capsules to make for similar appearance of DPH and placebo) and was in charge of code for drug administration. DPH was taken by subjects 100 mg t.i.d.; placebo capsules were provided on the same schedule.

Conditions

The assignment of each S to conditions was done randomly. Also, Wechsler Adult Intelligence Scale, Wechsler Intelligence Scale for Adolescents and Adults, Form I and Form II, were administered on a random basis. Psychoperceptual tests as Critical Flicker Fusion, IPAT Anxiety Scales, and Coloured Progressive Matrices were assigned accordingly.

Treatment of Data

A "t" test was employed for difference of repeated measures where drug retests were compared to the base-line placebo and later placebo condition to give an average baseline score. The code for drug administration was not broken until all subjects had completed all conditions.

RESULTS AND DISCUSSION

Preliminary inspection of the supporting tests did not reveal any obvious differences between drug and placebo testings, and "t" tests for the Coloured Progressive Matrices, Critical Flicker Fusion, and IPAT Anxiety Scale were not significant. Further, as to possible "normalizing" effects an analysis of

TABLE 21-I
A COMPARISON OF WECHSLER IQ & SUBJECT RESULTS OF 20 SUBJECTS
ON DPH AND PLACEBO TREATMENT

Subtest	d	Sd	t actual	Significance level (one-tailed)
VSIQ	6.15	5.79	4.63	.0005
PSIQ	4.60	7.21	2.79	.01
FSIQ	6.48	6.22	4.53	.0005
Info	.73	1.54	2.086	.05
Comp	1.23	2.09	2.56	.01
D. Span	.78	2.33	1.47	.1
Arith	1.33	2.51	2.29	.025
Simil	.08	2.39	1.45	.1
P. Arr	1.40	3.40	1.79	.05
P. Comp	.83	1.86	1.93	.05
Bl. Des	.28	1.88	.65	Not Significant
D. Sym	.55	2.03	1.17	.25

variance revealed there was less intersubtest variance under placebo conditions than under the drug.

In the above table, highly significant confidence levels are seen in the Verbal Scale IQ and Full Scale IQ scores with lesser significance appearing in the Performance Scale IQ. The significance level in the latter scale is viewed somewhat skeptically as this level could well be influenced by practice effects. The Full Scale IQ increase, of course, is a reflection of the great influence of Verbal Scale changes, as the Full Scale IQ score is a composite of the other two scales.

As several ethosuximide studies preceded this DPH study and the results being of such magnitude, the presence of extraneous variables need to be entertained. As to sources of bias, one must not only discuss appropriate cognitive measures but also the effect of the observer's expectations of the drug and the evaluation results. Expectations by the testor may be communicated to the S and influence his performance (commonly referred to as the "Rosenthal effect"). This point is raised since both testors had knowledge that the first testing was under placebo condition. In reviewing the findings of the Rosenthal study, however, it is not often remarked how relatively small an effect this turned out to be.[21] By raising the confidence level for data interpretation, as we have done here, these minor but recalcitrant sources of bias can be minimized.

The high significance of the Verbal Scale differences reveals a remarkable increase in verbal functions which can be attributed to the effects of DPH. Further, the significant subtest within the Verbal Scale is the Comprehension Subtest, which involves, among other things, discrimination in levels of thought and judgment in and about social situations. Whatever this subtest is thought to measure, the inter-modal relationships of the test are important here. In this particular subtest the items are given verbally by the examiner and received in the auditory sensory mode. Following in this sequence, is registration, integration, (including needed storage to organize thought processes) then expression. All these various functions would appear to be inextricably bound up with concentration. A clearly different type of task is demanded from the S in this subtest as compared to the constant visual stimulus inherent in the Performance Scale tasks. Perhaps this important factor of concentration is the communality underlying the subtests of the Verbal Scale. The findings in the present study are consistent with Haward's studies of the effects of DPH on concentration. Increases in verbal symbolic functions in this study following DPH are also strikingly similar to the results of this writer's studies on ethosuximide where verbal symbolic functions were selectively increased. This similarity merits further discussion.

The most recent study cited in the ethosuximide series (see Chap. 22) involved 125 consecutive psychological studies of children with learning problems, autonomic dysfunction, and with electrograms involving a spiking pattern. The premedication Wechsler score pattern for this group is one of relatively very low Verbal to high Performance Scale IQ. High subtest scores appeared in Comprehension, Similarities, and Object Assembly with low subtest scores appearing in Digit Symbol and Information. The last two subtests appear to underscore the learning problem as they deal with new learning, and storage of a fund of general knowledge. Further, the former subtest is a sensitive measure to improvement on ethosuximide while Information is one of the six Verbal Scale Subtests which improve after the drug.[16]

In this present DPH study, the Information score is significant and may be related to concentration as an end product, as it is a storage subtest. Concentration is intimately involved in the process of reception, storage, and recall. Perhaps the meaning of the increases seen in this study are twofold: that DPH improves concentration and that verbal-symbolic subtests are its most sensitive measures.

A suggestion for further studies on DPH and measured mental changes would be to introduce quantitative pharmaco-electroencephalography. By using frequency analyzer and digital computer methods this technique offers an exceptional outside criterion for psychological measurements since it has established that any drug which affects behavior produces changes in EEG (see Chap. 9).

A technique such as this may tell us something further about S's with minimal cortical brain dysfunction, some of whom are presently undetectable with usual visual readings. This refinement in measurement could also tell us why some so-called normal S's show large improvements on DPH while others do not. It might even tell us something about why S's do not get worse on DPH and why some of the non-responders seem to do better on placebo.

ACKNOWLEDGMENTS

The authors wish to express their gratitude to Sandra Weinman, M.S., who tested half of the subjects in this study; to Fred Pang, M.S., for the packaged preparations in the double-blind series; to Stephen Campbell, Ph.D. and Murray Binder, M.S., for statistical evaluation of these data; and to Lionel R. C. Haward, Dr. Psy., for his helpful suggestions.

REFERENCES

1. Bogoch, S., and Dreyfus, J.; *The Broad Range of Use of Diphenylhydantoin: Bibliography and Review.* The Dreyfus Medical Foundation, 1971.
2. Lindsley, D. B., and Henry, C. E.: The effect of drugs on behavior and the electroencephalograms of children with behavior disorder. *Psychosom Med, 4:* 140-149, 1941.
3. Brown, W. T., and Solomon, C. I.: Delinquency and the electroencephalograph. *Amer J Psychiat, 98:*499-503, 1942.
4. Walker, C. F., and Kirkpatrick, B. B.: Dilantin treatment for behavior problem children with abnormal electroencephalograms. *Amer J Psychiat, 103:*484-492, 1947.
5. Zimmerman, F. T.: Explosive behavior anomalies in children on an epileptic basis. *J Med., 56:*2537-2543, 1956.
6. Putnam, T. J., and Hood, O. E.: Project Illinois: A study of therapy in juvenile behavior problems. *Western Med,* July, 231-233, 1964.
7. Resnick, O.: The psychoactive properties of diphenylhydantoin: Experiences with prisoners and juvenile delinquents. *Int J Neuropsychiat, 3 (Suppl. 2):*530-548, 1967.
8. Baldwin, R., and Kenny, T. J.: "Learning disabilities." Special Child publication of the Seattle Sequin School, Inc., Vol. 2, 313, 1966.
9. Pincus, J. H., and Glaser, G. H.: The syndrome of 'minimal brain damage' in children. *New Eng J Med, 275:*27-35, 1966.
10. Chao, D., Sexton, J.A., and Davis, S.D.: Convulsive equivalent syndrome of childhood. *J Pediat, 64:*499-508, 1964.
11. Turner, W. J.: "The usefulness of diphenylhydantoin in treatment of non-epileptic emotional disorders:. *Int. J. Neuropsychiat., 3* (suppl 2) , 58-520, 1967.
12. Jonas, A. D.: The diagnostic and therapeutic use of diphenylhydantoin in the subictal state and non-epileptic dysphoria. *Int J Neuropsychiat, 3:*521-529, 1967.
13. Haward, L.R.C.: The effects of Sodium Diphenylhydantoinate and Pemoline upon concentration: A comparative study. in Smith, W. Lynn (Ed.) *Drugs and Cerebral Function.* Springfield, Thomas, 103-120, 1970.
14. Haward, L.R.C.: Effects of Sodium Diphenylhydantoinate on Concentration. *Bull Brit Psychol Soc,* 1969.
15. Smith, W. Lynn, Philippus, M.J., and Guard, H.L.: Psychometric study of children

with learning problems and 14-6 positive spike EEG patterns, treated with ethosuximide and placebo. *Arch Dis Child,* 43, Oct. 1968.

16. Smith, W. Lynn, and Weyl, T.C.: The effects of ethosuximide (Zarontin) ® on intellectual functions of children with learning deficits and cortical brain dysfunction. *Curr Ther Res, 10:*265-269, No. 6, June, 1968.

17. Smith, W. Lynn: Facilitating verbal-symbolic functions in children with learning problems and 14-6 positive spike EEG patterns with ethosuximide (Zarontin). In Smith, W. Lynn (Ed.) : *Drugs and Cerebral Function.* Springfield, Thomas, 121-133, 1970.

18. Guertin, W.H., Rabin, A.I., Frank, G.H., and Ladd, C.E.: Research with the Wechsler Intelligence Scales for Adults. *Psychol Bull, 59:*1-25, No. 1, January, 1962.

19. Smith, W. Lynn, and Lowrey, J.B.: Differential effects of cylandelate on psychological test performance in patients with cerebral vascular insufficiency, In Georg Thieme Verlag, Stuttgart, Stoecker, *et al* (Eds.) : *The Assessment of Cerebrovascular Insufficiency.* 1970.

20. Smith, W. Lynn: The effects of vasodilators on psychological test performance in patients with cerebrovascular insufficiency. In Smith, W. Lynn (Ed.) :*Drugs and Cerebral Function.* Springfield, Thomas, 252-260, 1970.

21. Rosenthal, R., and Jacobson, L.: *Pygmalion in the Classroom.* New York, Holt, Rinehart and Winston, 1968.

22. Buchanan, Robert A., M.D.: Parke, Davis and Co., Personal Communication, 1969.

PART VI

SYMPOSIUM PANEL: "NEUROPSYCHOPHARMACOLOGY TODAY"

Chapter 22

Neuropsychopharmacology Today

MODERATOR: GEORGE A. ULETT

BY WAY OF INTRODUCTION, let me say that I have asked all of the panel participants to prepare a brief statement which should include the following:

(1) A very brief summary of his own research.
(2) An indication of how his findings relate to other ongoing work in the field.
(3) An indication of what he thinks will be the most important breakthrough in this area in the future.

Certainly such speculation will bring some criticism and debate and stimulate discussion from other panel members and audience.

To begin the discussion, let me present my own bias. My own research has long focused in the EEG area, and I have been particularly concerned with quantification of the EEG. My recent interests have become a paper with my daughter Judith Ulett and Dr. Itil on changes in the EEG with smoking withdrawal which demonstrated slowing on deprivation and which reversed upon smoking, thus indicating the addictive nature of smoking; a paper with Dr. Akpinar and Dr. Itil using quantitative methods to demonstrate a specific fast EEG pattern correlating highly with hypnotizability, and a continuing focus of investigation with Dr. Itil on EEG quantitative methods in the field of psychopharmacology.

From my vantage point there have been three major revolutions in psychiatry. First, at the turn of the century, Sigmund Freud—dynamic psychiatry, psychoanalysis, etc. After the passage of two thirds of a century, however, there is evidence that classical psychoanalysis has had no major effect upon the vast problems of public psychiatry; and, indeed, during its heyday the great public mental hospitals of our country have become increasingly overcrowded. Although woefully ineffective from the public health point of view, this first psychiatric revolution left a positive legacy in terms of a humanitarian approach to the mentally ill, milieu and group experiences, together with some new approaches to brief psychotherapy.

The second psychiatric revolution is now upon us. This one, psychopharmacology, is producing more tangible results. Starting near the half-century mark, the use of psychoactive drugs has been a prime factor in reducing the state hospital population across the country by a factor of one third and has made it possible to treat thousands more as outpatients. Psychopharmacology is so vital to psychiatry that Dr. Itil, in our laboratories, has a continuing major program in this area concerned with the relationship between psychoactive drugs and the EEG. We have become convinced that electronic and computer techniques for frequency analysis of the EEG are essential in this kind of work.

Advent of the psychotropic drugs has served as an important motivation for research of the type reported here in the last few days. Some of the research discussed at this conference may well lead us to knowledge of basic etiology and hence to a rational science of therapeutic psychiatry.

Although I hope this will be true, the timing of important discoveries in medicine is unpredictable, and so we may have to utilize our existing tools for some years yet.

While awaiting the ultimate research breakthrough, we must continue to work on a day-to-day basis and still meet the growing need for thousands of additional patients who are seeking help for their mental illness. The key question is how can we deliver quality mental health services in the far greater amount needed with our present limited resources and shortages of personnel. If the public health estimate of "one in ten" persons needing psychiatric care is anywhere near accurate, we still have nearly 80 percent of the job left undone.

And so it would seem that there must come yet a third revolution in psychiatry, namely, new methods for the delivery of mental health care through automation, the use of the computer.

Since 1967 this has been a major preoccupation of the Missouri Division of Mental Health and the computer section of the Missouri Institute of Psychiatry. We have teams of professionals working as systems analysts for their own specialties—the social workers, for example, boiling down the usual social-work history to a two-page checklist; the psychologists, reducing the traditional four-hour battery to three simple tests that can be administered by a technician and scored and interpreted by the computer; psychiatrists, using a checklist mental status form that takes only three minutes to administer and the interpretation of which, by the computer, includes a diagnosis that correlates 60 percent with the traditional psychiatric case workup.

The hub of our network is a 360/50 IBM computer located in St. Louis and connected with out-state institutions by a network of terminals. In Missouri last year we handled the charts on thirty-six thousand patients. While our budget and the number of personnel available to us have reached a plateau, the work load is increasing about 10 percent a year. It is our belief therefore that total automation is the only way to solve this growing problem. As citizens interested in mental health, we can only applaud such a solution; as researchers we also see other benefits. The Missouri Standard System of Psychiatry (SSOP), will make available data not only for management control but also for research studies of treatment method, drug administration, and patient statistics on a size of patient sample never before possible. It is our hope and belief that this approach will clarify the semantics of psychiatry, promote a more scientific therapeutic approach, and make possible research that will help in solving some of the problems in the area of brain function that have been presented during the past few days by members of this panel.

So we hope that as a by-product of this system of psychiatry, we will gain a tremendous amount of information upon our patients, and perhaps this will contribute to the knowledge of cerebral function. So in a roundabout way, we came back to our our annual cerebral function symposium, and for this roundup session, I think I shall introduce the participants one at a time, alphabetically, and they may again follow this little format to tell who they are, what they are doing, something about their research, and how it fits into the overall picture.

First is Dr. Martin Adler, who is Associate Professor of Pharmacology in the Department of Pharmacology at Temple University.

Dr. Martin Adler: My particular interest in the field of neuropharmacology or psychopharmacology is focused primarily on the recovery of function following brain damage and the variables which affect such function following maximal recovery. As a pharmacologist, I have a special interest in the qualitative and quantitative responses to drugs in brain-damaged subjects.

The plasticity of the brain in the sense of compensatory mechanisms is truly remarkable and the recovery of function following injury to the brain is but one facet of such mechanisms. Yet, in the very process of compensation and even after compensation is complete, measurable changes have occurred. These changes may be of a subtle nature and measurable only by a battery of psychological tests or may be more gross, as in body tilt or alteration of gait. There are also probably changes which have not received much attention, such as altered responsiveness to centrally acting drugs. All people use drugs during their lives, and the brain-damaged individual is no exception. An altered level of neuronal activity is a frequent result of brain damage and may be seen at the time of insult, during the period of recovery, and even after maximal recovery is complete. With altered neuronal activity, one should not be surprised to see altered drug response. This might be of a magnitude so small that it is of academic interest only. On the other hand, clinically significant differences could result. As a case in point, our studies in animals have demonstrated that damage to certain sensory areas of the brain or damage to certain parts of the limbic system result in altered seizure thresholds to certain chemical agents, and such alterations vary both quantitatively and qualitatively as a function of time following the injury. In addition, the response to antiepileptics and certain other drugs also changes.

This leads me to speculate on certain aspects of the future of neuro-pharmacology and psychopharmacology. First, I see not only a continuation but an acceleration of a trend towards the absolutely essential practice of determining drug dosage on the basis of the individual, rather than an adherence to the traditional "usual" doses. This means a greater emphasis on dose-response relationships. Second, I foresee a period of greater research into the multitude of physiological and biochemical factors that affect drug response. Third, and perhaps most important, I believe that there will be an ever-increasing attempt at understanding the interactions between environmental factors, such as multiple sensory input and pathological conditions of the brain in regard to effective and optimal drug therapy.

Dr. Ulett: Very good, Dr. Adler, and thank you. Number two is Dr. Joseph Bogen. Dr. Bogen is the senior neurosurgeon of the Ross-Loos Medical Group in Los Angeles.

Dr. Bogen: Well, it comes as a surprise to me that I am supposed to tell what I do and why. I do neurosurgery. The reason that I work for the Ross-Loos Group, and I want to mention their name again, is that they allow me time for research. Ross-Loos was the first prepaid medical group in America, and the people who organized it in 1929 fought the establishment to stay in business. Now they are helping the establishment because they pioneered not only prepaid medical care but also arbitration agreements (in lieu of malpractice suits), which are now looked upon as one of the possible sources of saving the private practice of medicine.

I decided on neurosurgery when I was in medical school. I met Ron Myers (of the Myers and Sperry split-brain experiment) at Cal Tech, and we both agreed we wanted to go into neurology or neurosurgery because there were some investigations that just could not be done except with people. And it has actually turned out that way: What I have done for ten years now is spent most of my time, from an experimental point of view, either with the split-brain or hemispherectomy. This necessarily makes me what you might call an epileptologist, because these people are being treated for their benefit and usually the indication for the surgery is some form of epilepsy. I have become, in the course of this, a sort of amateur neuropsychologist and amateur electroencephalographer.

I am also becoming more and more an amateur evangelist because I have been crusading for a theory. I will mention that of the five or six people who presently subscribe to this theory, two are sociologists who just received a grant to find out if right and left in politics is indeed related to right and left in the head. At any rate, there is hope for this hypothesis, which I call "Neowiganism," and I would like to go over it with you now.

The essentials of this theory and its implications were first developed by A. L. Wigan in a book called *The Duality of the Mind* published in 1844. Wigan was first led to his theory by the postmortem observation of a man whom he had known well before the man's sudden death from unrelated causes. At autopsy, one cerebral hemisphere was found to be totally absent. Wigan was not only astounded by this finding, but had the wits to see its meaning: Only one hemisphere is required to have a mind or to be a person. Evidently then, the cerebrum is present in duplicate as are the kidneys or the lungs; the brain is not a single organ of two halves, but actually a closely apposed pair. Therefore, Wigan concluded that if only one cerebrum is required to have a mind, possession of two hemispheres (the normal state) makes possible or perhaps even inevitable the possession of two minds; and however synchronous these two minds may be most of the time, there must inevitably be some occasion when they are discrepant. This provides an anatomicophysiologic basis for that division of self, that internal struggle which is characteristic of so much of mankind's ill health and unhappiness. This magnificent speculation was accorded very little notice at the time.

In the past few years the duality of the mind has become a much more appealing view because of the remarkable accumulation of evidence supporting it. We now know that the fundamental fact adduced by Wigan was correct. Indeed it is hardly arguable; there is now an overwhelming abundance of evidence from both experimental and clinical hemispherectomy to support his observation. His conclusion that possession of two hemispheres means a capacity for two minds is not only rational but, however opposed it may be to common sense, it is now experimentally proven by the split-brain studies. The only way to avoid this conclusion is to start arguing about what Mind is, and that is the way out usually taken by people who find this conclusion unacceptable. My own opinion is that the results of the split-brain experiments have converted Wigan's conclusion from speculation to a repeatedly demonstrable fact.

What Wigan did not know, as it was not recognized by neurologists until the 1860's, is that speaking, reading, and writing are largely the function of but one hemisphere, the left one in the majority of persons. The past few years have seen the appearance of a great wealth of evidence for the theory that when the left hemisphere is dominant with respect to what Jackson called "propositional" function, the other hemisphere is dominant for a variety of capacities which can for convenience be subsumed under the term "appositional." Whereas the two hemispheres of a cat or monkey may sustain the existence of two duplicate minds, the lateralization typical of man requires that the two minds must necessarily be discrepant. "Neowiganism" means that each of us is possessed of two minds which differ in content, possibly even in goals, but most certainly in respect to mode of organization.*

The evolutionary advantage of having two different minds is obvious; possession of two independent problem-solving organs increases mightily the likelihood of a creative solution to a novel problem. At the same time there is an enormous increase in the likelihood of internal conflict. And so we have man, the most innovative of species and, at the same time the most at odds with himself.

This neuropsychological theory can be extended to afford a neurosociologic interpretation of cultural differences. For example, along with the aforementioned sociologists, I have come to believe that any cultural pattern represents a mix in various proportions of right and left hemispheric values. Investigations suggested by this approach are presently concerned with the demonstration that certain aptitudes or interests assignable to either hemisphere can be correlated with various demographic data. The theory predicts, in part, that individuals of the majority culture (M) will tend to favor verbal, logical, sequential, and analytic methods to solve problems, whereas members of the minority culture (m) will rely more on nonverbal, metaphoric, simultaneous (gestalt), and intuitive approaches. The usefulness of this approach will be judged principally on the extent to which significant differences are found between (M) and (m) and on questions chosen on the basis of neurologic findings regarding hemispheric specialization, which is why we call it "neurosociology."

With respect to the future of neuropsychopharmacology, we may note that if the two brains are different, drugs may act differently upon each of them. This must be considered, therefore, in all applications of drugs to humans with two brains. With respect to humans who have only one brain (following hemispherectomy), the effect of drugs on those who retain the left as compared with those who retain the right could be just as interesting as the psychological testing of these two groups. Presumably, infantile hemiplegics will show less pharmacologic difference than the tumor patients just as the infantile hemiplegics show less psychological differences.

In conclusion I should like to state again the facts, and outline what seems to me the really big question remaining. First of all, it takes only one hemisphere to have a mind. Secondly, possession of two hemispheres can clearly sustain the activity of two separate spheres of consciousness following commissurotomy. What remains in doubt is the question: Does splitting

---

*See Bogen, J. E.: The other side of the brain. II: An appositional mind. *Bull Los Angeles Neurol Soc, 34:*135-162, 1969.

the brain surgically create a duality of consciousness or duality of mind, or is it merely an experimental maneuver that makes it possible to demonstrate a duality that was previously present? You have this in every experiment; that is, it can be argued that the result or outcome is produced by the technique, rather than actually revealing the underlying physiology. For example, in an experiment to measure blood pressure one could ask: Is the blood pressure high because it was high before, or did you raise the blood pressure when you stuck a needle in the artery? I believe the duality was present before and that the commissural section does not create duality of mind, but merely makes it possible for us to demonstrate it. If the latter interpretation is correct, we can understand why ordinary self-consciousness is insufficient for the whole man, and why the full realization of human potential requires that each of us be devoted to a better understanding of our other selves.

Dr. Ulett: Thank you. Doctor Keith Conners is Director of the Child Development Laboratory at the MGH and is Associate Professor of the Department of Psychology at Harvard Medical School.

Dr. Conners: My interests have been in the biological bases of learning and behavioral development in children. I was fortunate in my early work to become associated with the unique tools provided for such questions by the applications of psychopharmacologic intervention through my collaboration with the studies of Dr. Leon Eisenberg. The earlier work convinces us that the various psychotropic drugs not only had a profound impact on the behavior and life style of children and their families, but also on their ability to learn.

However, although one can demonstrate that drugs change behavior and learning in groups of children, the individual variation in the group is always more impressive than the group effects. Obviously, a diagnostic difference, as between neurotic and hyperkinetic children, makes a considerable difference on the results of drug treatment, but this diagnostic classification is at the most a superficial typology based on manifest symptomatology and tells us nothing about underlying variations in the state of the CNS or the etiology of the disorders. Moreover, within a diagnostic category one still finds that there are very large individual differences in response to treatment.

One method of approach to such issues is the development of methods of assessment at a nonsymptomatic level that give promise of isolating basic dimensions, such as physiological parameters, birth history, and developmental deviations. One approach that we have found promising is the analysis of bioelectric activity as measured by cortical evoked potentials. These appear to discriminate between different categories of children and to show interesting, if somewhat complex, response to drugs. We plan particularly to pursue the lateral assymetries in evoked potential response as these are related to clinical symptoms and type of learning disorders, since the degree and type of lateralization may eventually shed light on important CNS developmental trends.

What I have presented in my paper is largely concerned with the attempt to use behavioral profiles, based on psychological tests, and parent and teacher ratings of behavior, to establish homogeneous subtypes of children. It seems to me that diagnostic heterogeneity is the major stumbling block to progress in the understanding of drug effects and CNS dysfunction in children. The one method we have tried is an empirical clustering technique, but other statistical models are available and should be tried.

The findings clearly indicate that heretofore nonsignificant drug effects are revealed in certain groups. They also indicate that the groups are different in at least one physiological dimension (evoked response amplitudes, and lateral assymetries) not used in the classification procedure, thus to some extent providing an external validation of the clustering procedure. Much work remains to be done in isolating other physiological differentiae for the groups defined by this method and other methods before we can arrive at a clear specification of the etiology for the different groups. On clinical grounds we are convinced that there are significant biological differences among the group of children loosely labeled as "minimal brain dysfunction" disorders. Both the pharmacologic and evoked potential measures may help to provide some operational definition at a *direct* level of brain dysfunction, rather than relying on behavioral inferences about underlying CNS pathology.

Dr. Ulett: Thank you, Dr. Conners. Doctor Walter Essman is Professor of Psychology and Biochemistry. I am not quite sure how these fields mix, but they do mix very well in Doctor Essman, Department of Psychology at Queens College, City University of New York.

Dr. Essman: Thank you. In trying to survey all the various aspects of psychopharmacology and the question of cerebral function, I seem to suffer from an identity crisis. I just cannot seem to find one label that I can adequately pin on myself and find that it describes either what I do or where my interests lie. Unfortunately, most of the labeling that is done in this field seems to be done on the basis of methology. If one does one's experiments in a test tube, one becomes a biochemist; if one scores psychological tests, one may be a psychologist, or if one prescribes in a clinical situation a psychoactive drug, chances are he may be a psychiatrist. I think more and more, these labels, that seem to be more in accord with methodology than with actual interest or practice, may be breaking down and I do not know how or in what direction; I really thought I would make some observations that relate to my own work, as far as the possible future of this field is concerned and in so doing bring in some of my own interests.

Specifically, I think I can best describe my own interests as being related to the question of brain function, and I think this interest spans everything from the brain as a whole functioning organ to regional cellular, subcellular, and molecular levels of functioning that go on occasionally, and probably much more than we care to attend to in the case of drug effects.

With respect to some of these comments I jotted down on drug effects and possible issues that might bear some further consideration, one thing that has occurred to me—and it is certainly not an original thought with me; I have seen this written about; I have heard it discussed—is the question of the interaction of drugs with endogenous substrates, specifically in the central nervous system, but not necessarily so. In other words, what I mean here is that we have heard from what Dr. Kety has said that there are a variety of agents that, among other things, change the level and turnover of many of the biogenicamines, but specifically, as he mentioned; of norepinephrine. The possible interaction of a drug with substrates, that might possibly hold some role as mediators of transmission or mediators of excitatory or inhibitory functions in the brain, seems a very relevant consideration that we might attend to. More specifically, we might consider substrate interactions in the brain. That is, interactions that may, for example, be initiated by a drug or drug metabolite, and this has come to light in one respect in some of our work, with respect to the interaction of one biogenicamines means, serotonin, 5'-hydroxytryptamine and ribonucleic acid. Doctor Bittman will have much more to say on the physical side of this interaction, but generally, what we have observed is that there is an inverse relationship between this specific biogenicamine and this nucleic acid that occurs when agents causing the release of serotonin in the brain are administered, and more generally, where electroconvulsive shock over an acute period is administered, this same relationship holds. It seems to predominate, by the way, in the hypothalamus and structures that make up the limbic system. The change in amine level that we have just mentioned carries with it a whole series of consequences that have, I think, important behavioral, biochemical, and pharmacological considerations that go along with them, such as their ability to reduce the synthesis of proteins, specifically the synthesis of proteins at the nerve ending, to reduce the level of total protein in several areas of the brain, and to initiate ionic changes at various cellular and subcellular sites within the nervous system. I think these changes raise questions as to drug metabolism and what will, for example, drug metabolism may hold if we know that there are electrolyte changes which such drugs themselves impose. For example, what do we really know about the metabolism of drugs as imposed on altered electrolyte conditions in the central nervous system. We know very little about this area.

There is also the question of tissue binding, and this is an issue that I think is an old one, particularly in the case of phenothiazines and the relationship between dosage, onset of effect, duration of effect, and the biochemical changes that attend such conditions.

Finally, I might just give some attention to the issue of the associative phenomena as produced at a cellular or molecular level with drugs that have some behavioral effect. We know that a variety of cholinergic drugs and several of the barbiturates are capable of producing what behaviorally, as well as neuropharmacologically, may be defined as dissociated, or dissociative behavior, that is an altered state wherein the stimulus conditions that prevail are quite different from those that prevail during the nondrug or postdrug state. It would be extremely interesting to have some further information about what sort of changes go on at a cellular level and how other drugs, and particularly not those typically categorized within the psychoactive pharmacopeia, produce changes of this sort and what these may mean, both behaviorally at a basic level and more generally, behavior at a therapeutic level.

Dr. Ulett: Walter, thank you. Dr. Turan Itil is Professor and Associate Chairman (Research) University of Missouri School of Medicine, Missouri Institute of Psychiatry in St. Louis.

Dr. Itil: In spite of tremendous advances made in biological psychiatric research, only a few of those methods are utilized in the field of psychopharmacology. Clinical pharmacology and biochemistry are being used in psychopharmacology, but basically to detect and/or prevent side effects or other undesirable psychotropic drug reactions. These methods have not been successful in either predicting the clinical efficacy of drugs or classifying the patient population in order to establish profiles for the most effective drug treatment for particular patients.

While investigating the pain phenomenon, we observed that some antihistaminic drugs (promethazine) and novocaine had a distinct therapeutic effect on pain syndromes of primarily thalamic and hypothalamic origin (Bente and Itil, 1953). In searching for objective parameters to establish the type of central effect of these compounds in man, we concluded that electroencephalography (EEG) was the best available method. As known, Berger, who developed the EEG, described in detail its use in the differentiation of drugs with central inhibitory and excitatory effects. However, knowing that the bioelectrical activity as recorded from the scalp with conventional recording techniques represents only a very small portion of the total bioelectrical process of the central nervous system (CNS) and that the drug level found in the CNS is only a small portion of the amount administered has made the scientific community cautious concerning the findings and interpretations of drug-induced EEG changes. As a consequence this method has been poorly utilized for determining the central effectiveness of drugs despite the fact that it is still the only simple method of investigating continuous brain function.

Our chlorpromazine study demonstrated that the EEG is indeed an objective method of assessing the mode of action of a psychotropic compound (Bente and Itil, 1954), as evidenced by the fact that despite the many advances in drug research in the last sixteen years, none of our findings published in the first study have required revision. Since that time, we have used the EEG (a) for diagnosis and subclassification of psychiatric disorders (Itil, 1964); (b) for predicting the outcome of treatment (resting EEGs but particularly pentothal-activated EEGs and all-night sleep patterns indicated that therapy-resistant schizophrenic patients have different brain functions than responsive schizophrenics) (Itil, 1964; Itil, unpublished data); and (c) for the classification of psychotropic drugs. It was possible to classify psychotropic drugs using EEG parameters exclusively and this corresponded closely to that based on clinical observation (Itil, 1961; Itil, 1968). In recent years, using different kinds of EEG quantification methods we reaffirmed the usefulness of this method in psychopharmacology as have several investigators such as Fink, Goldstein, Ulett, Pfeiffer, and Sugerman, etc. The technique of "quantitative pharmacoelectroencephalography" (see paper in this book) which we developed in recent years using analog frequency analyzer and digital computer methods of EEG analysis and statistical procedures is probably one of the most recent advances in new psychotropic drug evaluation. Using this method it was possible to correctly predict the type and the effective dosage ranges of three different new compounds.

The study of visual, auditory, and somatosensory evoked responses in psychiatric populations (Shagass, 1964) and psychotropic drug evaluations (Shagass *et al.*, 1968, Saletu *et al.*, 1970) is another objective physiological method which unfortunately has found limited use in psychopharmacology research.

Attempts to evaluate objectively the behavior of psychiatric patients and the development of different types of rating scales have been highly rewarding for psychopharmacology research. In order to study resistant and responsive schizophrenics patients, we developed several rating scales to assess psychopathology (Itil and Keskiner, 1966), behavior in an occupational therapy situation (Kimes *et al.*, 1967), motor behavior (Deibert *et al.*, 1966, see

Itil, 1969), psychosomatic changes (Itil and Keskiner, 1966), and physical and laboratory alterations (Holden *et al.*, 1968). Based on these relatively objective behavioral assessments, it is possible to correlate physiological data and behavior. The methodology of the clinical psychiatrist has undoubtedly been influenced by the techniques used in psychopharmacology. Drug research today should be free from subjectivity as much as possible and should be based on objective methods available for psychiatric and physiological evaluation of patients.

Dr. Ulett: Thank you, Dr. Itil. Now we will hear from Dr. Marvin Jaffe, Neurologist at the Stroke Research Center, Philadelphia General Hospital, and Instructor in Neurology, Jefferson Medical College.

Dr. Jaffe: During my talk on Wednesday, I reviewed the methods of cerebral blood flow now in general use and possible applications. As you recognize, these methods are very rigorous, uncomfortable, and carry the morbidity attendant to carotid puncture.

New approaches, which will be promising, include the development of an inhalation technique, using radioactive Xenon and more sophisticated computer analysis to correct for the errors introduced by this method.

The application of the radioactive oxygen method, which will permit simultaneous cerebral blood flow and cerebral metabolism studies, will also open new areas to research in brain physiology.

As I pointed out in my formal presentation, more emphasis must be placed in the correlation of the physiological data, with functional measures, both clinical and psychological, in order to determine if the "trick" which we do, increasing cerebral blood flow, is indeed of value in improving the patient.

Dr. Ulett: Thank you, Dr. Jaffe. Doctor Marcel Kinsbourne is the Associate Professor of Pediatrics and of Neurology and a lecturer in Psychology at Duke University Medical School in Durham, North Carolina.

Dr. Kinsbourne: In my discussion of methodology, I indicated my views as to which are the most difficult aspects of developmental studies. Exacting as may be the problems of schedule for trial of drug or other treatment, and difficult as it may be to select accurately defined and relevant subject groups, these aspects present problems far less serious than does the choice of appropriate behavioral measures. Nonspecific and misleading indices of behavior account for a substantial wastage of human and economic resources in the area of therapy and rehabilitation. On the one hand, experimenters are misled into initiating treatments for real life situations to which they are in fact by no means applicable. On the other hand, they are led to reject potentially effective treatment on the basis of irrelevant and heterogeneous behavioral measures. Significant advances in drug and other therapy are often hampered by the use of inapplicable tests usually of an umbrella type in which significant changes are drawn out by a mass of responses to irrelevant items. It is in the area of psychological assessment that major advances most need to be made, and I would suggest when these have been made, a new psychometry will arise, conceptually rather different from that of the present.

Test validity is the bugbear of psychometry. Does the test measure anything over and above subjects' performance on the particular items it happens to contain? Does it in any sense cast light upon a wider subset of the total spectrum of performances within the human behavioral repertoire? Factor analysis addresses itself to this question. The search is on for tests which are "factor pure." A contaminated measure is progressively refined until a factor pure task crystallizes out.

This approach is basically empirical and, like empirical research in general, unnecessarily circuitous and arduous. It totally ignores the impressive body of knowledge accumulated by experimental psychologists about the range of capabilities of the human organism. Many of the rigorous procedures in the experimental literature seem likely to approximate "factor pure" measures of basic cerebral processes. It is a misconception to suppose that these procedures are necessarily time consuming, or that only young adults majoring in psychology are capable of acting as subjects for the experimental measurement of channel capacity, acquisition of information and of skill and the like. We have been impressed by the reliable and patient performance of old people and of the brain damaged on such procedures, when they are approached in a sympathetic manner and the task is explained clearly and patiently. In principle, a test method, if properly designed, should be applicable to diverse populations. That being the case, there is a distinct advantage in cutting across conventional professional categories and applying the method to diverse populations; an exercise in comparative psychometry.

When performance of a specially selected group deviates from the norm, the question arises, does this deviation characterize the group in some unique fashion or is it nonspecific in that other clinically or developmentally deviant groups would have shown similar deficit? Thus, if old people score poorly on memory task, does this indicate a cognitive weakness specific to that developmental stage, or would many other conditions of impaired cerebral competence yield similar performance? While for some pragmatic purposes it is sufficient to establish the deficit without inquiring into its specificity, the researcher into processes of maturation and of disintegration of the brain must interest himself in partitioning those deficits which are nonspecific from those which uniquely characterize the population under investigation. An appropriate research strategy then is to define multiple deviant populations each of which on overall achievement measure score approximately the same on the cognitive task and then analyze in detail the various operations that contribute to that performance so as in each case to specify that operation which is performance limiting and determine whether what limits performance in one group is the same as what limits performance in another. We therefore anticipate that in the future psychometric measures will consist of simple, definable, and quantitative tasks applicable to a wide range of individuals differing in developmental and cognitive status, so that it will become possible to establish for each individual a profile of his abilities which bears some meaningful relationship to the limited set of operations of which the human brain is capable. Such measures would ultimately give a direct account of the function efficacy of the underlying neural substrate and permit the establishment of brain behavior relationship at a level of precision which is at present rarely achieved.

Dr. Ulett: I want to thank you, Dr. Kinsbourne. Doctor Don Klein is Director of Research at Hillside Hospital in New York.

Dr. Klein: There has been a good deal of talk about a number of my interests already. I am glad to see my interests so widely shared. The outstanding major difficulties that I am having right now are not so much scientific as administrative, and I do wish that we had more administrators like Doctor Ulett.

The point I am trying to make is this—I am interested in trying to refine the heterogeneity of human behavior and the particular subdividing approach that I have used is the psychopharmacological method. My idea is that if you expose a lot of people with all sorts of peculiarities of thinking, feeling, behaving, etc., to a medication and you get a wide variety of responses, that it is a good simple-minded beginning to think that the people that are showing similar drug response patterns may have something similar wrong with them; that is there is a basic underlying psychopathophysiology that is causing them to respond similarly to this drug.

Now, it follows that we have to do a number of things, that as I think came out in my talk today, are not too simple. You have to be able to describe exactly, objectively, and reliably things like patterns of psychopathology. You also have to be able to describe, and this is a much more difficult problem, patterns of change, that is not only patterns of psychopathology but changes in the pattern over time—but I think that can be licked. But then what you need is rather large numbers of subjects who can be treated and studied in a uniform way, and that gets to be very difficult. A previous speaker was saying there was a difference between the patients who respond well to medication and the patients that do not. Well that is exactly the sort of thing I am interested in. If you are working with chronic schizophrenics, there are a fairly ample supply of chronic schizophrenics around, except that to try to find a chronic schizophrenic who has not received fourteen treatments before and who is not actually a chronic residual drug-fast schizophrenic is no simple matter.

The particular study I did involved some 350 patients assigned randomly to imipramine, chlorpromazine, and placebo. I think it is probably one of the largest single drug studies performed in one hospital. I had also the tremendous fortunate opportiunity to be able to have studied all these patients during the entire course of their experimental treatment. Now, that is unusual, and I do not say it in any tribute to me and my personal endeavors as much as to the administrative setup at Hillside Hospital that would allow me to do such a thing, because most hospitals will not allow that much of an "interference" with the sacrosanct treatment process as Hillside allowed and supported.

For instance, when the NIMH want to study the effects of phenothiazines in relatively acute schizophrenics they could not do it at any single hospital; they had to do it in nine hospitals and they had to develop methods for systematically assessing the patients in all the different hospitals and then by computerized techniques melding the results and getting comparisons. Now, the people at NIMH deserve the most enormous amount of credit for having launched and carried out this tremendous program which, nonetheless, actually finished up with only a few more than a couple of hundred patients in it, and as they will readily admit, an enormous amount of measurement error because the studies were being carried out under such different circumstances, by such different people, with such different degrees of training, etc.

My point is that to try to subdivide people by treating them and then studying the various patterns of treatment response, requires numbers upwards of several hundreds. If, as I believe, I can discern at least fourteen different change patterns in response to the major psychotropic agents and then I want to be able to compare the initial characteristics of the people in the various change patterns reliably, I need very big numbers.

Now, how am I going to get several hundred patients that I can treat uniformly, over long enough period of time, to do these systematic investigations? The answer is, I cannot—under the present organization of psychopharmacological research in the United States, which consists of a number of small centers where the research is essentially an appendage of the service and treatment responsibility of the hospital. We have gotten to the point where we know the drug works; we are now trying to find the right drug for the right person. However, we are having tremendous difficulty getting the differential indications for drugs because we need much larger samples, studied in one place, by uniform methods.

What this calls for is quite a different administrative structure. That is, what the country needs, what science needs, what psychopharmacology needs to make further progress in this area is to set up mission-oriented research hospitals. That is, for instance, let us say you had a situation where you had a two hundred-bed hospital, which was devoted to the study of acute schizophrenia, and it was set up and known as the research hospital for acute schizophrenia. Patients would come there on a voluntary basis; by the way there is no lack of voluntary acute schizophrenics, they do not have to be committed. The patient would understand that by coming in to that hospital they would be entered into a research program, where the attempt would be made to find out whether one or another medication was particularly valuable to them. Then after the study was completed, which would probably be a matter of a couple of months in most studies of this sort, if they had not gotten better they would receive the best sort of treatment that we have available and be entered permanently on the follow-up after care clinic of this facility. That would be their reward for offering themselves as research subjects in this fashion; they would be paid in the form of continuing high level care.

Now, this would enable us to answer many questions, about which we do not have the foggiest notions. For instance, we have been working with Thorazine® now for almost twenty years. We still do not know when or if you should stop the medication. If you have treated an acute schizophrenic and he is out of his episode, should you stop the medication? Nobody knows; nobody has ever done the study. Dave Engelhart and his group have come close to it in some of their studies on chronic schizophrenics, but for acute schizophrenia it is still a complete mystery.

We have no studies on the prophylaxis of acute schizophrenia. We do not have any long-term longitudinal intensive studies. What I am saying for acute schizophrenia applies in spades for the affective disorders and triple spades for the character disorders and neuroses.

It would be a moderately expensive undertaking, but I think the costs-benefit ratio would be considerably higher than that of the present support of bits and pieces programs and projects, giving only limited answers. This is not because of lack of ingenuity on the part of the scientists. If anything, the scientists have remarkable ingenuity considering the administrative limitations under which they work. But if you had a two hundred-bed research hospital with an average four-month length of stay—enough time, I think, to study most schizophrenics pretty thoroughly, treat them in a uniform fashion, get them on their feet, out and follow them, in two years you would have studied one thousand two hundred patients in a uniform fashion. That two years would be a well-spent two years. Unfortunately, we just do not have the setup for it, and unless the federal government does a 180 degree turn and takes off like a rocket we are not going to have that sort of a setup for quite a while. Of course my utopian wish is that we had several such facilities for every major psychiatric syndrome, that is, acute schizophrenia, chronic schizophrenia, mania, depression, drug abuse, retardation, alcoholism, geriatrics, etc.

Dr. Ulett: Thank you, Don. Doctor Aaron Smith is Director of the Neuropsychological Laboratory, Department of Physical Medicine and Rehabilitation, University of Michigan Medical School in Ann Arbor. Doctor Smith.

Dr. Aaron Smith: Please note that my following remarks have been developed in collaboration with Dr. Jonathan E. Walker. Long ago, even before there were tranquilizers, a remarkable English neurophysiologist observed: "We should think it a very misleading research if a pharmacologist were to set himself to determine the mode of action of a drug on the human economy before he ascertained whether the animal on which he proposed to experiment exhibited symptoms of being similarly affected by the drug as man himself." (Ferrier, 1878, p. 20).[11]

Although I am a neuropsychologist-come-lately on the drug research scene (Walker, Albers, Tourtellotte, Henderson, Potvin, and Smith),[12] this first experience, a double-blind study of effects of amantadine on higher and lower level cerebral functions in patients with Parkinson's disease gave me some appreciation of the persisting complex problems in neuropsychopharmacological research suggested by Ferrier almost a century ago.

The problems of physiological matching, including determinations of interspecies and intraspecies variations in the relevant biochemistry of experimental animals are especially important for definitions of toxicity as well as for assessments of the efficacy of drugs prescribed to alleviate disorders of specific physiologic systems in man. The importance of animal experimentation for correlations of changes in brain chemistry and behavior is obvious. The development of techniques for isolation of viable neurons and identification of neurotransmitters offer fertile new approaches to the animal neuropharmacologist.[13]

For various reasons, behavioral effects of drugs in humans have been more difficult to define. One reason is a tendency to design the experiments in terms of gross psychiatric dimensions rather than quantifiable behavioral outputs. Another is the tendency of humans to try to please the investigator, and basic (animal) scientists have justly criticized many studies on this basis. Another problem is the difficulty encountered in obtaining normal adult volunteers for drug studies, hence the tendency to use addicts, criminals, and terminally ill patients.

However, we should like here to urge the use of humans in carefully designed neuropsychopharmacological investigations. First, the results are immediately applicable to man. Predictions of behavioral effects in man from animal experimentation are notoriously unreliable, and usually rest on complicated training schedules and restricted behavioral outputs. Man is the most intelligent animal, and after a simple set of instructions can perform an enormous number of tasks involving many different types of behavior in a short period of time. Use of a double-blind crossover technique minimizes experimenter bias and the natural desire of experimenters to observe and report positive findings. Evaluation of drugs in humans can be more rapid, comprehensive, predictive, and reproducible than animal experimentation. Animals, of course, cannot report how drugs make them feel. In the final analysis, such studies are often less expensive.

The value of a large battery of quantitated behavioral tests is obviously of critical importance in determining central nervous system effects in man. For example, the drug amantadine seems to exert a quite selective beneficial effect in Parkinsonism on those tests which measure coordination and gait, with no marked effect on vision, strength, speed of movement, reaction time, sensation, or cognitive functions.

Although animal experiments may indicate toxicity levels, they are obviously unsuitable for assessing designed (or possibly unexpected) side effects of various drugs on human language, and the "higher" verbal and nonverbal reasoning capacities. Ultimately, the effect of any drug on higher and lower level cerebral functions is eventually determined by the results of repeated trials in man. The validity and sensitivity of measures of sensory, motor, mental, and language functions are therefore of critical importance in assessment of effects of drugs.

The development of a standardized battery of objective tests of motor, sensory, and other neurologic functions that are variously assessed in clinical neurological examinations (Tourtellotte *et al.*, 1965),[14] and specially selected test batteries (designed to differentiate effects of brain insults on the sensory and motor modalities involved in standardized psychological tests, from effects on the higher mental functions the tests are designed to measure) of neuropsychological functions are therefore of special value in studies of effects of various drugs on cerebral functions.

In instances where changes in specific higher or lower level cerebral functions have been clearly demonstrated, the "mode of action" and the specific or general nature of effects of the drug are of obvious theoretical and practical importance. Just as in effects of brain lesions or hemispherectomy, the nature of the underlying processes producing specific or general changes in cerebral functions may be inhibitory or facilitatory. In reviewing previous studies of effects of drugs on motor symptoms and mental functions, the different ranges (general versus specific) and modes (inhibitory versus facilitatory) of action are suggested in studies of Parkinsonism.

A study of effects on higher functions of different medications reportedly relieving the symptoms of Parkinsonism, reported poorer performances by the medicated patients than controls. Although Talland[15] reported the evidence was not conclusive, he attributed the reduced mental capacities of the treated group to conventional medications used. The diminution of tremors and general symptoms in Parkinson patients and concurrently reduced "higher" functions thus suggests that the "mode of action" of the medications was a slight general inhibitory effect, resulting in reductions of a wide range of cerebral functions.

Conversely, other studies using L-dopa have reported marked reductions of Parkinsonism symptoms associated with significant improvement in tests of verbal and nonverbal higher functions in most patients,[16-19] and a relatively high proportion with severe emotional disorders.[10-12] The severe emotional disorders tended to subside when L-dopa dosages were reduced. A general facilitatory effect on these types of behavior seems indicated by these findings.

The double-blind study of amantadine revealed a significant but seemingly less marked reduction in Parkinsonism symptoms, than that reported in studies of L-dopa, with significant improvement in only those neuropsychological tests involving manual dexterity and visuomotor coordination. Although the absence of changes in other mental tests indicates more selective effects of amantadine than L-dopa or earlier conventional medication, the appearance of hallucinations in high dosages suggest the mode of action of amantadine may also be facilitatory.

The above suggested interpretations of the findings in a selected sample of studies of effects of different medications on higher and lower functions of patients with parkinsonism may be gratuitous. Albeit, they also suggest that detailed standardized tests of neurological functions such as the CQNE and specially designed neuropsychological test batteries can provide comprehensive and objective measures of higher and lower level cerebral functions for determining the efficacy and the nature of side effects of pharmacologic agents.

Dr. Ulett: Thank you, Aaron. That brings us finally to Dr. Lynn Smith, our host and the gentleman whom we must thank for a very interesting and productive session out here in this fine part of the world. Lynn.

Dr. Lynn Smith: Before I talk about my own particular interests and goals

I would like to make one comment as the symposium's chairman and that is my hope that the symposium may, in the future, be able to bring to you more *process* studies. Perhaps the underlying processes are implicit in some of the studies presented at this year's meeting and last, but I would like to see more explicit elaborations on drug action. For example, how about a drug to regulate a patient's level of narcissism? I think real progress will have been made when we can provide a compound that will enable the depressed person to participate in the "goodies" within his milieu, thereby actively lifting his self-esteem, or wounded narcissism, enabling the patient himself to deal effectively with his depressed condition. On the other end of the continuum is the narcissitic person, who, although not in pain psychologically, could benefit from a preparation to make the great love affair with self less satisfying in order to make for an increased awareness of others which would lead to more accurate interpersonal reality perceptions. Perhaps more clearly an illustration of underlying process treatment is seen in the various drugs which facilitate learning as they appear to integrate an underlying process of irregular discharge expressed in shifting attention. The phenothiazines are thought by some to provide an integration process to the various ego functions whereby the schizophrenic is able to gradually work out of his psychotic solution for a more realistic one.

During last year's meeting I was compelled to present some of my research in the learning facilitator and vasodilator drugs in order to complete these respective sections.[23] I am continuing to research these areas and would like to relate some of my further observations. First, in my studies of ethosuximide (Zarontin®) on children with learning problems and 14-6 cps positive spike EEG's, I have concentrated on some 125 consecutive cases in an age group between seven and fifteen years of age, and am curious whether there may emerge an actual neuropsychological expression in the intelligence scales (Wechsler) of these children with learning problems, 14-6 cps EEG's, and high incidence of accompanying autonomic dysfunction as headache and/or stomach ache. The pattern seen in this group is a very low verbal to high performance scale IQ (10 to 45 pts differential), with high subtest scores in Comprehension, Similarities, and Object Assembly but with low subtest scores in Information and Digit Symbol. This particular pattern may be a more global reflection of the spike pattern *per se,* however, as it is seen to some extent in the other various related EEG nomenclatures involving spiking. The controls for comparison are extremely difficult to come by in order to validate this suggested neuropsychological expression as children with learning problems are not encouraged by their schools to get EEG's and of course those without learning problems who may have 14-6 cps EEG's are an even more elusive group to come by. At any rate, this suggested neuropsychological profile is different from any of the clinical entities outlined by Wechsler, *i.e.* organic, obsessive, hysteric, schizophrenic, psychopath, etc. Similar to Doctor Metcalf's ontogenic observation of the 14-6 cps group (see Metcalf and Jordan) , we have noticed this neuropsychological expression tends to emerge and disappear before and after onset of puberty.

I had the pleasure of presenting a paper on the effects of vasodilators at a symposium on the "Assessment of Cerebral Vascular Insufficiency" at the Würzburg University Medical School in Germany last March.[25] At this meeting I was very impressed with the work of the British geriatricians, neurosurgeons, and psychologists, especially their ability to work out programmed procedures for handling their psychological test data. Later, while lecturing at the University of Leeds in England I discovered one English psychologist's fascinating psychological test approach to studying the elderly. I could give you some concrete illustrations of the test items, but to save time, let me say that they are unique in that they get well into the patient's framework and what is important and meaningful to the patient then becomes the basis for the test items for assessing patient's reception, storage, and recall. I mention this one example of meaningful testing items because these test items are absolutely basic to valid assessment of drug efficacy. Psychologists in the States, I am afraid, continue to employ far too many minor tests in their research without recognizing or developing these few major subtests so crucially important to assessing changes.

As this panel draws to a close, and most of this year's program for that matter, I want to take this opportunity to thank all the panelists, and Dr. Ulett who helped organize and served as panel moderator, for their timely and informative papers and comments. Also, my appreciation to those in the audience who participated in these stimulating discussions. My one regret is that because of mechanical failure we were unable to preserve the entire second part of this discussion which contained good controversy. But again, thanks for a most stimulating and meaningful symposium.

Dr. Ulett: I want to underscore Dr. Lynn Smith's last comments and add to "stimulating and meaningful" a most successful meeting, and a highly informative and interdisciplinary exchange.

REFERENCES

1. Bente, D., and Itil, T. M.: Periphere Anäathesie und Schmerzgeschehen. *Acta Neuroveg, 7:*258-262, 1953.
2. Bente, D., and Itil, T. M.: Zur Wirkung des Phenothiazin körpers Megaphen auf das menschliche Hirnstrombild. *Arzneimittel—Forschung, 4:*418-423, 1954.
3. Itil, T. M.: Elektroencephalographische Studien Bei Psychosen und Psychotropen Medikamenten. *Ahmet Sait Matbaasi,* Istanbul, 1964.
4. Shagass, C., and Schwartz, M.: Evoked potential studies in psychiatric patients. *Ann NY Acad Sci, 112:*526-542, 1964.

5. Shagass, C.: Pharmacology of evoked potentials in man. In Efron, D. H. *et al.* (Eds.) : *Psychopharmacology: A Review of Progress 1957-1967*. Washington, D. C., U. S. Government Printing Office, 1968.

6. Saletu, B., Saletu, M., Itil, T. M., and Jones, J.: Somatosensory evoked potential changes during thiothixene treatment in schizophrenic patients. Prepared for The American EEG Society Meeting in Washington, D. C., September 17-19, 1970.

7. Itil, T., and Keskiner, A.: Psychopathological and Psychosomatic Rating Scales, Psychiatric Research Foundation of Missouri. Publication no. 12, 1966.

8. Kimes, M., Holden, J. M. C., Keskiner, A., and Itil, T. M.: Occupational Therapy Rating Scale, Psychiatric Research Foundation of Missouri, Publication no. 11, 1967.

9. Itil, T. M.: Quantitative analysis of "motor pattern" in schizophrenia. In Sankar, D. V. (Ed.) : *Schizophrenia, Current Concepts and Research*. 1969, pp. 210-219.

10. Holden, J. M. C., and Itil, T. M.: The application of automated techniques in assessing psychotropic drug-induced side effects. *Amer J Psychiat, 125:*154-161, 1968.

11. Ferrier, D., *The Localization of Cerebral Disease*. London, Smith, Elder and Co., 1878.

12. Walker, J. E., Albers, J. W., Tourtellotte, W. W., Henderson, W. G., Potvin, A. R., and Smith, A.: *A Quantitative Evaluation of Amantadine in the Treatment of Parkinson's Disease*. (In press) .

13. Efron, D. H.: *Psychopharmacology: A Review of Progress 1957-1967*. U. S. Government Printing Office Publication no. 1836, 1968.

14. Tourtellotte, W. W., Haerer, A. F., Simpson, J. F., Kuzma, J. W., and Sikorski, J.: Quantitative Clinical Neurological Testing. *New York Acad Sci, 122:*480-505, 1965.

15. Talland, G. A.: Cognitive Function in Parkinson's Disease. *J Nerv Ment Dis, 135:* 196-205, 1962.

16. Boshes, B., and Arbit, J.: A controlled study of the effect of L-dopa upon selected cognitive and behavioral functions. *Trans Am Neurol Ass, 1970* (to be published) .

17. Blonsky, R. E.: Second Annual Symposium, The United Parkinson Foundation, Chicago, 1969, pp. 10-19.

18. Beardsley, J. V., and Puletti, F.: Personality (MMPI) and cognitive (WAIS) changes by Parkinson's patients after L-dopa treatment. *Pro Midwestern Psychol Ass*, April 29, 1970.

19. Meier, M. J., and Martin, W. E.: Measurement of behavioral changes in patients on L-dopa. *Lancet, i:*352, 1970.

Author Index

Subject Index

A

Abbott Laboratories, xv, 237

Acalculia, 192

Acetylcholine
  as chemical transmitter, 305
  behavioral state alterations through use of ACH, 291
  bound, 306, 307
  endogenous ACH, 314
  free, 307
  "hot" pool, 314
  in brain (ACH), 299, 305
    concentration, 284
    changes in levels after ECS, 282, 283
    in cytoplasm of cell bodies and axons, 306
    in mitochondria, 306, 312
    influence of barbituates, 308
    labile bound, 307, 313
    nicotine treatment effect, 284
    radioactive, 310, 312-14
      relationship of ACH turnover, 309
      resistance to cholinesterases, 305
      stable-bound, 307, 315
    subcellular distribution, 308, 314
    synaptosomal ACH, 310, 313, 314, 316
    synthesized, 315, 316
    tests of three pool hypothesis, 308
      turnover of vesicular acetylcholine, 311, 312
      vesicular decrement, 284, 308, 310, 313, 314

Acetylcholinestrase, 284

ACTH, 299

Actinomycin, 322

Adenyl Cyclase, 300

Adrenergic system, 296-98
  stimulation of, 301

Age decrement in performance, 112, 113

Agonist versus antagonist, 28

Agrophobic adults, 201, 218, 219
  diagnosed as
    anxiety-neurotic, 201
    phobic-anxiety, 201, 215
    phobic-anxiety depersonalized, 201

Albany Medical Center, 8

Alcohol, use for chronic anticipatory anxiety, 256

Alkaline phosphatase, 232

Alpha activity, 71, 74, 76, 77, 141, 145, 147, 151, 153, 154, 157, 158, 160, 162

Amantadine effect on Parkinson's disease, 371-73

American Heart Association, 86

American Medical Association, 246

The American Psychiatric Association Diagnostic and Statistical Manual of 1952, 248
  Revision, 1968, 248

Amine, xiii
  biogenic, xiii
  endogenous, 290
  importance in neural systems, 97

Aminophylline, 102

Amnesia in mice, effect of ECS and nicotine, 275-78, 281, 282, 285, 286

AMP, cyclic, 300

Amphetamines, 238, 291, 292, 300
  amusca, 50
    motor, 50
    sensory, 50

Amygdale, 168, 169

Anabasine, nicotine studies of mice, 281, 282

Analog frequency analyzer, 148, 153, 164

Anemia, after treatment with methyldopa, 322

Anesthesia, 15, 16
  local, 15

Anger, reduction with chlorpromazine, 263, 265

Angina pectoris, 87

Angiography, 92, 100, 102, 103

Anhedonia, 218

Animal curators, 28

Animal studies in comparison to human brain function, 65

Annual Cerebral Function Symposium, xiii, xiv

Anosognosia, 50

ANOV, 157

Anthropoid apes, 28

Anticholinergic reaction type, 147

Anticonvulsant drugs, 56, 59, 345, 346

Anticonvulsive treatment, 69

Antidepressant drugs, 215

Antigravity muscles, 28

in the brain, 291

peripheral, 288, 292

Synaptic efficacy, 294

transmission, 307, 311

vesicles, 306, 307, 311, 313, 316

Syntax, 39

Synthesis of proteins, at the nerve ending, 363

T

Tactile exploration in mammals, snout and face oriented, 29

perception, 29

sensation, 29

Taxonomic eclassification, 186

quantitative procedures, 186, 187

Telencephalon, 289, 300

Temporal lobe removals and effect on expressive speech, 30, 32

Temporal parietal lobe removal and its effect, 31, 32

Terminal phoneme in Wepman test, 116

Tetrabenazine, 293

Thalamus, 9, 10, 23, 24, 32, 33, 69, 70

anterior dorsal, 9

anterior superior, 112

infarction, 22

posterior dorsal, 10

Theta waves, 76, 160

Thioridazine

compared with placebo for deep sleep, 73, 74, 78

EEG activity, 76

drug treatment of childhood psychosis, 227-32

effect on subcortical substrates, 79

induced changes in two hemispheres, 71, 72

inhibitory influence, 77

study of effects on computer resting and sleep, 71

study using EEG analysis, 149

Thiothixene, 148

Thorazine, 228, 370

Thromboembolic, 104

Thrombosis, 22

Thrombus (lysis), 86, 87, 100

Thymoleptic reaction type, 147, 148

Tissue acidosis, 100-102

Tofranil, 209

Toxicity of drugs in psychotic children, 233

Tranylcypromine used with ECS, 278

Tricyclics, 215

Trifluperidol, 148

Trifluoperazine, drug treatment of childhood psychosis, 227, 228, 230, 231

Triple-blind drug study, 242

Trimethylamine (TMA), nicotine studies of mice, 285, 286

Tubercles, olfactory, 168

Typological classification of patients and drug response, 186

Tyrosine, 320

Tumors, 6, 30, 37-57, 60, 63, 64, 92 *see* Hemispherectomy

vascular effect on cerebral blood flow, 94

Twin-brained species other than man and results of hemispherectomy, 63

U

Ungulates, 28, 29

U. K. Medical and Science Research Councils, 316

Urinary sodium, 20

"U Series" drugs, mental retardation, 236

U. S. P. H. S. (NINDS-postdoctoral fellowship), 316

V

Van Syke Apparatus, 91

Vascular disease, 92, 102, 104

abnormality, 100

occlusions, 103

stenosis, 100

Vascularization, secondary, 84

Vasoconstrictor treatment, 102, 104

Vasodilating agents, 98

drugs, 100, 102, 103

Vasodilators, 104

Vasodilatation, 100, 101, 102

Vasoparalysis, 100, 101

Vein

jugular, 91

occlusion, 22

Ventricular system, 30, 31

Ventriflexion, 11, 14

Ventriflexor tone, 16

Verbal effects of removal of nondominant hemisphere, commands, 21

comprehension, 21

Vesicular membrane

turnover compared to vesicular acetylcholine, 311, 312

Vesicles, 314

Vestige organ, 40

Vibratory sense, 19

Vision, 29

Visual

acuity, 46, 63

cortex, 29